Clinical Management of Gastrointestinal Stromal Tumor

Kaixiong Tao • Hui Cao
Editors

Clinical Management of Gastrointestinal Stromal Tumor

PMPH
PEOPLE'S MEDICAL PUBLISHING HOUSE

Springer

Editors
Kaixiong Tao
Gastrointestinal Surgery
Wuhan Union Hospital
Wuhan, China

Hui Cao
Gastrointestinal Surgery
Renji Hospital
Shanghai, China

ISBN 978-981-99-9391-8 ISBN 978-981-99-9392-5 (eBook)
https://doi.org/10.1007/978-981-99-9392-5

This Springer imprint is published by the registered company Springer Nature Singapore Pte Ltd.
The registered company address is: 152 Beach Road, #21-01/04 Gateway East, Singapore 189721, Singapore

Contents

Part I Surgical Management of Gastrointestinal Stromal Tumors

1 **Laparoscopic Management of Gastrointestinal Stromal Tumors** 3
Tao Wang, Ming Wang, Gan Mao, Jie Jia, and Hui Cao

2 **Laparoscopic Combined with Endoscopic Management of Gastrointestinal Stromal Tumors** 9
Xinyu Zeng, Ming Wang, Qian Shen, Huikuan Chu, and Gang Zhao

3 **Da Vinci Robotic Management of Gastrointestinal Stromal Tumors** 17
Tao Wang, Ming Cai, and Yanbing Zhou

4 **Endoscopic Management of Gastrointestinal Stromal Tumors** 21
Qi Jiang, Zhen Ding, Jiaxian Yu, Lei Tu, and Yingjiang Ye

Part II Preoperative Treatment of Gastrointestinal Stromal Tumors

5 **Rectal Gastrointestinal Stromal Tumors with Preoperative Treatment** 31
Yao Lin, Youwei Kou, Chengguo Li, Xing Liu, and Jiren Yu

6 **Giant Abdominal Gastrointestinal Stromal Tumors with Preoperative Treatment** 39
Lei Yang, Xiaodong Gao, and Kuntang Shen

7 **Preoperative Treatment of Duodenal Gastrointestinal Stromal Tumors** 43
Yongzhou Huang, Yuan Yin, and Zhiqiang Ma

8 **Avapritinib Therapy for Preoperative Treatment of Gastrointestinal Stromal Tumors with *PDGFRA* Mutation** 47
Bo Ni, Linxi Yang, and Kaixiong Tao

9 **Preoperative Treatment of Rectal-Vaginal Septum Gastrointestinal Stromal Tumors** 53
Wenchang Yang, Zhidong Gao, and Yingjiang Ye

Part III Uncommon Pathological Types of Gastrointestinal Stromal Tumors

10 **Small Hypermitotic Gastrointestinal Stromal Tumors** 63
Jianbo Lyu, Xin Chen, and Yong Li

11 **Mitotic Extremely High Gastrointestinal Stromal Tumors** 69
Pei Zhou, Zhen Xiong, and Kaixiong Tao

12 **Neurofibromatosis Type 1 Associated Gastrointestinal Stromal Tumors** 75
Yao Lin, Xiangyu Zeng, Chengguo Li, Zhidong Gao, and Jian Li

13 **Succinate Dehydrogenase Deficient GIST** 83
Peng Zhang, Weizhen Liu, Yuqiang Du, and Bo Zhang

14 ***KIT* Mutant Gastrointestinal Stromal Tumors with Lymphatic Metastasis** 93
Yongzhou Huang, Xiangyu Zeng, and Ye Zhou

15 **Gastrointestinal Stromal Tumors with *PDGFRA* Exon 18 D842V Mutation** 99
Liwu Zeng, Peng Zhang, and Kailin Cai

16 **Multiple Gastrointestinal Stromal Tumors** 105
Peng Zhang, Yuan Yin, Xinyu Zeng, Qun Zhao, and Jun Zhang

17 **Hereditary Gastrointestinal Stromal Tumors** 113
Xiaoqi Li, Linxi Yang, and Gang Zhao

Part IV Gastrointestinal Stromal Tumors with Other Malignant Tumors

18 **Intermediate-Risk Gastrointestinal Stromal Tumor with Advanced Gastric Cancer** 119
Tianlong Ling, Haibo Qiu, and Leping Li

19 **Gastrointestinal Stromal Tumors with Kidney Cancer** 125
Chen Huang, Ruizhi Zhang, and Yong Li

Part V Targeted Therapy for Gastrointestinal Stromal Tumors

20 **Gastrointestinal Stromal Tumors Progression During Adjuvant Therapy** 133
Tianlong Ling, Ming Wang, and Xianfa Wang

21 **Gastrointestinal Stromal Tumors Recurrence After Stopping Adjuvant Therapy** 139
Xiaoqi Li, Wenze Wan, and Han Liang

22 **Low Risk Rectal Gastrointestinal Stromal Tumors Recurrence 12 Years After Surgery** 145
Xiaoqi Li, Cong Li, and Zekuan Xu

23 **Surgery Combined with Targeted Therapy in Advanced Gastrointestinal Stromal Tumors** 149
Chun Zhuang, Ming Wang, Haibo Qiu, and Ye Zhou

24 **Avapritinib Therapy in Advanced Gastrointestinal Stromal Tumor with *PDGFRA* Mutation** 161
Xiaoqi Li, Xinli Ma, and Gang Zhao

25 **Therapy for Advanced Gastrointestinal Stromal Tumors** 165
Xinli Ma, Ming Wang, Kuntang Shen, Xinhua Zhang, Bo Ni, Linxi Yang, and Hui Cao

26 **Management of Targeted Drug Adverse Reaction** 179
Bo Ni, Jian Li, and Lin Shen

Part VI Management of Patients with Special Gastrointestinal Stromal Tumors

27 Senile Gastrointestinal Stromal Tumors with Coronary Heart Disease 185
Chun Zhuang, Tianlong Ling, and Guoqing Liao

28 Gastric Gastrointestinal Stromal Tumors with Gastroparesis After Surgery 191
Lin Tu, Peng Zhang, and Junbo Hu

29 Gastrointestinal Stromal Tumors with Brain Metastases 197
Lin Tu, Tao Chen, and Zhigang Jie

30 Gastrointestinal Stromal Tumors with Giant Liver Metastases 203
Linxi Yang, Tianlong Ling, and Kaixiong Tao

Part VII Management of Misdiagnosed Gastrointestinal Stromal Tumors

31 Small Intestine Gastrointestinal Stromal Tumor Misdiagnosed as Gynecological Tumor 209
Lin Tu, Youwei Kou, and Jinbo Gao

32 Castleman Disease Misdiagnosed as Gastrointestinal Stromal Tumor 215
Chen Huang, Chun Zhuang, and Yulong He

33 Other Primary Malignant Tumors Misdiagnosed as Recurrent Gastrointestinal Stromal Tumor 219
Bo Ni, Lin Tu, Chen Huang, Xin Wu, Wenchang Yang, Weizhen Liu, and Hui Cao

Editors and Contributors

Editor in Chief

Kaixiong Tao Department of Gastrointestinal Surgery, Union Hospital, Tongji Medical College, Huazhong University of Science and Technology, Wuhan, China

Hui Cao Department of Gastrointestinal Surgery, Renji Hospital, Shanghai Jiaotong University School of Medicine, Shanghai, China

Compile Secretary

Peng Zhang Department of Gastrointestinal Surgery, Union Hospital, Tongji Medical College, Huazhong University of Science and Technology, Wuhan, China

Ming Wang Department of Gastrointestinal Surgery, Renji Hospital, Shanghai Jiaotong University School of Medicine, Shanghai, China

Review Experts

Hui Cao Department of Gastrointestinal Surgery, Renji Hospital, Shanghai Jiaotong University School of Medicine, Shanghai, China

Gang Zhao Department of Gastrointestinal Surgery, Renji Hospital, Shanghai Jiaotong University School of Medicine, Shanghai, China

Yanbing Zhou Department of Gastrointestinal Surgery, The Affiliated Hospital of Qingdao University, Qingdao, China

Yingjiang Ye Department of Gastrointestinal Surgery, Peking University People's Hospital, Beijing, China

Jiren Yu Department of Gastrointestinal Surgery, The First Affiliated Hospital of Zhejiang University School of Medicine, Hangzhou, China

Kuntang Shen Department of Gastrointestinal Surgery, Zhongshan Hospital, Fudan University, Shanghai, China

Zhiqiang Ma Department of Gastrointestinal Cancer, Arion Cancer Center, Beijing, China

Kaixiong Tao Department of Gastrointestinal Surgery, Union Hospital, Tongji Medical College, Huazhong University of Science and Technology, Wuhan, China

Yong Li Department of Gastrointestinal Surgery, Guangdong Provincial People's Hospital, Guangzhou, China

Jian Li Department of Gastrointestinal Oncology, Peking University Cancer Hospital & Institute, Beijing, China

Bo Zhang Department of Gastrointestinal Surgery, Huaxi Hospital, Sichuan University, Chengdu, China

Ye Zhou Department of Gastric Surgery, Fudan University Cancer Hospital, Shanghai, China

Kailin Cai Department of Gastrointestinal Surgery, Union Hospital, Tongji Medical College of Huazhong University of Science and Technology, Wuhan, China

Jun Zhang Department of Gastrointestinal Surgery, The First Affiliated Hospital of Chongqing Medical University, Chongqing, China

Leping Li Department of Gastrointestinal Surgery, Shandong Provincial Hospital, Jinan, China

Yong Li Department of General Surgery, The Fourth Hospital of Hebei Medical University, Shijiazhuang, China

Xianfa Wang Department of General Surgery, Sir Run Run Shaw Hospital, affiliated with the Zhejiang University School of Medicine, Hangzhou, China

Han Liang Department of Gastric Surgery, Tianjin Medical University Cancer Institute & Hospital, Tianjin, China

Zekuan Xu Department of Gastric Surgery, The First Affiliated Hospital with Nanjing Medical University, Nanjing, China

Lin Shen Department of Gastrointestinal Oncology, Peking University Cancer Hospital & Institute, Beijing, China

Guoqing Liao Department of Gastrointestinal Surgery, Xiangya Hospital, Central South University, Changsha, China

Junbo Hu Department of Gastrointestinal Surgery, Tongji Hospital, Tongji Medical College, Huazhong University of Science and Technology, Wuhan, China

Zhigang Jie Department of General Surgery, The First Affiliated Hospital of Nanchang University, Nanchang, China

Jinbo Gao Department of Gastrointestinal Surgery, Union Hospital, Tongji Medical College, Huazhong University of Science and Technology University, Wuhan, China

Yulong He Digestive Diseases Center, The Seventh Affiliated Hospital of Sun Yat-sen University, Shenzhen, China

Case Providers

Ming Wang Department of Gastrointestinal Surgery, Renji Hospital, Shanghai Jiaotong University School of Medicine, Shanghai, China

Jie Jia Department of Gastrointestinal Surgery, Union Hospital, Tongji Medical College, Huazhong University of Science and Technology, Wuhan, China

Huikuan Chu Department of Gastroenterology, Union Hospital, Tongji Medical College, Huazhong University of Science and Technology, Wuhan, China

Ming Cai Department of Gastrointestinal Surgery, Union Hospital, Tongji Medical College, Huazhong University of Science and Technology, Wuhan, China

Zhen Ding Department of Gastroenterology, Union Hospital, Tongji Medical College, Huazhong University of Science and Technology, Wuhan, China

Lei Tu Department of Gastroenterology, Union Hospital, Tongji Medical College, Huazhong University of Science and Technology, Wuhan, China

Youwei Kou Department of Gastrointestinal Surgery, Shengjing Hospital of China Medical University, Shenyang, China

Xing Liu Department of Colorectal Surgery, Fujian Medical University Union Hospital, Fuzhou, China

Xiaodong Gao Department of General Surgery, Zhongshan Hospital, Fudan University, Shanghai, China

Yuan Yin Department of Gastrointestinal Surgery, West China Hospital, Sichuan University, Chengdu, China

Linxi Yang Department of Gastrointestinal Surgery, Renji Hospital, Shanghai Jiaotong University School of Medicine, Shanghai, China

Zhidong Gao Department of Gastrointestinal Surgery, Peking University People's Hospital, Beijing, China

Xin Chen Department of Gastrointestinal Surgery, Union Hospital, Tongji Medical College, Huazhong University of Science and Technology, Wuhan, China

Zhen Xiong Department of Gastrointestinal Surgery, Union Hospital, Tongji Medical College, Huazhong University of Science and Technology, Wuhan, China

Xiangyu Zeng Department of Gastrointestinal Surgery, Union Hospital, Tongji Medical College, Huazhong University of Science and Technology, Wuhan, China

Weizhen Liu Department of Gastrointestinal Surgery, Union Hospital, Tongji Medical College, Huazhong University of Science and Technology, Wuhan, China

Peng Zhang Department of Gastrointestinal Surgery, Union Hospital, Tongji Medical College, Huazhong University of Science and Technology, Wuhan, China

Qun Zhao Department of General Surgery, The Fourth Hospital of Hebei Medical University, Shijiazhuang, China

Haibo Qiu Department of Gastric Surgery, Sun Yat-sen University Cancer Center, Guangzhou, China

Ruizhi Zhang Department of Gastrointestinal Surgery, Union Hospital, Tongji Medical College, Huazhong University of Science and Technology, Wuhan, China

Wenze Wan Department of Gastrointestinal Surgery, Union Hospital, Tongji Medical College, Huazhong University of Science and Technology, Wuhan, China

Cong Li Department of Colorectal Surgery, Sun Yat-sen University Cancer Center, Guangzhou, China

Xinli Ma Department of Gastrointestinal Surgery, Renji Hospital, Shanghai Jiaotong University School of Medicine, Shanghai, China

Xinhua Zhang Department of Gastrointestinal Surgery, The First Affiliated Hospital of Sun Yat-sen University, Guangzhou, China

Jian Li Department of Gastrointestinal Oncology, Peking University Cancer Hospital & Institute, Beijing, China

Tianlong Ling Department of Gastrointestinal Surgery, Renji Hospital, Shanghai Jiaotong University School of Medicine, Shanghai, China

Tao Chen Department of General Surgery, Nanfang Hospital, Southern Medical University, Guangzhou, China

Chun Zhuang Department of Gastrointestinal Surgery, Renji Hospital, Shanghai Jiaotong University School of Medicine, Shanghai, China

Lin Tu Department of Gastrointestinal Surgery, Renji Hospital, Shanghai Jiaotong University School of Medicine, Shanghai, China

Xin Wu Department of General Surgery, The First Medical Center, Chinese PLA General Hospital, Beijing, China

Translators

Tao Wang Department of Gastrointestinal Surgery, Union Hospital, Tongji Medical College, Huazhong University of Science and Technology, Wuhan, China

Gan Mao Department of Gastrointestinal Surgery, Union Hospital, Tongji Medical College, Huazhong University of Science and Technology, Wuhan, China

Xinyu Zeng Department of Gastrointestinal Surgery, Union Hospital, Tongji Medical College, Huazhong University of Science and Technology, Wuhan, China

Qian Shen Department of Gastrointestinal Surgery, Union Hospital, Tongji Medical College, Huazhong University of Science and Technology, Wuhan, China

Qi Jiang Department of Gastrointestinal Surgery, Union Hospital, Tongji Medical College, Huazhong University of Science and Technology, Wuhan, China

Jiaxian Yu Department of Gastrointestinal Surgery, Union Hospital, Tongji Medical College, Huazhong University of Science and Technology, Wuhan, China

Yao Lin Department of Gastrointestinal Surgery, Union Hospital, Tongji Medical College, Huazhong University of Science and Technology, Wuhan, China

Chengguo Li Department of Gastrointestinal Surgery, Union Hospital, Tongji Medical College, Huazhong University of Science and Technology, Wuhan, China

Lei Yang Department of Gastrointestinal Surgery, Union Hospital, Tongji Medical College, Huazhong University of Science and Technology, Wuhan, China

Yongzhou Huang Department of Gastrointestinal Surgery, Union Hospital, Tongji Medical College, Huazhong University of Science and Technology, Wuhan, China

Bo Ni Department of Gastrointestinal Surgery, Renji Hospital, Shanghai Jiaotong University School of Medicine, Shanghai, China

Wenchang Yang Department of Gastrointestinal Surgery, Union Hospital, Tongji Medical College, Huazhong University of Science and Technology, Wuhan, China

Jianbo Lyu Department of Gastrointestinal Surgery, Union Hospital, Tongji Medical College, Huazhong University of Science and Technology, Wuhan, China

Pei Zhou Department of Gastrointestinal Surgery, Union Hospital, Tongji Medical College, Huazhong University of Science and Technology, Wuhan, China

Peng Zhang Department of Gastrointestinal Surgery, Union Hospital, Tongji Medical College, Huazhong University of Science and Technology, Wuhan, China

Yuqiang Du Department of Gastrointestinal Surgery, Union Hospital, Tongji Medical College, Huazhong University of Science and Technology, Wuhan, China

Liwu Zeng Department of Gastrointestinal Surgery, Union Hospital, Tongji Medical College, Huazhong University of Science and Technology, Wuhan, China

Xiaoqi Li Department of Gastrointestinal Surgery, Renji Hospital, Shanghai Jiaotong University School of Medicine, Shanghai, China

Tianlong Ling Department of Gastrointestinal Surgery, Renji Hospital, Shanghai Jiaotong University School of Medicine, Shanghai, China

Chen Huang Department of Gastrointestinal Surgery, Renji Hospital, Shanghai Jiaotong University School of Medicine, Shanghai, China

Chun Zhuang Department of Gastrointestinal Surgery, Renji Hospital, Shanghai Jiaotong University School of Medicine, Shanghai, China

Xinli Ma Department of Gastrointestinal Surgery, Renji Hospital, Shanghai Jiaotong University School of Medicine, Shanghai, China

Lin Tu Department of Gastrointestinal Surgery, Renji Hospital, Shanghai Jiaotong University School of Medicine, Shanghai, China

Linxi Yang Department of Gastrointestinal Surgery, Renji Hospital, Shanghai Jiaotong University School of Medicine, Shanghai, China

Part I

Surgical Management of Gastrointestinal Stromal Tumors

Laparoscopic Management of Gastrointestinal Stromal Tumors

1

Tao Wang, Ming Wang, Gan Mao, Jie Jia, and Hui Cao

Keywords

Gastrointestinal stromal tumor · Surgery · Laparoscopy Jejunum

1.1 Case 1 A 64-Year-Old Man with GIST Who Underwent Laparoscopic Surgery

Tao Wang and Ming Wang

1.1.1 Introduction

Surgical resection is the preferred treatment for locally resectable gastrointestinal stromal tumor (GIST). Surgery should follow the principles of complete tumor resection, avoiding tumor rupture, and ensuring negative histological margins. Open surgery was previously the dominant treatment for gastric GIST. In recent years, with the advancement of surgical technology and equipment and the promotion of minimally invasive procedures, laparoscopic surgery has become more widely used in the treatment of GIST, especially gastric GIST [1].

1.1.2 Case Background

A 64-year-old man presented to the local hospital with repeated dull pain and discomfort in the right upper abdominal quadrant. A CT scan of the chest showed: a small streak shadow in both pulmonary lobes, a little bilateral pleural effusion, enlarged lymph nodes in the mediastinum and right hilar calcification foci, multiple cysts in the liver, gallbladder stones, and a space-occupying lesion in the left upper abdominal quadrant. In light of these findings, further examination was recommended. Subsequently, gastroscopy and abdominal enhanced CT were performed. Gastroscopy revealed a submucosal bulge with a diameter of 4.5 cm in the fundus of the stomach, which was suspected to be a GIST. Enhanced CT revealed a space-occupying lesion at the bottom of the stomach, approximately 5.5 cm × 5.0 cm in size (possible GIST); multiple cysts in the liver; multiple stones in the gallbladder; and multiple cysts on both kidneys. During the course of the disease, the patient had no discomfort such as nausea, vomiting, constipation, diarrhea, hematemesis, or melena. The patient was admitted to the hospital for further treatment.

1.1.2.1 Past History and Family History

The patient was previously healthy and reported no drug allergies. The patient's parents were alive, and there was no similar medical history within the family.

1.1.2.2 Physical Examination

The abdomen was flat, without gastric or intestinal pattern and peristaltic waves. The abdomen was soft, without tenderness, rebound tenderness, or palpable mass, and bowel sounds were normal.

1.1.2.3 Auxiliary Examination

Gastroscopy A submucosal bulge, suspected to be GIST, 4.5 cm in diameter, was seen in the fundus of the stomach.

T. Wang · G. Mao · J. Jia (✉)
Department of Gastrointestinal Surgery, Union Hospital, Tongji Medical College, Huazhong University of Science and Technology, Wuhan, China
e-mail: wangtaojx@hust.edu.cn; maogan@hust.edu.cn

M. Wang (✉) · H. Cao
Department of Gastrointestinal Surgery, Renji Hospital, Shanghai Jiaotong University School of Medicine, Shanghai, China

K. Tao, H. Cao (eds.), *Clinical Management of Gastrointestinal Stromal Tumor*, https://doi.org/10.1007/978-981-99-9392-5_1

Superficial atrophic gastritis with erosion and duodenal papilla erosion was observed. The pathology showed moderate chronic active inflammation of the mucosa with the formation of lymphoid follicles.

Abdominal CT A space-occupying lesion was found at the fundus of the stomach, considered to be a possible GIST. Furthermore, multiple cysts in the liver, multiple stones in the gallbladder, and multiple cysts in both kidneys were observed (Fig. 1.1).

Initial Diagnosis
1. Fundus GIST
2. Gallbladder stones with cholecystitis
3. Multiple cysts in the liver

1.1.3 Therapy

1.1.3.1 Case Analysis

The patient was an elderly man, who visited the hospital following the accidental finding of a gastric fundus mass in the course of diagnosing and treating gallbladder stones. Imaging and gastroscopy suggested the possibility of GIST in the fundus of the stomach. The patient was generally in good condition, and the tumor was deemed to be resectable. No metastasis was found, and surgery could be performed. Since the gastric tumor was located in the fundus of the stomach, it was suitable for laparoscopic surgery, and laparoscopic cholecystectomy could also be performed at the same time. Postoperative treatment was to be based on the results of pathology and genetic testing.

1.1.3.2 Treatment

The patient underwent laparoscopic gastric tumor resection with cholecystectomy on October 17, 2018. The gallbladder was approximately 7.0 cm × 5.0 cm × 3.0 cm in size. The gallbladder wall was rough, and the gallbladder contained three mixed stones, all of which were approximately 1 cm in diameter. The common bile duct was not dilated. A tumor with a diameter of 5 cm was found on the upper portion of the greater curvature of the stomach, protruding into and out of the gastric cavity. The mass originated from the submucosa, and there was no swelling of the peri-gastric lymph nodes. After the fundus and upper part of the stomach were fully freed during the operation, the tumor was removed using a linear cutting and closing device (Fig. 1.2). The excised tumor was placed in an extraction bag and the umbilical incision was extended to allow for the removal of the specimen.

1.1.3.3 Postoperative Pathology and Genetic Testing

Pathological Diagnosis Gastric GIST, 5.5 cm × 5.0 cm × 5.0 cm in size, mitotic count 4/50 HPF (Fig. 1.3).

Immunohistochemistry CD117 (+), DOG-1 (+), CD34 (+), SMA (−), S-100 (−), Ki-67 (Li: 3%), SDHB (+).

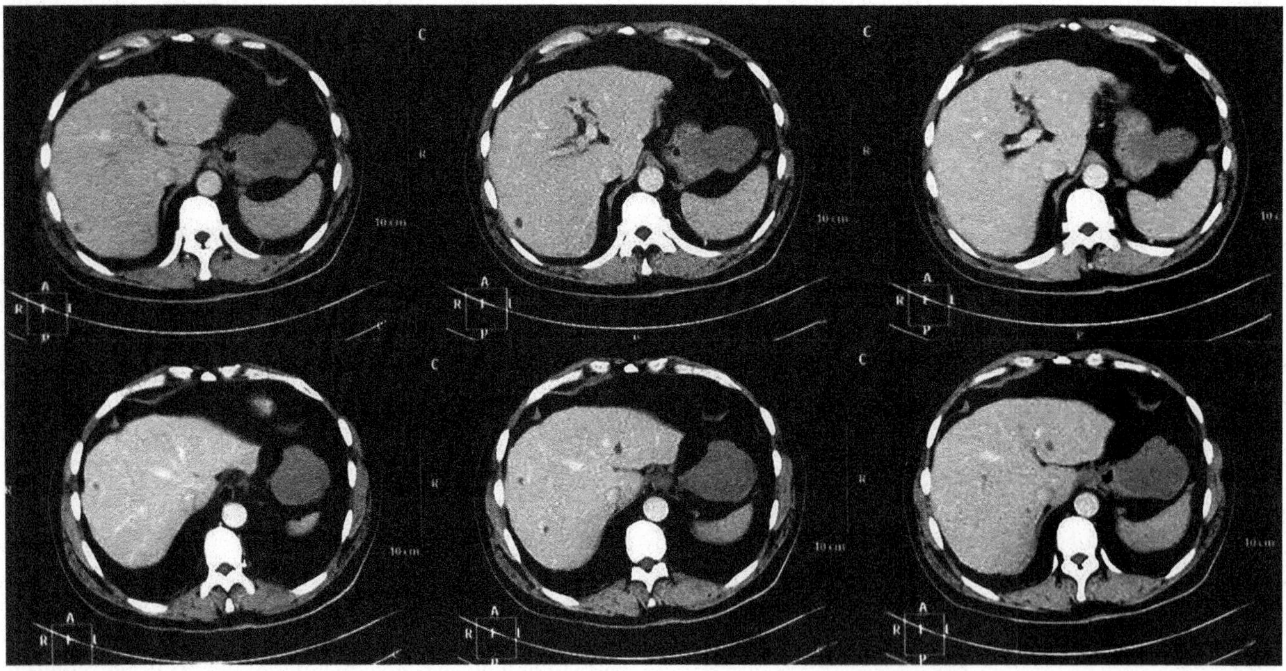

Fig. 1.1 A space-occupying lesion of the gastric fundus

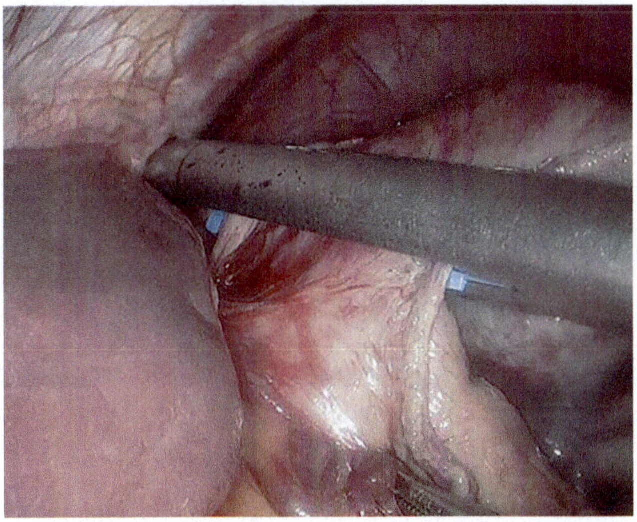

Fig. 1.2 Complete tumor resection with a laparoscopic linear cutting stapler

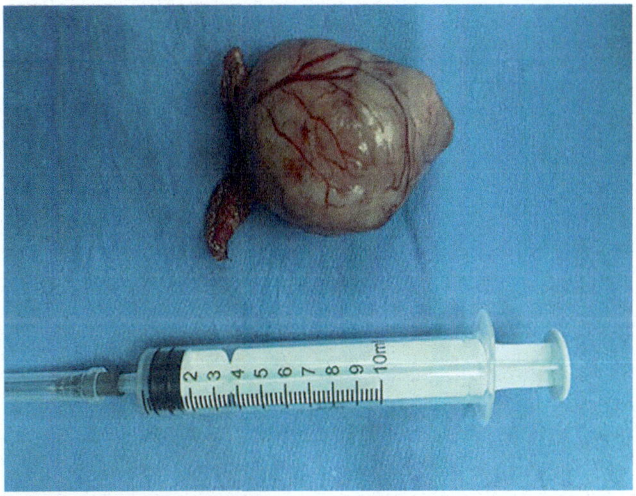

Fig. 1.3 Gross specimen

Genetic Testing A heterozygous mutation was found on exon 11 of *KIT*, 559GTT>GAT. This mutation caused the encoded amino acid to be converted from valine to aspartic acid. The 9, 13, and 17 exons of *KIT* and the 12 and 18 exons of *PDGFRA* were all wild type.

1.1.4 Prognosis

The patient followed a liquid diet for 3 days after surgery and was discharged 5 days after surgery. The pathological examination results confirmed the diagnosis of GIST with a moderate risk of recurrence. During outpatient follow-up, the patient received 400 mg/d imatinib as adjuvant therapy, the general condition of the patient was good and there were no obvious side effects. After taking imatinib for 1 year, the drug was discontinued. During the regular follow-up for 39 months after the operation, no recurrence or metastasis of GIST occurred in the patient.

1.2 Case 2 A Case of Laparoscopic Surgery for Jejunal GIST

Gan Mao and Jie Jia

1.2.1 Introduction

The growth of jejunoileal GIST is relatively insidious, and small asymptomatic GIST is rarely found based on clinical manifestations. Jejunoileal GIST has a high malignant potential [2]. Therefore, surgical resection should be actively performed. Laparoscopic surgery is safe and feasible for small GIST (those with a diameter of ≤5 cm), when the tumor is relatively free [3]. In addition, laparoscopic techniques are of great value for judging the position of GIST in the small bowel during operation.

1.2.2 Case Background

The patient, a 52-year-old man, had tarry stool, twice a day, with no obvious cause, which started 1 week ago. This was accompanied by nausea and vomiting. He was admitted to the hospital for treatment.

1.2.2.1 Past History and Family History

The patient reported that he was usually in good health and had no history of allergies. The patient's parents were in good health and there was no similar medical history in the family.

1.2.2.2 Physical Examination

The abdomen was flat and soft, without palpable masses. The liver and spleen are not palpable below the costal margin, and there was no tenderness or rebound tenderness. There was also no percussion pain in the kidney area, or shifting dullness, and bowel sounds were normal.

1.2.2.3 Auxiliary Examination

Blood Routine WBC 4.70 × 10^9 /L, RBC 5.37 × 10^{12}/L, Hb 142 g/L, PLT 216 × 10^9/L, NEUT% 59.1%, LY% 32.2%.

Blood Biochemistry TBil 9.2 μmol/L, DBil 4.5 μmol/L, TP 78.0 g/L, ALB 50.9 g/L, Cre 88.1 μmol/L, BUN 3.12 mmol/L, Na^+ 141.2 mmol/L, K^+ 4.53 mmol/L, Cl^- 96.7 mmol/L.

Abdominal CT A whole abdomen scan with enhanced CT on December 14, 2018, showed that the segmental wall of the jejunum in the left lower abdomen was thickened, with a range of approximately 3.4 cm × 3.0 cm. Enhanced CT showed obvious enhancement of the lesion. The adjacent serosal surface was smooth, and there were no obviously enlarged lymph nodes around the lesion. The results were suggestive of GIST. No other abnormalities were detected (Fig. 1.4).

Initial Diagnosis Jejunal GIST.

1.2.3 Therapy

1.2.3.1 Case Analysis

The patient was a middle-aged man who presented to the doctor with tarry stools for a week. After completing the relevant examinations, the preliminary diagnosis was considered to be a GIST in the jejunum which was approximately 3.4 cm × 3.0 cm in size. Because the tumor did not appear to invade the surrounding organs or tissues and had a small diameter, it was suitable for laparoscopic resection. Postoperative treatment was to be guided based on the results of pathology and genetic testing.

1.2.3.2 Treatment

The patient underwent preoperative preparation following the concept of enhanced recovery after surgery (ERAS) as well as underwent laparoscopic exploration and jejunal tumor resection on December 20, 2018. Intraoperative exploration revealed that the tumor was located at the jejunum, 100 cm away from Treitz ligament, with a size of approximately 4.0 cm × 3.0 cm. A laparoscopic linear cutting stapler was used to resect the jejunum with a margin of 1 cm from the tumor. The tumor was placed in an extraction bag, and extracted through the umbilical incision. Subsequently a side-to-side jejunal anastomosis was performed to close the intestinal cavity. Absorbable thread was intermittently sutured to reinforce the anastomosis. The laparoscopic access points were sutured and the operation was deemed successful. The operation time was 60 min, and the intraoperative blood loss was approximately 20 mL (Figs. 1.5 and 1.6).

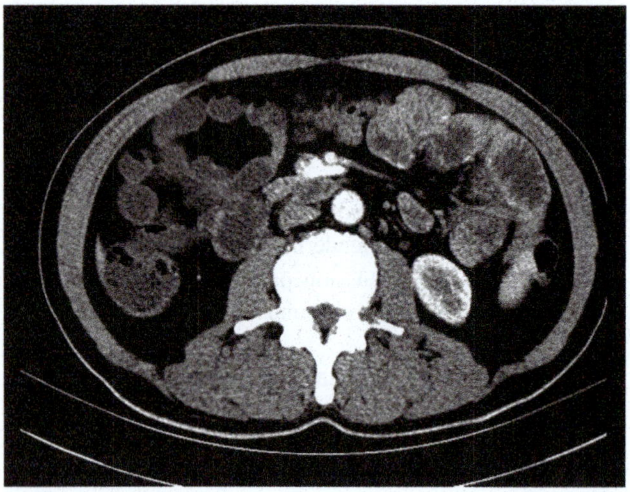

Fig. 1.4 The jejunal tumor

1.2.3.3 Postoperative Pathology and Genetic Testing

Pathological Diagnosis Jejunal GIST. The size of the mass was 3.5 cm × 2.0 cm, mitotic count 5/50 HPF. According to the modified National Institutes of Health (NIH) risk classification the tumor was low risk.

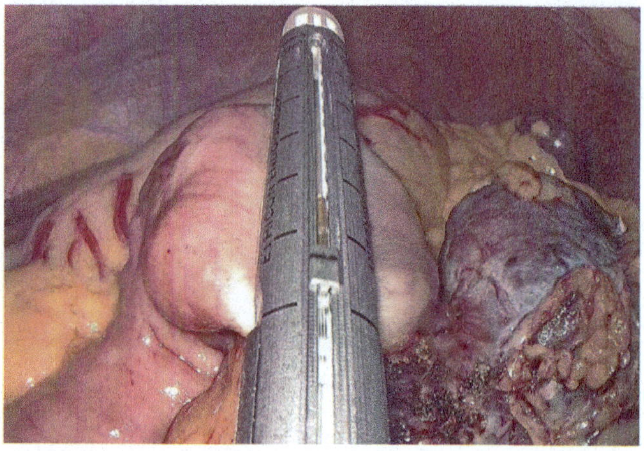

Fig. 1.5 Dissection of the proximal jejunum

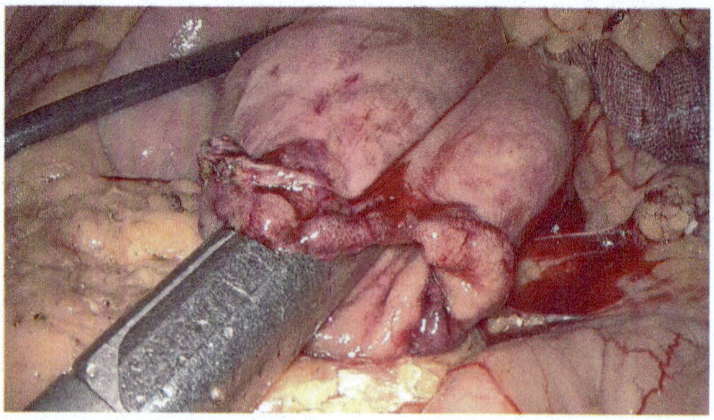

Fig. 1.6 Side-to-side anastomosis of jejunum

Immunohistochemistry CD117 (+), DOG-1 (+), CD34 (+), SMA (−), S-100 (−), Ki-67 (Li: <5%).

Genetic Testing Heterozygous mutation in exon 11 of *KIT*, the mutation type was p.Y570_P573dup; exon 12 and 18 of *PDGFRA* were wild type.

1.2.4 Prognosis

The patient recovered well after the operation and was discharged on the fifth postoperative day. No targeted drug therapy was administered after the operation as the tumor was classified as low-risk. As of January 2022, the patient had been followed up for 37 months without recurrence.

1.2.5 Experience of Diagnosis and Therapy

1.2.5.1 The Feasibility and Controversy of Laparoscopic Surgery for GIST

In the past, laparotomy was the primary surgical procedure performed for the treatment of gastric GIST. Since GIST rarely metastasizes through a lymphatic route, it is generally sufficient to ensure a negative margin by wedge resection [4]. Therefore, in recent years, the updated guidelines have supported the application of laparoscopic surgery for gastric GIST and gradually relaxed the indications [1, 5]. However, tumor rupture is still an independent, poor prognostic factor for GIST [6]. Once a tumor ruptures into the abdominal cavity, the risk of recurrence is extremely high. Therefore, the possibility of GIST tumor being fragile and easy to rupture limits the application of laparoscopic surgery. Chinese consensus guidelines for GIST highlights that that these indications should be strictly controlled when choosing laparoscopic surgery to treat GIST, and the operation should be carefully regulated [5]. Laparoscopy is not recommended for patients with large tumors, difficult operations, or those who require combined organ resection.

1.2.5.2 Basic Principles of Laparoscopic Surgery for GIST

Laparoscopic surgery for GIST also follows the basic principles of open surgery. The principle of "less contact, less squeezing" should be followed during the operation, and care should be taken to avoid tumor rupture and spreading, leading to abdominal implantation or blood metastasis. Therefore, it is necessary to use an extraction bag after resection. Removing the tumor in small portions to allow for minimally invasive surgery with small incisions should be avoided as this can affect the pathological evaluation after surgery.

1.2.5.3 Laparoscopic Surgery Treatment Strategies for GIST in Different Locations

The current guideline consensus is that laparoscopic techniques are recommended for GIST with small tumor diameters and when the tumor is located in a favorable anatomical location (such as the anterior wall of the stomach, the greater curvature of the stomach, jejunum, or ileum). However, no prospective clinical research has been conducted to determine whether relatively small GIST, located in difficult anatomical sites (such as posterior gastric wall, lesser curvature of the stomach, near the cardia, near the pylorus), are also suitable for laparoscopic surgery. From the limited retrospective research data and clinical practice in our hospital, it is safe and feasible to perform laparoscopic surgery for some gastric GIST in difficult anatomical locations [7], but there are certain differences for surgical treatment strategies based on different anatomical regions and size restrictions. It is more suitable to close the gastric cavity using manual rather than instrumental suturing after resection, and the dual-mirror technique is recommended.

1.3 Expert Comments

Hui Cao

Laparoscopic treatment strategies vary depending on the size, anatomical location, and different gross growth patterns of GIST. For example, a GIST on the greater curvature and fundus of the stomach can often be resected with an intracavitary cutting closure device. While for a GIST on the minor curvature, adjacent to the cardia or pylorus, it is more difficult to use an intracavitary cutting closure device for resection, and closure often requires involvement of a portion of local gastric wall. Manual suturing after resection requires greater surgical skills for the surgeon and identifying the location of small GIST that completely protrude into the cavity may need to rely on intraoperative gastroscopy.

Compared to open surgery, laparoscopic surgery has the advantages of small incisions, better vision, less bleeding, and less pain [8]. However, GIST are brittle and prone to rupture, and the postoperative recurrence rate will be greatly increased. Therefore, whether laparoscopic surgery can be used for GIST with large diameters or complex anatomical locations is still controversial. Surgeons who have received rigorous training in laparoscopic techniques need to fully evaluate the difficulty of tumor resection and the risk of tumor rupture during the perioperative period while focusing on minimally invasive surgery and choose the best surgical method to maximize patient benefits.

References

1. von Mehren M, Randall RL, Benjamin RS, Boles S, Bui MM, Ganjoo KN, George S, Gonzalez RJ, Heslin MJ, Kane JM, Keedy V, Kim E, Koon H, Mayerson J, McCarter M, McGarry SV, Meyer C, Morris ZS, O'Donnell RJ, Pappo AS, Paz IB, Petersen IA, Pfeifer JD, Riedel RF, Ruo B, Schuetze S, Tap WD, Wayne JD, Bergman MA, Scavone JL. Soft tissue sarcoma, version 2.2018, NCCN clinical practice guidelines in oncology. J Natl Compr Cancer Netw. 2018;16(5):536–63. https://doi.org/10.6004/jnccn.2018.0025.
2. Dematteo RP, Gold JS, Saran L, Gönen M, Liau KH, Maki RG, Singer S, Besmer P, Brennan MF, Antonescu CR. Tumor mitotic rate, size, and location independently predict recurrence after resection of primary gastrointestinal stromal tumor (GIST). Cancer. 2008;112(3):608–15. https://doi.org/10.1002/cncr.23199.
3. Liao CH, Yeh CN, Wang SY, Fu CY, Tsai CY, Liu YY, Cheng CT, Yeh TS. Surgical option for intestinal gastrointestinal stromal tumors--perioperative and oncological outcomes of laparoscopic surgery. Anticancer Res. 2015;35(2):1033–40. https://ar.iiarjournals.org/content/35/2/1033.long
4. Güller U, Tarantino I, Cerny T, Schmied BM, Warschkow R. Population-based SEER trend analysis of overall and cancer-specific survival in 5138 patients with gastrointestinal stromal tumor. BMC Cancer. 2015;15:557–68. https://doi.org/10.1186/s12885-015-1554-9.
5. Li J, Ye Y, Wang J, Zhang B, Qin S, Shi Y, He Y, Liang X, Liu X, Zhou Y, Wu X, Zhang X, Wang M, Gao Z, Lin T, Cao H, Shen L, Chinese Society of Clinical Oncology Csco Expert Committee On Gastrointestinal Stromal Tumor. Chinese consensus guidelines for diagnosis and management of gastrointestinal stromal tumor. Chin J Cancer Res. 2017;29(4):281–93. https://doi.org/10.21147/j.issn.1000-9604.2017.04.01.
6. Blay JY, Kang YK, Nishida T, von Mehren M. Gastrointestinal stromal tumours. Nat Rev Dis Primers. 2021;7(1):22. https://doi.org/10.1038/s41572-021-00254-5.
7. Xiong Z, Wan W, Zeng X, Liu W, Wang T, Zhang R, Li C, Yang W, Zhang P, Tao K. Laparoscopic versus open surgery for gastric gastrointestinal stromal tumors: a propensity score matching analysis. J Gastrointest Surg. 2020;24(8):1785–94. https://doi.org/10.1007/s11605-019-04318-6.
8. Hu J, Or BH, Hu K, Wang ML. Comparison of the post-operative outcomes and survival of laparoscopic versus open resections for gastric gastrointestinal stromal tumors: a multi-center prospective cohort study. Int J Surg. 2016;33(Pt A):65–71. https://doi.org/10.1016/j.ijsu.2016.07.064.

Laparoscopic Combined with Endoscopic Management of Gastrointestinal Stromal Tumors

2

Xinyu Zeng, Ming Wang, Qian Shen, Huikuan Chu, and Gang Zhao

Keywords

Gastrointestinal stromal tumors · Laparoscopy surgery Endoscopic surgery · Laparoscopy · Endoscopy Cooperation

2.1 Case 3 A 41-Year-Old Woman with GIST Who Underwent Laparoscopic and Endoscopic Cooperative Surgery

Xinyu Zeng and Ming Wang

2.1.1 Introduction

Laparoscopic and endoscopic cooperative surgery has emerged as a minimally invasive surgical technique for GIST in recent years. In the past, when laparoscopy was performed alone, it was not easy to detect small lesions (tumor diameter <2 cm) due to the lack of fine tactile sensation [1]. In addition, due to the limitation of laparoscopic instruments, it is more difficult to assess the posterior wall of the gastroduodenum and intraluminal tumors during exploration, which easily leads to the omission of lesion resection and procedure conversion to laparotomy [2]. In this case, intraoperative gastroscopy to locate the lesion was particularly necessary to ensure the smooth progress of laparoscopic surgery. In addition, as GIST lesions found under gastroscopy generally originate from the muscularis propria, the risks of treatment using gastroscopy alone are greater, and the operation time is increased. The use of laparoscopy can assist endoscopic procedures, through timely detection and management of complications arising from endoscopic resection, therefore increasing surgical safety and efficiency [3]. Laparoscopic and endoscopic cooperative surgery combines the advantages of laparoscopy and endoscopy, counteracts the disadvantages of laparoscopy or endoscopy alone, and further expands the scope of application for minimally invasive surgical techniques.

2.1.2 Case Background

A 41-year-old woman presented with abdominal distension accompanied by nausea without vomiting, dizziness, headache, fatigue, and blackouts after eating greasy food in July 2018. Upon coughing, the patient produced a small amount of white sputum, but the patient did not report hemoptysis, chest pain, chest tightness, or other symptoms. The patient had a normal high-salt diet. The patient then visited a local hospital on August 10, 2018. Gastroscopy showed atrophic gastritis, a local gastric bulge (this was described as a submucosal lesion and endoscopic ultrasonography was recommended) and antral polypoid change. Gastric mucosal biopsy pathology showed chronic non-atrophic gastritis (acute active stage) in the antrum and *Helicobacter pylori* (HP) infection. Anti-HP treatment was administered at another hospital, and the patient's subjective symptoms were relieved 2 weeks later. For further treatment, the patient visited Renji Hospital, Shanghai Jiaotong University School of Medicine. On August 20, 2018, ultrasonic gastroscopy showed possible gastric GIST. On August 25,

X. Zeng · Q. Shen
Department of Gastrointestinal Surgery, Union Hospital, Tongji Medical College, Huazhong University of Science and Technology, Wuhan, China
e-mail: zengxy@hust.edu.cn; m202175880@hust.edu.cn

M. Wang (✉) · G. Zhao
Department of Gastrointestinal Surgery, Renji Hospital, Shanghai Jiaotong University School of Medicine, Shanghai, China

H. Chu (✉)
Department of Gastroenterology, Union Hospital, Tongji Medical College, Huazhong University of Science and Technology, Wuhan, China
e-mail: 2012XH0827@hust.edu.cn

K. Tao, H. Cao (eds.), *Clinical Management of Gastrointestinal Stromal Tumor*, https://doi.org/10.1007/978-981-99-9392-5_2

2018, contrast-enhanced CT of the stomach revealed a mass in the lesser curvature of the stomach, which appeared to be of submucosal origin, suspected to be a large GIST; multiple microcysts in the liver; and gallbladder adenomyosis. A small amount of bilateral pleural effusion was identified. Since the onset of the disease, the patient had normal stools, good sleep and diet, and a weight loss of 2.5 kg within 1 month.

2.1.2.1 Past History and Family History

The patient was previously healthy, and reported no history of drug allergy; her parents were in good health, and there was no similar medical history in the family.

2.1.2.2 Physical Examination

The patient's vital signs were stable. The abdomen was flat, and no gastrointestinal or peristaltic waves were observed. The abdomen was soft, with no tenderness, rebound pain, or palpable mass in the abdomen. Bowel sounds were normal.

2.1.2.3 Auxiliary Examination

Ultrasonic Gastroscopy A bulging lesion was observed on the posterior wall of the upper gastric body. The lesion appeared as a hypoechoic mass at the bulge, had a uniform internal echo, originated from the fourth layer and protruded into and out of the gastric cavity (Fig. 2.1).

Gastric Contrast-Enhanced CT A mass was observed in the lesser curvature of the gastric body, and the CT findings indicated that it was of submucosal origin. A possible diagnosis of GIST was considered, based on a combination of endoscopic and pathological findings. The CT also revealed multiple microcysts in the liver, and gallbladder adenomyosis. A small amount of bilateral pleural effusion could also be seen (Fig. 2.2).

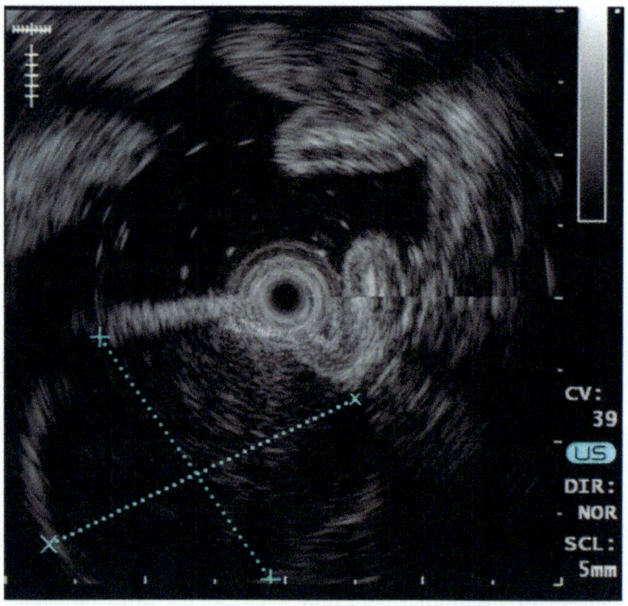

Fig. 2.1 Endoscopic ultrasonography indicated that the gastric bulge originated in the fourth layer and protruded into and out of the cavity

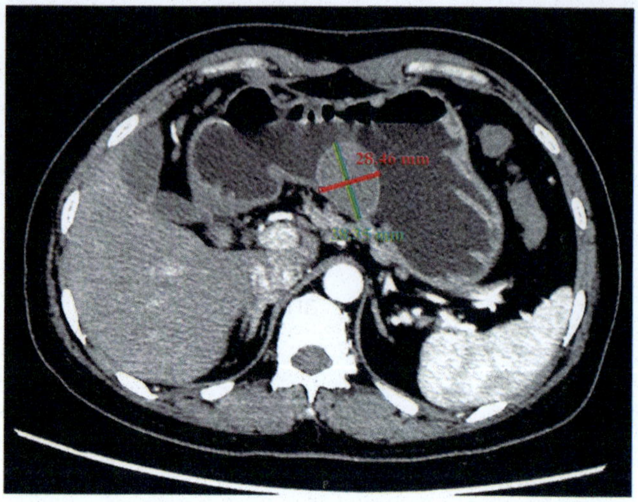

Fig. 2.2 CT revealed a mass in the lesser curvature of the gastric body

2.1.3 Therapy

2.1.3.1 Case Analysis

The patient was a middle-aged woman who presented with abdominal distension after eating. Imaging and endoscopic ultrasonography revealed the possibility of GIST in the lesser curvature of the gastric fundus. The patient was in good general condition, the tumor was determined to be resectable, and no metastasis was seen. Based on the patient characteristics, surgical treatment was recommended, and postoperative treatment should be guided by the results of pathology and genetic testing.

2.1.3.2 Treatment

The patient underwent laparoscopy and gastroscopy for gastric tumor resection on August 30, 2018, and a gastrointestinal surgeon and gastroenterologist performed surgery together. Intraoperatively, endoscopy showed a submucosal tumor with a diameter of 4 cm in the posterior wall of the lesser curvature of the gastric body, it was an intraluminal growth, with no invasion of the gastric mucosa or serosa (Fig. 2.3). There was a calcified fat nodule with a diameter of 1 cm palpable in the lesser omental bursa, but no enlargement of perigastric lymph nodes, and no metastases in the liver, pelvic cavity, or peritoneum. The endoscope was placed through the mouth to explore the tumor, and a submucosal water injection was performed at the tumor margin (Fig. 2.4). Under endoscopic guidance, an ultrasonic scalpel was used to incise the serosa of the gastric wall 1 cm from the tumor margin, and the full thickness of the gastric wall was incised along the outside of the tumor capsule to completely remove the tumor (Fig. 2.5). The gastric wall defect was intermittently sutured in full thickness with 3-0 absorbable suture and the gastric wound was examined by intraoperative gastroscopy. Some mucosal defects on the wound were endoscopically reinforced with titanium clips (Fig. 2.6). The excised tumor was placed in a specimen bag and removed through the umbilical incision (Fig. 2.7).

2.1.3.3 Postoperative Pathology and Genetic Testing

Pathological Diagnosis GIST (4.0 cm × 3.0 cm), mitotic count <5/50 HPF. Fatty necrotic fibrotic nodules were present.

Immunohistochemistry Tumor cells were CD117 (+), DOG-1 (+), CD34 (+), SDHB (+), S-100 (−), SOX10 (−), STAT6 (−), Ki-67 (Li: 1%), ALK (−), and β-catenin (−).

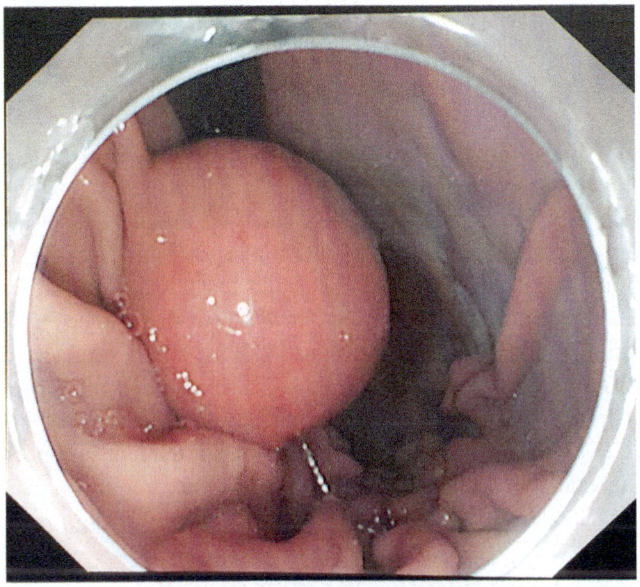

Fig. 2.3 Intraoperative endoscopic exploration of the tumor

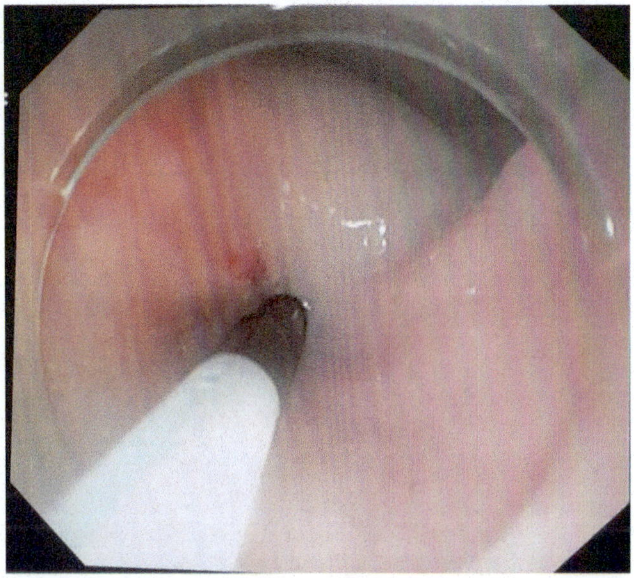

Fig. 2.4 Intraoperative endoscopic submucosal water injection at the edge of the tumor

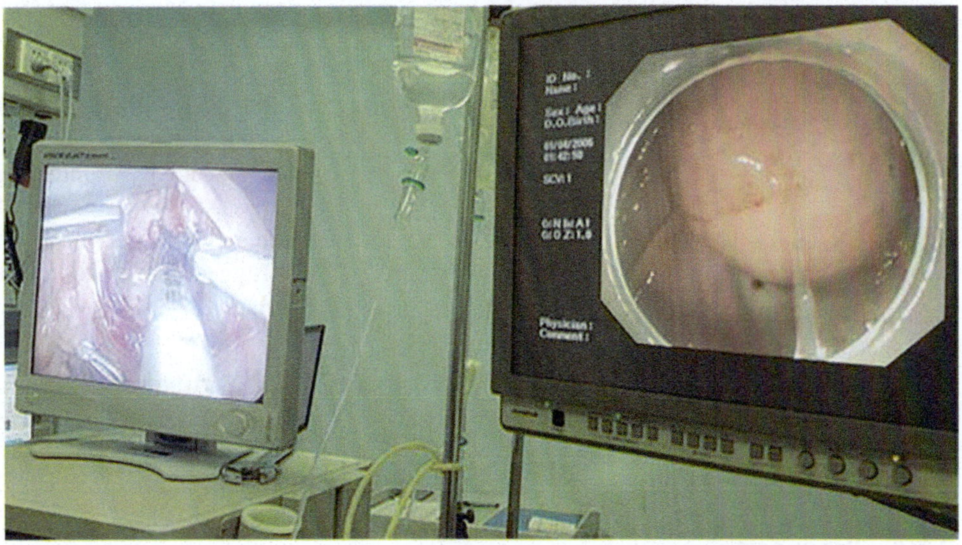

Fig. 2.5 Laparoscopic tumor resection was performed by the surgeon under intraoperative endoscopic surveillance

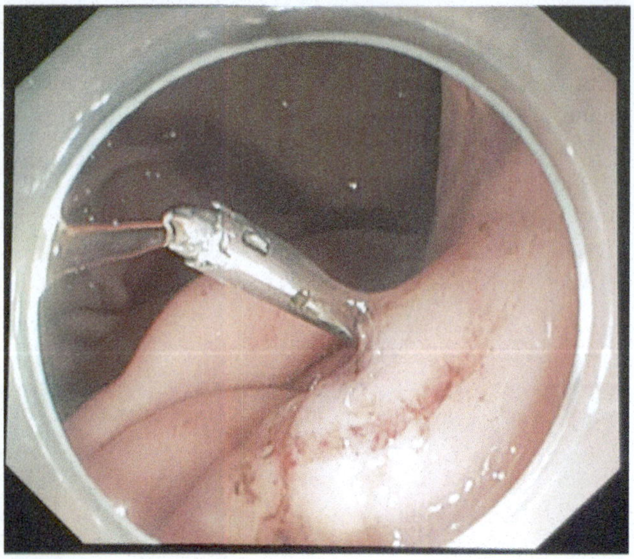

Fig. 2.6 Endoscopic titanium clips for supplementary clamping of mucosal wounds

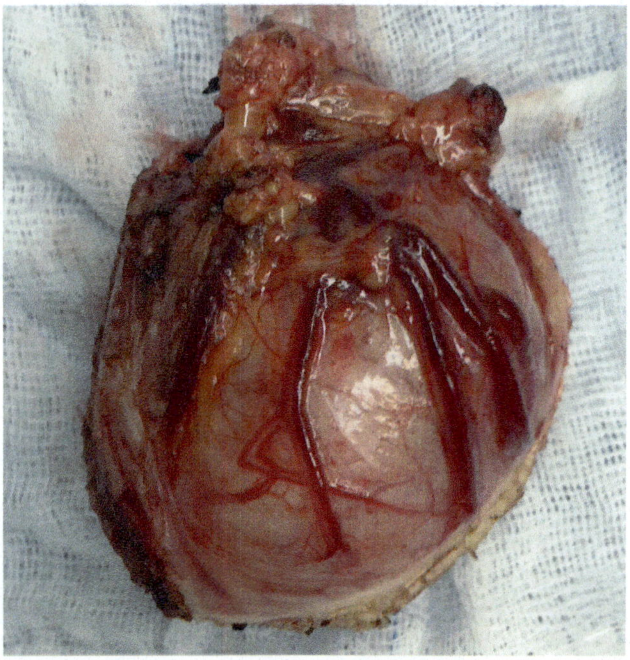

Fig. 2.7 The gross specimen

Genetic Testing The sequencing analysis showed heterozygous mutation in exon 11 of *KIT* at codon 557, TGG > AGG, and the encoded amino acid was changed from tryptophan to arginine. Exons 9, 13, and 17 of *KIT* and exons 12 and 18 of *PDGFRA* were wild type.

2.1.4 Prognosis

The patient was discharged on a liquid diet 3 days after surgery. Pathology confirmed the diagnosis of gastric GIST with a low risk of recurrence according to the modified NIH risk classification. The patient was advised to seek regular follow-up, and reported no complaints of discomfort on telephone follow-up in mid-December 2018.

2.2 Case 4 A 73-Year-Old Man with GIST Who Underwent Laparoscopic and Endoscopic Cooperative Surgery

Qian Shen and Huikuan Chu

2.2.1 Case Background

A 73-year-old man was admitted to hospital to investigate a loss of appetite for over 3 months. On July 30, 2021, positron emission tomography (PET)-CT showed a nodular shadow of gastric soft tissue density protruding beyond the gastric contour, there was increased metabolic local foci, and further increased delayed imaging, which was considered to be indicative of a large GIST. On August 6, 2021, contrast-enhanced CT of the stomach showed a soft tissue nodule in the lesser curvature of the gastric wall, which was also consistent with a GIST. Since the onset of the disease, the patient had poor appetite, normal sleep, daily unformed stool, frequent urgent urination, physical weakening, and weight loss of 2 kg.

2.2.1.1 Past History and Family History

The patient had been diagnosed with diabetes more than 4 years previously and reported irregular medication usage, and irregular blood glucose monitoring. He reported no drug allergies. Both parents were deceased and the causes of death were unknown, but there was no similar medical history in the family.

2.2.1.2 Physical Examination

The patient's vital signs were stable. The abdomen was flat, and no gastrointestinal pattern or peristaltic waves were seen. There was no abdominal tenderness, no rebound tenderness or guarding, without any palpable mass. The shifting dullness was negative, and bowel sounds were normal.

2.2.1.3 Auxiliary Examination

PET-CT A nodular shadow of gastric soft tissue density, protruding outside the gastric contour, with elevated local metabolism was observed. This was considered to be a possible GIST (Fig. 2.8).

Gastric Contrast-Enhanced CT Soft tissue nodules on the lesser curvature of the gastric wall were observed. A possible diagnosis of GIST was considered.

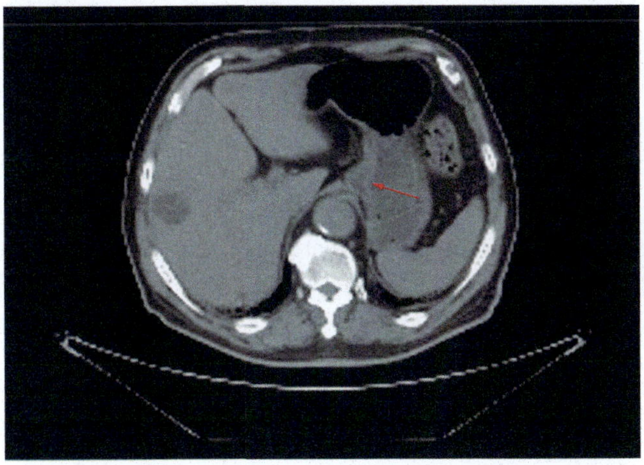

Fig. 2.8 Preoperative CT showed the extragastric soft tissue mass

2.2.2 Therapy

2.2.2.1 Case Analysis

The patient was an elderly man who presented with loss of appetite for more than 3 months. Following the initial examinations, the patient's preliminary diagnosis was GIST. Treatment with surgical resection was considered because the tumor did not invade the surrounding organ tissues. Combining laparoscopy with endoscopy allowed the advantages of both procedures to be utilized. Locating the lesions intraoperatively using gastroscopy can ensure smooth progress of laparoscopic surgery. Additionally, the use of laparoscopy can assist endoscopic surgery, through timely detection and treatment of complications arising from endoscopic resection. Therefore, it was recommended that the patient undergo combined laparoscopic and endoscopic surgery.

2.2.2.2 Treatment

Preoperative examination revealed no obvious surgical contraindications, and the patient underwent combined laparoscopy and gastroscopy for gastric tumor resection on August 25, 2021. Laparoscopic exploration of the abdominal peritoneum, pelvic cavity, liver, and other organs showed no metastases, and no mass was observed in the anterior gastric wall. The gastrocolic ligament was incised laterally from the gastroepiploic vascular arch, the posterior gastric wall was explored, and pancreatic adhesions observed in the posterior gastric wall were separated. Endoscopic and laparoscopic views showed that the tumor was located in the lesser curvature of the posterior gastric wall and was approximately 1.5 cm × 2 cm in size, with a smooth surface and clear boundary (Fig. 2.9). The intraoperative diagnosis was of a GIST, exhibiting as a posterior gastric wall mass. The gastric body mass was resected with a portion of the posterior wall. The adherent omental tissue near the tumor on the lesser curvature of the posterior wall of the gastric body was separated, the tumor was completely removed by clamping and firing a 45 mm blue nail linear cutter stapler into the gastric wall at the root of the tumor, and the gastric wall incision was reinforced using barbed suture embedding (Figs. 2.10 and 2.11). Tumor specimens were removed in specimen bags.

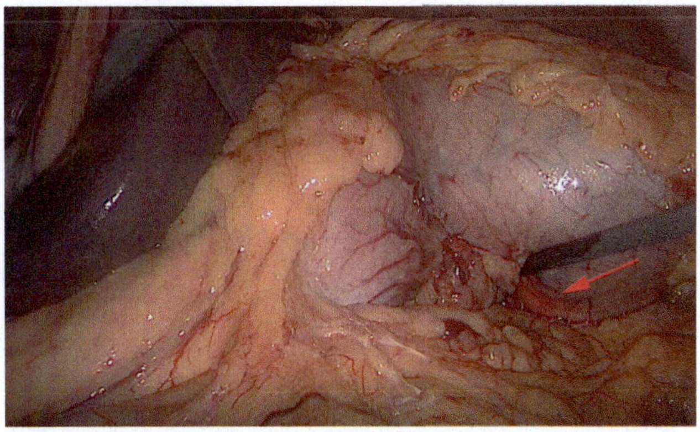

Fig. 2.9 Intraoperative endoscopic exploration of the tumor with clear endoscopic guidance through the gastric wall

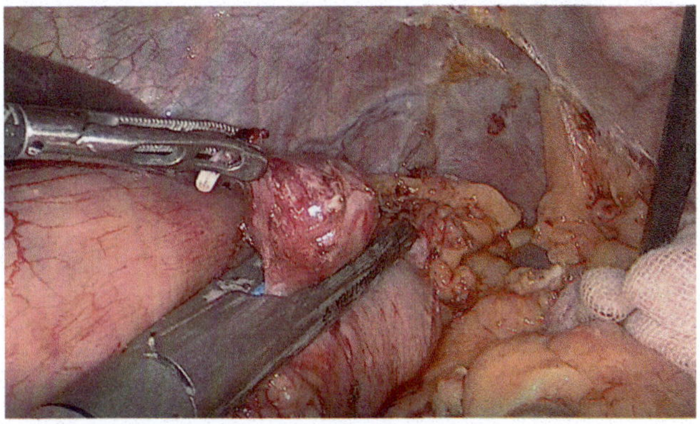

Fig. 2.10 Tumour resection using combined endoscopy and laparoscopy

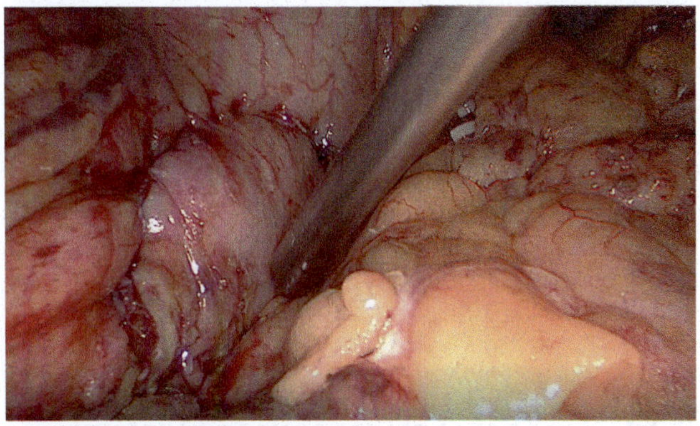

Fig. 2.11 Incision suture

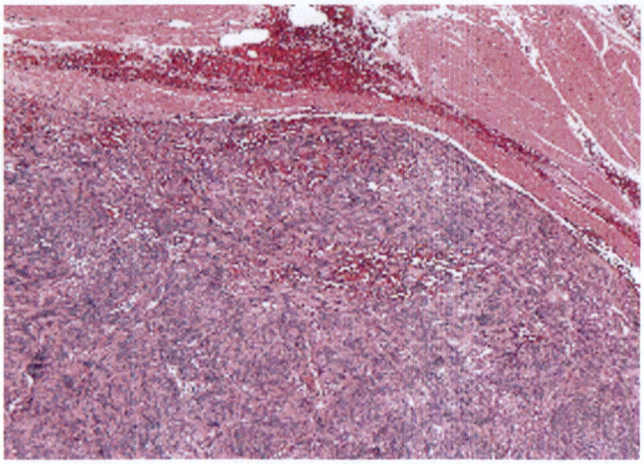

Fig. 2.12 Postoperative pathological diagnosis: GIST, mainly composed of spindle cells

2.2.2.3 Postoperative Pathology and Genetic Testing

Pathological Diagnosis Gastrointestinal stromal tumor (1.5 cm × 1.5 cm in size), with mitotic count less than 5/50 HPF, classified as very low risk according to the modified NIH risk classification. (Fig. 2.12).

Immunohistochemistry CD117 (+), CD34 (+), DOG-1 (+), SMA (−), S100 (−), ALK (−), SDHB (+), Ki-67 (Li: 3%).

Genetic Testing Genetic testing was not performed for this patient as there was a very low recurrence risk.

2.2.3 Prognosis

The patient recovered well after the surgery. The abdominal drainage tube was removed, and the patient did not report any particular discomfort. The patient was discharged from hospital 6 days after surgery. As of January 30, 2022, there was no recurrence.

2.2.4 Experience of Diagnosis and Therapy

2.2.4.1 The Advantages of Laparoscopic and Endoscopic Cooperative Surgery in the Treatment of GIST

GIST originate from the muscularis mucosae or muscularis propria of the gastric wall, and can protrude intraluminally or extraluminally [4]. Locating GIST, especially small GIST, prior to laparoscopy is a problem that afflicts clinicians. Even after preoperative examination using gastroscopy, endoscopic ultrasound, and CT, it is still likely to be difficult to detect the lesion during surgery, especially with the lack of tactile feedback during laparoscopic surgery. The advantages of laparoscopy combined with gastroscopy for locating a mass intraoperatively are very obvious. By using laparoscopic magnification and gastroscopic examination, lesions can be quickly and accurately located [5].

Both endoscopic therapy and laparoscopic surgery inevitably have some limitations for the treatment of GIST. The limitations of endoscopic treatment alone are the following: (1) Endoscopic treatment is difficult to perform for gastric GIST that is large or located in the fundus or cardiac. (2) It is difficult to safely and completely remove gastric GIST which originates from the muscularis propria endoscopically as this is rich in blood supply. Additionally, endoscopic therapy usually relies on energy cutting, but it is difficult to find the balance point of energy cutting, so the risk of complications such as bleeding and perforation is relatively high. This is also the main reason leading to conversion to laparotomy. (3) It is difficult to comprehensively determine the depth of invasion of a gastric GIST under direct endoscopic vision, and there is a possibility of leaving positive resection margins. The main limitations for laparoscopic surgery alone are as follows: (1) It is very difficult to locate the tumor when laparoscopy is used alone to treat intraluminal gastric GIST, especially small GIST. due to the lack of tactile feedback in laparoscopic surgery; (2) Laparoscopic resection for GIST close to the cardia and pylorus may lead to postoperative stenosis; (3) Wedge resection using a cutter stapler often removes excessive normal gastric wall tissue, and occasionally leaves positive resection margins. However, laparoscopic and endoscopic cooperative surgery can effectively avoid the above shortcomings.

With the support of intraoperative endoscopy, surgeons can not only accurately locate, but also observe whether tumor resection is complete and avoid excessive resection of normal tissue. Additionally, endoscopy can aid in the timely detection of complications such as intraluminal bleeding after resection and suturing, poor closure and stenosis after closure and these complications can be dealt with using laparoscopic surgery. Additionally, if perforation is caused by endoscopic surgery, this can be repaired immediately. Laparoscopic observation can allow for timely detection of thermal damage that cannot be identified endoscopically and timely repair or gastric wall reinforcement, which can avoid postoperative delayed perforation, thus increasing the safety and effectiveness of surgery and improving the postoperative quality of life.

2.2.4.2 Key Points of Attention in the Implementation of Laparoscopy and Endoscopic Cooperative Surgery

As an emerging surgical diagnosis and treatment technique, there are some key points to be aware of when performing laparoscopic and endoscopic cooperative surgery: (1) In the process of tumor resection, care should be taken to avoid touching the tumor with the endoscope or laparoscope to prevent abdominal implantation metastasis caused by tumor rupture; (2) As little air as possible should be injected into the gastric cavity to reduce the tension of the gastric wall, without affecting the observation or operation, to improve the ease of laparoscopic operation and reduce the occurrence of postoperative abdominal distension; (3) The endotracheal tube can be easily loosened or removed during gastroscopic surgery, and anesthesia should be closely observed to prevent accidents; (4) Attention should be paid to the principle of asepsis when inserting the endoscope to avoid contaminating the surgical area; (5) The laparoscopic light source should be temporarily turned off after inserting the endoscope to avoid affecting endoscopic observation. After the lesion is preliminarily located using the laparoscope according to the position of the endoscopic light source, the corresponding serosal surface should be lightly touched with dissecting forceps to ensure accurate localization; (6) During the implementation of laparoscopic and endoscopic cooperative surgery, the choice of surgical approach should be determined based on the tumor characteristics. Generally, gastroscopy should be used to evaluate the lesion and then the specific resection method can be determined; (7) The purpose of laparoscopic surgery combined with endoscopic surgery is to perform a more minimally invasive surgery, but each step of the procedure must be performed meticulously, and it is necessary to minimize the incidence of complications and avoid reoperation due to intraoperative or postoperative bleeding, anastomotic leakage, and other complications.

2.3 Expert Comments

Gang Zhao

With the improvement of people's health awareness and the popularization of endoscopy, more and more small gastric GIST are found in physical examinations. Although most gastric GIST <2 cm can be followed up regularly without surgery, surgical intervention needs to be considered for gastric GIST ≥2 cm in size, small GIST with unfavorable endoscopic ultrasound factors, and small GIST which are observed to grow rapidly during follow-up [6]. There are still great controversies in the treatment of small gastric GIST using endoscopic resection alone, mainly focusing on the possible risks such as incomplete resection and complications such as bleeding and perforation, while laparoscopic resection alone also has some limitations in the treatment of small gastric GIST, especially for intraluminal tumors that are difficult to accurately locate.

Combined laparoscopic and endoscopic procedures plays an important role in the treatment of small GIST as the technique integrates the advantages of the two techniques, improves and avoids shortcomings, greatly improves the safety of laparoscopic and endoscopic techniques, and expands the scope of application [7]. Laparoscopy can detect bleeding and perforation and provide treatment with suturing, greatly reducing the difficulty of endoscopic surgery. Intraoperative bleeding can be accurately located endoscopically, and this information can be used to guide the appropriate extent of surgery and reduce surgical trauma.

At present, the greatest obstacle to the popularization and development of laparoscopically combined techniques is the difficulty in arranging cooperation between various departments (such as surgery, gastroenterology, operating room, anesthesiology). It is believed that with the establishment and improvement of multidisciplinary collaborative diagnosis and treatment mechanisms, combined laparoscopy techniques will play an increasingly important role in the diagnosis and treatment of small GIST [8].

References

1. Meng Y, Li W, Han L, Zhang Q, Gong W, Cai J, Li A, Yan Q, Lai Q, Yu J, Bai L, Liu S, Li Y. Long-term outcomes of endoscopic submucosal dissection versus laparoscopic resection for gastric stromal tumors less than 2 cm. J Gastroenterol Hepatol. 2017;32(10):1693–7. https://doi.org/10.1111/jgh.13768.
2. Hiki N, Yamamoto Y, Fukunaga T, Yamaguchi T, Nunobe S, Tokunaga M, Miki A, Ohyama S, Seto Y. Laparoscopic and endoscopic cooperative surgery for gastrointestinal stromal tumor dissection. Surg Endosc. 2008;22(7):1729–35. https://doi.org/10.1007/s00464-007-9696-8.
3. Qiu WQ, Wang M, Zhuang J, Shen ZY, Xue HB, Shen L, Ge ZZ, Shen YY, Liu Q, Cao H. Clinical analysis of laparoscopic and endoscopic cooperative surgery in the treatment of gastric gastrointestinal stromal tumor: report of 46 cases. Zhong Hua Wei Chang Wai Ke Za Zhi. 2012;15(3):240–2. https://doi.org/10.3760/cma.j.issn.1671-0274.2012.03.013.
4. Blay JY, von Mehren M, Blackstein ME. Perspective on updated treatment guidelines for patients with gastrointestinal stromal tumors. Cancer. 2010;116(22):5126–37. https://doi.org/10.1002/cncr.25267.
5. Bédard EL, Mamazza J, Schlachta CM, Poulin EC. Laparoscopic resection of gastrointestinal stromal tumors: not all tumors are created equal. Surg Endosc. 2006;20(3):500–3. https://doi.org/10.1007/s00464-005-0287-2.
6. Chien CH, Chien RN, Yen CL, Fang KM, Liu CJ, Lin CL, Chang JJ, Chen LW, Lee TS, Chen SW, Hu CC, Chang LC. The role of endoscopic ultrasonography examination for evaluation and surveillance of gastric subepithelial masses. Chang Gung Med J. 2010;33(1):73–81. http://cgmj.cgu.edu.tw/3301/330109.pdf
7. Balde AI, Chen T, Hu Y, Redondo NJD, Liu H, Gong W, Yu J, Zhen L, Li G. Safety analysis of laparoscopic endoscopic cooperative surgery versus endoscopic submucosal dissection for selected gastric gastrointestinal stromal tumors: a propensity score-matched study. Surg Endosc. 2017;31(2):843–51. https://doi.org/10.1007/s00464-016-5042-3.
8. Mullady DK, Tan BR. A multidisciplinary approach to the diagnosis and treatment of gastrointestinal stromal tumor. J Clin Gastroenterol. 2013;47(7):578–85. https://doi.org/10.1097/MCG.0b013e3182936c87.

Da Vinci Robotic Management of Gastrointestinal Stromal Tumors

3

Tao Wang, Ming Cai, and Yanbing Zhou

Keywords

Gastrointestinal stromal tumor · Stomach · Robotic surgery

3.1 Case 5 A 36-Year-Old Man with Gastric GIST Who Received Da Vinci Robotic Surgery

Tao Wang and Ming Cai

3.1.1 Introduction

The Da Vinci surgical robot system consists of three parts, including the doctor's console, imaging system, and bedside robotic arm system. Compared to traditional laparoscopic surgery, the Da Vinci surgical robot has clearer imaging, a larger movement angle of the robotic arm, and more flexible operational capabilities. At the same time, the Da Vinci robotic surgical system can also filter physiological vibrations, making surgery more precise [1]. Research by Desiderio et al. shows that robotic surgery is safe and feasible to remove GIST [2]. Therefore, the Da Vinci surgical robot is reliable for GIST surgery.

T. Wang · M. Cai (✉)
Department of Gastrointestinal Surgery, Union Hospital, Tongji Medical College, Huazhong University of Science and Technology, Wuhan, China
e-mail: wangtaojx@hust.edu.cn; caiming918@hust.edu.cn

Y. Zhou
Department of Gastrointestinal Surgery, The Affiliated Hospital of Qingdao University, Qingdao, China

3.1.2 Case Background

The patient, a 36-year-old man, was found to have mass lesions in the fundus of the stomach during a physical examination at a local hospital on September 14, 2016. On September 20, 2016, he was admitted to the Department of Gastrointestinal Surgery, Union Hospital, Tongji Medical College, Huazhong University of Science and Technology. An ultrasound gastroscopy revealed a slightly hypoechoic mass in the gastric submucosa. He was diagnosed with a gastric fundus mass in the outpatient clinic and was admitted to the hospital.

3.1.2.1 Past History and Family History

He reported no history of allergies; his parents were alive and there was no similar medical history in his family.

3.1.2.2 Physical Examination

The abdomen was flat and soft; no masses were palpable; the liver and spleen were not palpable below the costal margin, and there was no tenderness or rebound tenderness. There was no percussion pain in the kidney area. There was no shifting dullness, and bowel sounds were normal.

3.1.2.3 Auxiliary Examination

Blood Routine WBC 4.90×10^9/L, RBC 5.45×10^{12}/L, HB 161 g/L, PLT 218×10^9/L, NEUT% 61.1%, LY% 30.2%.

Blood Chemistry TBil 11.2 μmol/L, DBil 3.8 μmol/L, TP 80.0 g/L, ALB 52.9 g/L, Cre 91.1 μmol/L, BUN 4.12 mmol/L, Na^+ 142.2 mmol/L, K^+ 4.33 mmol/L, Cl^- 98.8 mmol/L.

Tumor Markers No abnormalities.

K. Tao, H. Cao (eds.), *Clinical Management of Gastrointestinal Stromal Tumor*, https://doi.org/10.1007/978-981-99-9392-5_3

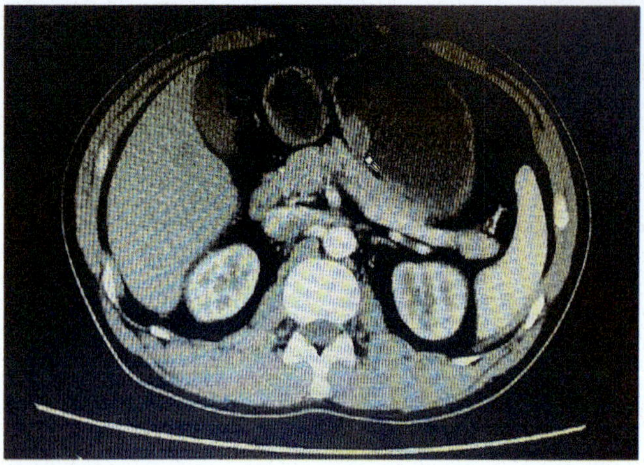

Fig. 3.1 Enhanced CT revealed the tumor of the lesser curvature

Abdominal CT Enhanced abdominal CT in September 2016 showed an approximately 2.3 cm × 1.2 cm mass at the lower curvature of stomach. The CT value of the plain scan was about 50 HU. The CT value of the arterial and venous phases after enhancement was about 74 and 80 HU, respectively. The internal density of the mass was uneven; the boundary of the lesion was clear; the adjacent serosal surface was smooth; the surrounding fat gap was clear, and there were no obvious swollen lymph nodes. The diagnosis was possibly GIST. No other abnormalities were detected (Fig. 3.1).

Initial Diagnosis Space-occupying lesion of the gastric fundus, possible GIST.

3.1.3 Therapy

3.1.3.1 Case Analysis

The patient was a middle-aged man who consulted the doctor due to a physical examination revealing a gastric fundus mass. After completing the relevant examinations, the initial diagnosis was of a (gastric) GIST. The tumor was located on the lesser curvature of the stomach and was approximately 2.3 cm × 1.2 cm in size. Because the mass did not invade the surrounding organs and tissues, surgical resection was considered an appropriate first-line treatment. Robotic surgery can provide magnified, three-dimensional high-definition images controlled by the surgeon, making it easier to distinguish the relationship between tissues and organs, and reducing damage to surrounding normal tissues. Because the tumor was adjacent to the cardia, the patient had higher requirements for minimally invasive surgery to avoid affecting the function of the cardia after the operation, and it was recommended that the patient undergo robotic surgery.

3.1.3.2 Treatment

The patient underwent preoperative preparation under the guidance of an enhanced recovery after surgery (ERAS) program and underwent robot-assisted abdominal cavity exploration and gastric tumor resection on September 27, 2016. Intraoperative gastroscopic exploration revealed that the tumor was located in the posterior wall of the stomach near the cardia and was approximately 2.0 cm × 1.0 cm in size. An incision was made in the omentum on the greater curvature to expose the tumor in the posterior wall of the stomach, and an additional incision was made in the anterior wall of the stomach opposite the tumor. The gastric wall was cut with a laparoscopic linear cutting stapler 1 cm from the tumor, and the tumor was completely resected. The tumor was placed in a specimen bag and the bag opening was ligated with silk thread. The specimen was removed through an incision near the umbilicus. The stomach wall was reinforced with absorbable thread, and the incision around the umbilicus was sutured. The operation was successful, with an operative time of 60 min, and intraoperative blood loss was approximately 10 mL (Figs. 3.2, 3.3, 3.4 and 3.5).

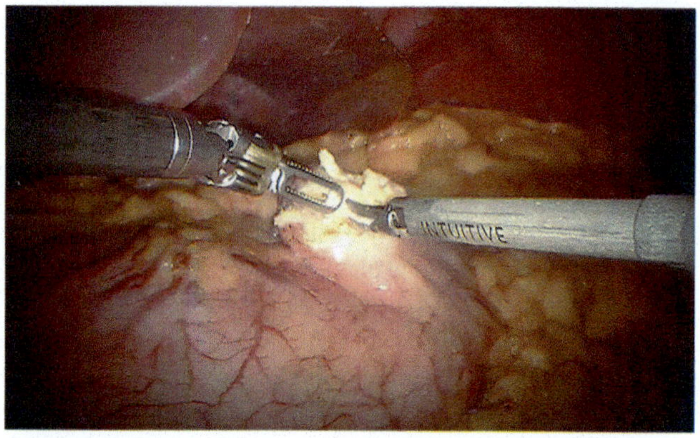

Fig. 3.2 An incision was made in the anterior wall of the stomach

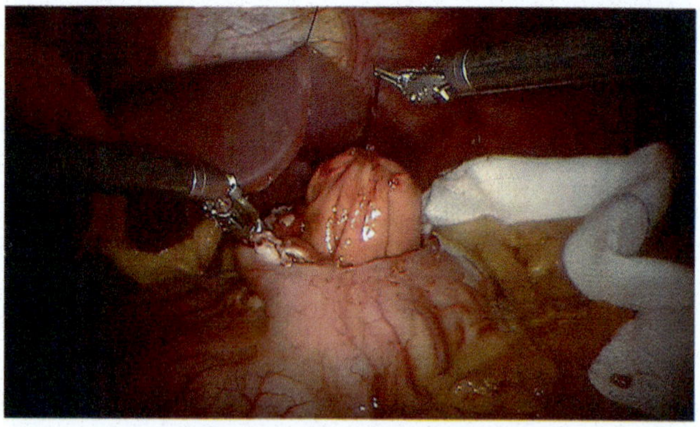

Fig. 3.3 Silk thread was used to lift the tumor

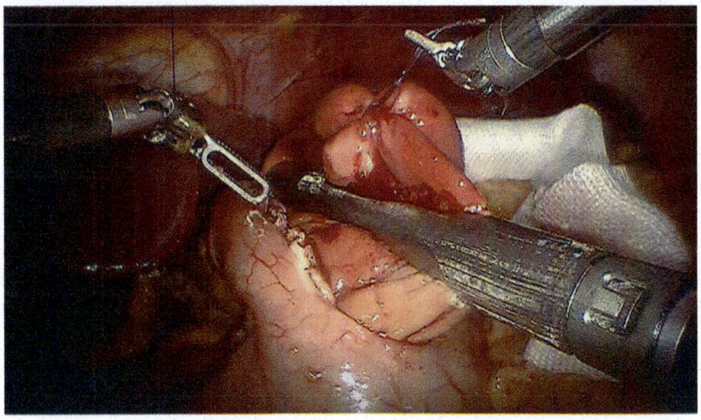

Fig. 3.4 The tumor was removed with a linear cutting stapler

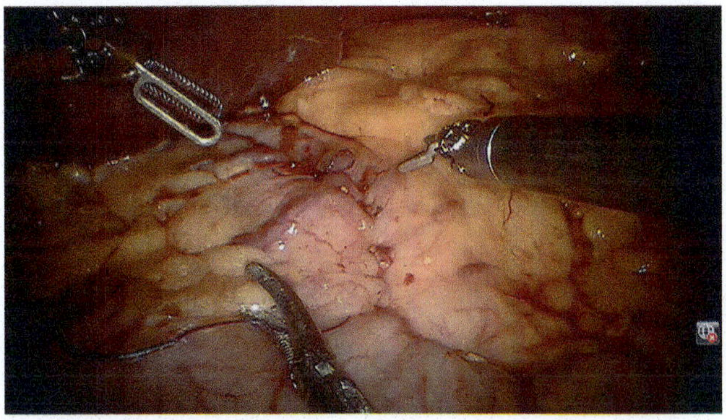

Fig. 3.5 Absorbable thread was used to suture the stomach wall

3.1.3.3 Postoperative Pathology and Genetic Testing

Pathological Diagnosis Gastric GIST (1.9 cm × 1.7 cm × 1.0 cm), mitotic count less than 5/50 HPF. According to the modified NIH risk classification, the tumor was very low risk.

Immunohistochemistry CD117 (+), DOG-1 (+), CD34 (+), SMA (−), S-100 (−), Ki-67 (Li < 5%).

Genetic Testing Mutations were detected in exon 11 (p.P573_P585dup) and 13 (P.V654A) of *KIT*, and exons 12 and 18 of *PDGFRA* were all wild-type.

3.1.4 Prognosis

The patient began flatus 24 hours postoperatively. On the first postoperative day, the gastrointestinal decompression tube and urinary catheter were removed, and the patient began to drink water and out of bed. On the second day, there was no bloating or discomfort, and enteral nutrition was given. On the 3rd day, the patient was given a semi-liquid diet. On the 4th day postoperative, the drainage tube was removed, and routine blood, liver and kidney function, procalcitonin, and C-reactive protein tests were normal. The patient was subsequently discharged from the hospital.

As the postoperative risk was very low risk, no targeted drug therapy was administered. As of January 2022, after 63 months of follow-up, the patient has survived and is disease-free.

3.1.5 Experience of Diagnosis and Therapy

At present, the surgical team of Professor Kaixiong Tao of the Department of Gastrointestinal Surgery, Union Hospital of Tongji Medical College, Huazhong University of Science and Technology has performed robotic surgery on more than 20 patients with GIST, and all patients have a good prognosis. Based on the experience of our center in successfully implementing robotic resection of GIST, we believe that robotic surgery has the following advantages: the robotic arm of the surgical robot is fixed, providing a three-dimensional and high-definition surgical field of vision, which can enlarge the surgical field when required; The Da Vinci robotic instrument arm operates without tremor and can move freely in seven directions, ensuring fine operations in a narrow surgical space; during the Da Vinci robotic surgery, the surgeon adopts a comfortable sitting position to reduce fatigue and the incidence of errors. Additionally, remote surgery can be performed by connecting a Da Vinci robot to the Internet. However, to date, Da Vinci robotic surgery has not been widely implemented in GIST for economic reasons.

The robotic surgery system breaks through the limitations of traditional surgery and laparoscopic surgery and improves the surgical accuracy for GIST treatment to a new level. Compared to laparoscopic surgery, robotic surgery is more minimally invasive, reduces the probability of postoperative complications for patients, and speeds up the postoperative recovery [3].

In this case, we combined ERAS protocols with the minimally invasive advantages of Da Vinci robotic surgery to reduce surgical stress and complications and accelerate postoperative recovery. The specific steps for implementing ERAS for GIST are the following: (1) Preoperative education: Inform patients and their families of the necessity of implementing ERAS; (2) Intestinal preparation: Intestinal preparation is not routine, but 800 mL of 10% glucose solution is taken orally 10 h before surgery, followed by 400 mL of 10% glucose solution 2 h before anesthesia; (3) Anesthesia plan: systemic combined with epidural block; (4) Use insulation blanket to control body temperature, and fluid input intraoperatively; (5) Postoperative analgesia: analgesia methods such as transversus abdominis plane nerve block and local incision infiltration may be used; (6) Encourage a small amount of water intake after anesthesia, encourage getting out of bed within 24 h after the operation, and remove the urinary catheter within 48 h.

The patient was discharged 4 days after surgery in this case, suggesting that the robotic surgery combined with the ERAS program was safe and effective, and can shorten the patient's recovery time, promote the recovery of the patient's gastrointestinal function after surgery, and improve the perioperative comfort of the patient.

3.2 Expert Comments

Yanbing Zhou

The Da Vinci robot has become a surgical platform familiar to and frequently used by surgeons and can provide more accurate and high-quality surgical treatments for patients. Da Vinci robotic surgery has many advantages over traditional minimally invasive techniques. For example, the surgical field of view can be magnified more than ten times and can present the surgeon with three-dimensional, high-definition images of the patient's body cavity, as well as extremely small blood vessels and nerves [4, 5]. Obviously, surgical instruments can simulate the flexible operation of the human wrist, filter out unnecessary vibrations, and exceed the accuracy of human hands. In the surgical application for GIST, robotic surgery has the advantages of the excellent 3D display, magnification of the surgical field, seven degrees of freedom of the robotic arm, the ability to perform fine anatomical operations and microscopic suturing, and can prevent damage to nerves and blood vessels [5]. Robotic surgery is more suitable for the surgical treatment of areas such as the cardia, pylorus, duodenum, pelvis, and rectum. Based on the biological behavior of GIST, preoperative imatinib adjuvant therapy and dynamic evaluation may be adopted for patients with tumors located in areas which are difficult to reach laparoscopically, local progression, and who may require potential expansion surgery, and surgery can be performed after the tumor is downgraded. Robotic surgery can increase the R0 resection rate without expanding the scope of surgery, and preserve organ functions to the greatest extent, including cardia, pyloric function, and even urination, defecation, and sexual function. Buchs et al. [6] took the lead in studying the safety of robotic GIST wedge resection and the short-term prognosis of patients, and the results showed that patients who underwent robotic surgery to remove gastric GIST recovered well after surgery, and there were no instances of patient relapse in the 18-month follow-up period. Solaini et al. [7] reported that the R0 resection rate and short-term prognosis of patients in the robotic surgery group were no different from those of patients in the laparoscopic surgery group. In addition, studies have shown that robotic surgery could extend the feasibility of a minimally invasive approach to patients requiring advanced suturing [2, 8]. This patient strictly followed the perioperative ERAS management principles, and the Da Vinci surgical robot system completely removed the cardia GIST and retained the gastric cardia function, without complications such as cardiac stenosis or reflux. The patient was followed up for 5 years and survived without recurrence, which was a successful model. At present, there are few reports on the application of robotic surgery for GIST, and the number of cases is small [9, 10]. Generally speaking, the surgery is more accurate, and the curative effect is not inferior to that of traditional laparoscopic surgery. However, the indications, clinical efficacy, outcome, and evaluation of health economics indicators for Da Vinci robotic GIST surgery still need to be verified by well-designed clinical studies.

References

1. de'Angelis N, Genova P, Amiot A, Charpy C, Disabato M, Belgaumkar AP, Chahrour A, Legou F, Azoulay D, Brunetti F. Robotic versus laparoscopic gastric resection for primary gastrointestinal stromal tumors >5 cm: a size-matched and location-matched comparison. Surg Laparosc Endosc Percutan Tech. 2017;27(1):65–71. https://doi.org/10.1097/SLE.0000000000000371.
2. Desiderio J, Trastulli S, Cirocchi R, Boselli C, Noya G, Parisi A, Cavaliere D. Robotic gastric resection of large gastrointestinal stromal tumors. Int J Surg. 2013;11(2):191–6. https://doi.org/10.1016/j.ijsu.2013.01.002.
3. Crippa J, Grass F, Dozois EJ, Mathis KL, Merchea A, Colibaseanu DT, Kelley SR, Larson DW. Robotic surgery for rectal cancer provides advantageous outcomes over laparoscopic approach: results from a large retrospective cohort. Ann Surg. 2021;274(6):e1218–22. https://doi.org/10.1097/SLA.0000000000003805.
4. Yamamoto H, Ebihara Y, Tanaka K, Matsui A, Nakanishi Y, Asano T, Noji T, Kurashima Y, Murakami S, Nakamura T, Tsuchikawa T, Okamura K, Shichinohe T, Hirano S. Robot-assisted thoracoscopic esophagectomy for gastrointestinal stromal tumor of the esophagus: A case report. Int J Surg Case Rep. 2021;86:106335. https://doi.org/10.1016/j.ijscr.2021.106335.
5. Jin D, Yao L, Yu J, Liu R, Guo T, Yang K, Gou Y. Robotic-assisted minimally invasive esophagectomy versus the conventional minimally invasive one: A meta-analysis and systematic review. Int J Med Robot. 2019;15(3):e1988. https://doi.org/10.1002/rcs.1988.
6. Buchs NC, Bucher P, Pugin F, Hagen ME, Morel P. Robot-assisted oncologic resection for large gastric gastrointestinal stromal tumor: a preliminary case series. J Laparoendosc Adv Surg Tech A. 2010;20(5):411–5. https://doi.org/10.1089/lap.2009.0385.
7. Solaini L, Cavaliere D, Fico V, Milone M, De Pascale S, Desiderio J, Vitali G, Parisi A, Fumagalli Romario U, De Palma GD, D'Ugo D, Ercolani G. Open versus laparoscopic versus robotic gastric gastrointestinal stromal tumour resections: A multicentre cohort study. Int J Med Robot. 2021;17(2):e2198. https://doi.org/10.1002/rcs.2198.
8. Zhao J, Wang G, Jiang Z, Jiang C, Liu J, Zhou J, Li J. Robotic Gastrotomy with intracorporeal suture for patients with gastric gastrointestinal stromal tumors located at cardia and subcardiac region. Surg Laparosc Endosc Percutan Tech. 2018;28(1):e1–7. https://doi.org/10.1097/SLE.0000000000000498.
9. Saumoy M, Guenthart B, Madanat L, Afaneh C, Kahaleh M. Robotic-assisted endoscopic full-thickness resection of a gastrointestinal stromal tumor: the tip of the iceberg. Endoscopy. 2018;50(8):E216–7. https://doi.org/10.1055/a-0624-1644.
10. Maggioni C, Shida A, Mancini R, Ioni L, Pernazza G. Safety profile and oncological outcomes of gastric gastrointestinal stromal tumors (GISTs) robotic resection: single center experience. Int J Med Robot. 2019;15(6):e2031. https://doi.org/10.1002/rcs.2031.

Endoscopic Management of Gastrointestinal Stromal Tumors

4

Qi Jiang, Zhen Ding, Jiaxian Yu, Lei Tu, and Yingjiang Ye

Keywords

Gastrointestinal stromal tumor · Surgery · Endoscopy Esophagus · Submucosal tunneling endoscopic resection

4.1 Case 6 A 68-Year-Old Woman with Cardia GIST Who Underwent Endoscopic Surgery

Qi Jiang and Zhen Ding

4.1.1 Introduction

Endoscopic submucosal dissection (ESD) developed from endoscopic mucosal resection (EMR) and involves cutting off the target lesion through submucosal injection with stained normal saline and high-frequency electrosurgical knife dissection to remove the lesion en bloc. The advantage of minimally invasive endoscopic surgery such as ESD and EMR is in maintaining the integrity of the gastric wall, which can effectively reduce the probability of postoperative anastomotic stenosis for cardia or pylorus GIST.

Q. Jiang · J. Yu
Department of Gastrointestinal Surgery, Union Hospital, Tongji Medical College, Huazhong University of Science and Technology, Wuhan, China
e-mail: jiangqijx@hust.edu.cn; yujx@hku-szh.org

Z. Ding (✉) · L. Tu (✉)
Department of Gastroenterology, Union Hospital, Tongji Medical College, Huazhong University of Science and Technology, Wuhan, China
e-mail: tulei@hust.edu.cn

Y. Ye
Department of Gastrointestinal Surgery, Peking University People's Hospital, Beijing, China
e-mail: yeyingjiang@pkuph.edu.cn

4.1.2 Case Background

The patient, a 68-year-old woman, presented to the local hospital, complaining of abdominal pain for 1 week. Upper GI endoscopy revealed a gastric fundus neoplasm and erosive gastritis. Anti-inflammatory and acid suppression treatment were administered, and supportive cares were performed. In November 2016, the patient was admitted to the Department of Gastrointestinal Surgery, Union Hospital, Tongji Medical College, Huazhong University of Science and Technology for further treatment. Endoscopic ultrasonography (Fig. 4.1) demonstrated a submucosal lesion in the greater curvature of the gastric cardia with normal mucosa and regular wall. The tumor echo was even, and it measured 2 cm × 2 cm with a continuous envelope. The neoplasm originated from the muscularis propria and was growing toward the lumen, which was considered as GIST.

4.1.2.1 Past History and Family History

The patient was previously healthy and reported no drug allergies. The patient's parents were deceased, and there was no similar medical history in the family.

4.1.2.2 Physical Examination

The patient's vital signs were stable, and the skin and mucous membranes were not yellowish or pale. The abdomen was flat, and no gastrointestinal or peristaltic waves were observed. The abdomen was soft with no tenderness, rebound tenderness, or palpable mass, and bowel sounds were normal.

4.1.2.3 Auxiliary Examination

Common Blood Count WBC 3.77 × 10^9/L, RBC 3.66 × 10^{12}/L, Hb 119 g/L, PLT 248 × 10^9/L, NEUT (%) 52.60, LY (%) 41.10.

K. Tao, H. Cao (eds.), *Clinical Management of Gastrointestinal Stromal Tumor*, https://doi.org/10.1007/978-981-99-9392-5_4

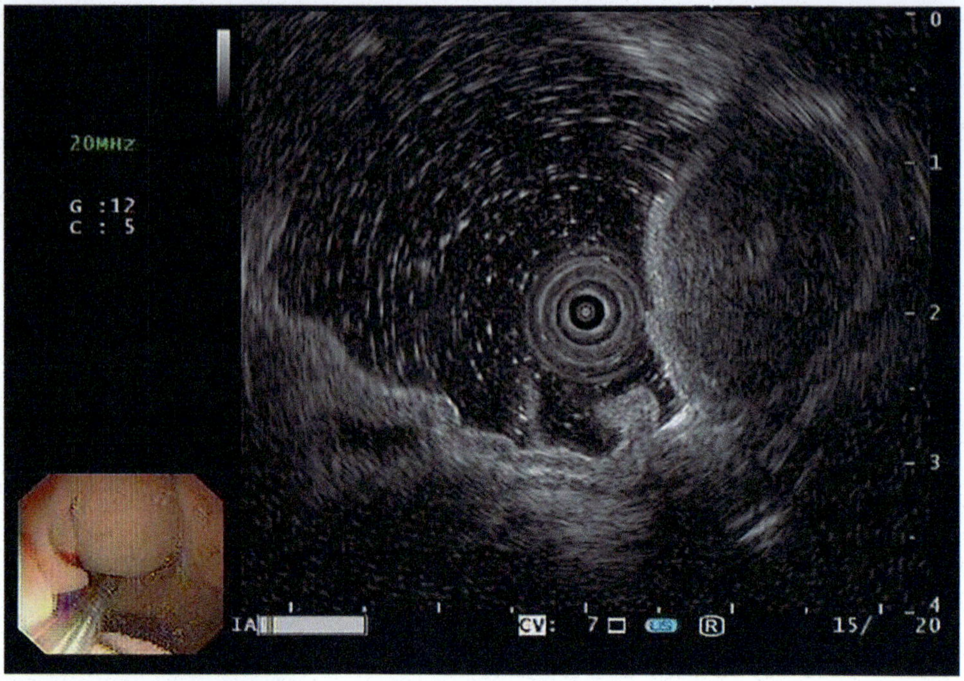

Fig. 4.1 Endoscopic ultrasound revealed a subepithelial lesion in the greater curvature of the gastric cardia

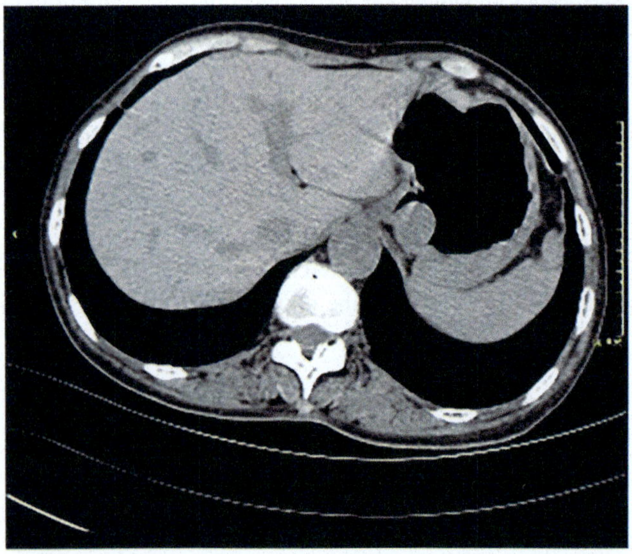

Fig. 4.2 Abdominal CT showed a space-occupying lesion in the cardia of the stomach

Serum Chemistry Profile No significant abnormalities.

Serum Cancer Biomarkers No significant abnormalities.

Abdominal CT A space-occupying lesion was identified in the cardia of the stomach, measuring 1.8 cm × 1.7 cm in size, with a regular wall and peri-gastric fatty space. No enlarged lymph node was detected. The mass was determined to be a gastric neoplasm, possibly a gastric GIST (Fig. 4.2).

4.1.2.4 Primary Diagnosis

1. Space-occupying lesion at the cardia of the stomach, possibly GIST
2. Erosive gastritis

4.1.3 Therapy

4.1.3.1 Case Analysis

The patient was an elderly woman with a complaint of abdominal pain for 1 week. The primary diagnosis was gastric GIST. The neoplasm was located on the gastric fundus adjacent to the gastric cardia, measuring 2 cm × 2 cm. According to the Chinese Consensus Guidelines for Diagnosis and Management of Gastrointestinal Stromal Tumor (2017 Edition), GIST located in sites such as the esophagogastric junction (EGJ) are indicated for surgery whenever found, as this can prevent tumor growth, which can make it difficult to preserve the function of gastric cardia. In such cases, ESD is preferred because using a laparoscopic cutting stapler may lead to postoperative anastomotic stenosis of the cardia.

4.1.3.2 Treatment

The patient underwent ESD in November 2016. Endoscopy was introduced for exploration after administration of general anesthesia. An elevated lesion measuring 2.0 cm in diameter was noted at the greater curvature of the gastric cardia. Procedures were as follows: (1) Argon Plasma Coagulation (APC) was performed to remark the margin of

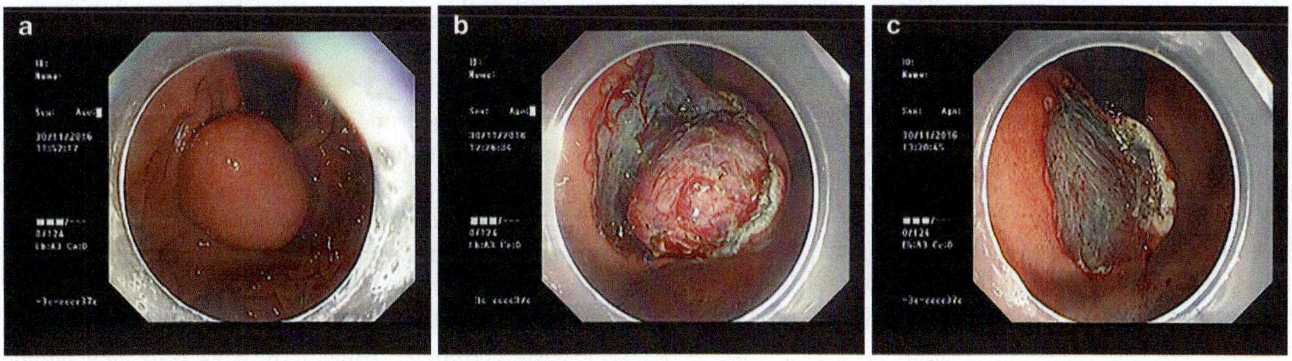

Fig. 4.3 Dissecting the junction between tumor and muscularis propria and resecting the tumor completely

the lesion; (2) After a submucosal injection of normal saline mixed with epinephrine and indigo carmine, marking dots were made lateral to the margin of the lesion; (3) The mucosal membrane of the tumor was dissected along the APC marking dots to expose the submucosal tumor; (4) The junction between the tumor and muscularis propria was dissected using a single-use electrosurgical knife and the tumor was completely resected for pathological examination (Fig. 4.3). No obvious perforation or active bleeding was seen in wound closure. The operative time was 85 min with 10 mL estimated blood loss.

4.1.3.3 Postoperative Pathology and Genetic Testing

Pathological Diagnosis Gastric cardia GIST, measuring 2.0 cm × 1.8 cm × 1.0 cm in size, mitotic count 7/50 HPF. According to the modified NIH classification, the tumor was moderate risk.

Immunohistochemistry CD117 (+), CD34 (+), DOG-1 (+), SMA (−), S-100 (−), Ki-67 (Li: < 5%).

Genetic Testing Mutation in exon 11 of *KIT*, the mutation type was c.1735_1737delGAT. Exons 9, 13 and 17 of *KIT* and exons 12 and 18 of *PDGFRA* were all wild type.

4.1.4 Prognosis

The patient fasted on the first postoperative day (POD) and followed a liquid diet on the second POD, with no reported symptoms of bleeding or abdominal pain. The patient followed a semi-liquid diet with no abnormalities and was discharged on the third POD. She did not receive adjuvant imatinib therapy for financial reasons. The patient was relapse free at 62–month postoperative follow-up in January 2022.

4.1.5 Experience of Diagnosis and Therapy

The location of the tumor in this case required special consideration. Dysfunction of the cardia would have been inevitable if traditional surgery was performed. Resection of the cardia can lead to numerous complications, including gastroesophageal reflux disease (GERD), and affects patients' quality of life. In this case, the patient did not experience side-effects or complications such as cardia stenosis or GERD, and the patient was free of relapse at the 62-month follow-up. This indicates that performing endoscopic GIST resection for carefully evaluated indications is safe and feasible in a high-volume medical center. Referring to the EGJ adenocarcinoma of Siewert's Classification and reports from domestic and foreign literature: most scholars define EGJ GIST as those in the area ranging from 2 cm proximal and distal to the cardia. The anatomical features of the EGJ, such as narrow lumen and a steep angle, make this area difficult to resect endoscopically. The particular features of this area may even increase the incidence of postoperative complications. Therefore, regions adjacent to the EGJ were considered a forbidden zone for endoscopic surgery in the past.

Additionally, resection in the cardia often causes severe gastroesophageal reflux, leading to unfavorable postoperative quality of life for patients. Therefore, to improve the postoperative quality of life, previous small sample studies performed ESD and endoscopic muscularis excavation (EME) on patients with EGJ GIST [1, 2]. The reported R0 resection rate of these study was 95.6–100%, and none of the patients experienced complications such as gastrointestinal stricture or GERD. None of the patients experienced local recurrence or distant metastasis during the 2-year follow-up period.

For asymptomatic gastric GIST with a diameter ≤2 cm, regular (6–12 months) endoscopic surveillance could be considered when adverse factors such as irregular borders, ulcers, strong echo, and heterogeneity are absent [3]. If patients present with clinical symptoms such as GI bleeding and abdominal pain, resection should be considered. For localized gastric GIST with a diameter >2 cm, treatment is as follows: (1) If there is no contraindication to surgery and complete resection is possible, surgical resection can be directly performed; (2) For tumors which are difficult to be resected or with high risk factors for surgery, such as combined organ resection or severely affected organ function, neoadjuvant imatinib should be considered, and surgery should be performed when the tumor has reduced in size. It was previously believed that a large sample size comparative study of mid- and long-term safety for ESD in the resection of GIST has not been performed, and thus routine ESD resection could not be recommended. With the development of endoscopic technology, reports of successful endoscopic ESD resection of GIST are increasing. The Chinese Consensus on Endoscopic Diagnosis and Management of Gastrointestinal Submucosal Tumors (Version 2018) stated that endoscopic submucosal excavation (ESE) is developed from ESD and is suitable for submucosal tumors (SMT) with a diameter ≥2 cm [4].

Although serious complications of ESD are rare, they can seriously affect the patient's prognosis and quality of life and physicians should be aware of these. Common complications of ESD are as follows: (1) Bleeding: the incidence of post-ESD bleeding is about 7% and most cases can be treated endoscopically. A study by Kim et al. [5] found that high-risk factors for bleeding after ESD included patient age ≤ 65 years, lesion diameter greater than 15 mm, and when the endoscopic physician has ≤5 years' experience. In addition, delayed postoperative bleeding is closely related to the tumor location. The incidence of bleeding is significantly higher for a lesion in the middle or lower 1/3 of the stomach compared to that of the upper 1/3 of the stomach; (2) Perforation: the incidence of perforation is 3.5–4.0%. High-risk factors for gastric perforation are lesions in the middle or upper part of stomach, ulcerated lesions, and large tumor. (3) Residual tumor and positive resection margins are mainly caused by preoperative failure to define tumor boundaries. Preoperative marking and design of the resection area can reduce the probability of residual tumor and local recurrence; (4) Stenosis: the incidence of stenosis after ESD is low. The cause of stenosis in most cases is reported to be excessive mucous membrane resection, which is more likely to occur for tumors located in the gastric antrum.

4.2 Case 7 A 51-Year-Old Man with Esophageal GIST Performed Endoscopic Surgery

Jiaxian Yu and Lei Tu

4.2.1 Introduction

Submucosal tunneling endoscopic resection (STER) is a technique where an artificial tunnel between the gastrointestinal mucous membrane and the muscularis propria is created. Through the tunnel, diagnosis can be made and treatment can be administered in the submucosa, muscularis propria, serosa, and even outside of the digestive tract. In contrast to the stomach, the esophagus is covered by an outer membrane instead of serosa, which increases the risk of esophageal perforation when performing ESD on a submucosal tumor originating from the esophageal muscularis propria. The advantage of STER is that titanium clips can be used to close the mucous membrane after resection of a lesion in the muscularis propria, ensuring the integrity of the mucous membrane and thus broadening the indications for endoscopic treatment. Additionally, the advantages of STER include better recovery after surgery, lower possibility of secondary chest and abdominal infection or digestive tract leakage, and shorter operation time [6, 7].

4.2.2 Case Background

The patient, a 51-year-old man, presented to the local hospital with a complaint of abdominal pain in the right upper quadrant for 2 days. Upper GI endoscopy revealed an elevated lesion in the mid-esophagus and chronic erosive gastritis. The patient was given supportive treatment, which did not significantly relieve his symptoms. In November 2016, the patient was admitted to the outpatient of Union Hospital, Tongji Medical College, Huazhong University of Science and Technology for further investigation. Upper GI endoscopy showed a smooth, elevated surface lesion measuring 1.1 cm in diameter, located 30 cm from the incisors. Endoscopic ultrasound (Fig. 4.4) revealed a 1.1 cm × 0.7 cm low echo lesion originating from the muscularis propria with a clear border. The patient was subsequently admitted to the Department of Gastroenterology.

4.2.2.1 Past History and Family History

The patient had undergone cholecystectomy for cholecystitis in 2012 and reported no drug allergies. The patient's parents were deceased, and there was no similar medical history in the family.

4.2.2.2 Physical Examination

The patient's vital signs were stable, and the skin and mucous membranes were not yellowish or pale. The abdomen was flat, and no gastrointestinal or peristaltic waves were observed. The abdomen was soft, with no tenderness, rebound tenderness, or palpable mass, and bowel sounds were normal.

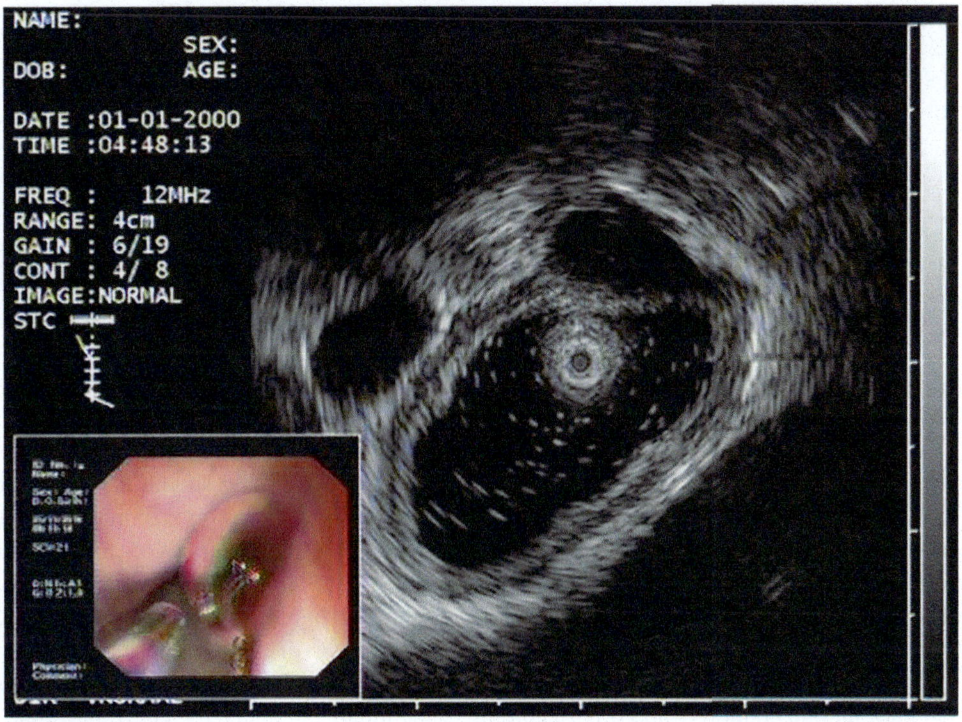

Fig. 4.4 Endoscopic ultrasound revealed a 1.1 cm × 0.7 cm low-echo lesion

4.2.2.3 Auxiliary Examination

Common Blood Count and Serum Chemistry Profile No significant abnormalities.

Esophageal CT A neoplasm with a diameter of 1 cm, located 30 cm from the incisor teeth at the mid-esophagus, growing toward the lumen was identified.

4.2.2.4 Primary Diagnosis

1. Elevated lesion in the esophageal muscularis propria, possibly GIST
2. Erosive gastritis
3. Prior history of cholecystectomy

4.2.3 Therapy

4.2.3.1 Case Analysis

The patient was a middle-aged man who complained of abdominal pain in the right upper quadrant for 2 days. The primary diagnosis was an elevated lesion in the esophageal muscularis propria, which was considered to be a possible GIST. Although the tumor was small (1.1 cm × 0.7 cm) and endoscopic ultrasound demonstrated the absence of adverse factors such as irregular border, ulceration, a strong echo and heterogeneity, the location of the tumor indicated that surgical resection or close follow-up should be considered. The patient had a strong desire for surgery. A multi-disciplinary team (MDT) evaluated the patient's case. Thoracotomy and thoracoscopic surgery have disadvantages such as large surgical trauma, slow recovery after surgery and inaccurate localization, but STER can resect the tumor en bloc and maintain the integrity of the esophagus. Therefore, we decided to perform STER for endoscopic resection of the esophageal elevated lesion.

4.2.3.2 Treatment

The patient underwent endoscopic resection of the esophageal elevated lesion using STER on December 1, 2016. Upper GI endoscopy demonstrated a flat submucosal lesion located 33 cm from the incisors. The surgical procedures were as follows: (1) The patient received tracheal intubation and general anesthesia in a left lateral decubitus position. (2) The residue and mucus in the esophageal cavity were cleared using irrigation and suction with a cap on the front end of the lens body. Indigo carmine was injected into the submucosa surrounding the tumor, and a location 4–5 cm proximal of the tumor was marked as an incision point. (3) A mixture of normal saline, indigo carmine, and epinephrine was used for repeated submucosal injections to the mucosa at the incision point (Fig. 4.5a). A Hook Knife was used to cut the mucosa, and the endoscope was introduced to the submucosa, forming a longitudinal tunnel in the muscularis propria and submucosa. The separation range was 2 cm beyond the tumor body and fully exposed the tumor (Fig. 4.5b). 4) The tumor was completely separated using the Hook Knife, and care was taken to protect the integrity of the tumor capsule and avoid damage to the esophageal adventitia (Fig. 4.5c). (5) After removing the tumor, the site was repeatedly irrigated to clean the bleeding point and the mucosal incision was closed

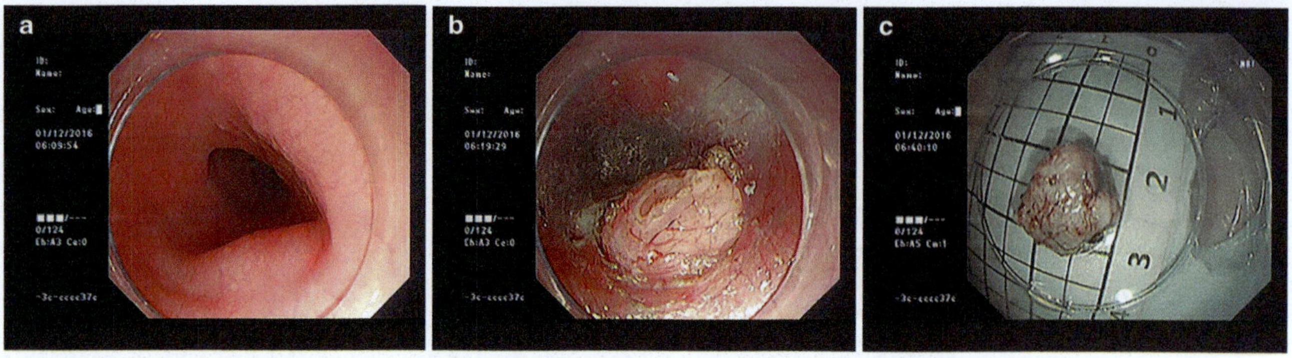

Fig. 4.5 Intraoperative images. (**a**) A submucosal mixture injection of normal saline, indigo carmine, and epinephrine repeated. (**b**) A longitudinal tunnel in the muscularis propria and submucosa. (**c**) The gross specimen

with a titanium clip. A gastric tube was placed after surgery. The operation time was 65 min, and the intraoperative bleeding was 15 mL.

4.2.3.3 Postoperative Pathology and Genetic Testing

Pathological Diagnosis Esophageal GIST (1 cm × 1 cm × 0.6 cm), mitotic count 0–1/50 HPF. According to the modified NIH classification the tumor was very low risk.

Immunohistochemistry CD117 (+), CD34 (+), SMA (−), S-100 (−).

Genetic Testing A mutation was detected in exon 11 of *KIT*, mutation type is p.V559D. The 9, 13 and 17 exons of *KIT* and the 12 and 18 exons of *PDGFRA* were all wild type.

4.2.4 Prognosis

The patient fasted on the first POD. The gastric tube and urinary catheter were removed and he followed a liquid diet on the second POD. The patient took in a semi-liquid diet and was discharged on the third POD. He did not receive adjuvant imatinib therapy as the pathological report classified the tumor as very low risk. At the 62-month follow-up in January 2021, the patient was relapse-free and did not present with complications such as esophageal stenosis or dysphagia.

4.2.5 Experience of Diagnosis and Therapy

Esophageal GIST only account for 0.66% of all GIST, and are most often found in the distal esophagus. Treatment should be considered based on the diameter, location and characteristics of the tumor, and options include endoscopic enucleation, STER, and laparoscopic or thoracoscopic resection, but the surgical indications for each technique have not yet been determined according to corresponding consensus and norms. Robb et al. reported that the surgical method should be selected based on the size of the tumor. For tumors <20 mm in diameter, ESD or STER is preferred; for tumor 20–65 mm in diameter, traditional thoracotomy or thoracoscopic tumor removal is preferred; for tumors 65–90 mm in diameter, tumor removal or esophagectomy is the first choice; for tumors >90 mm in diameter or with ulceration, esophagectomy is preferred [8]. The American Society for Gastrointestinal Endoscopy (ASGE) Guideline and the European Society of Gastrointestinal Endoscopy (ESGE) Guideline indicated that STER can be used for the resection of non-metastasized SMTs, with a diameter <40 mm, originating from the muscularis propria and located in the esophagus or stomach. Additionally, the distal esophagus, gastric cardia, lesser curve of the gastric body, and greater curve of the gastric antrum are more suitable to perform STER [9, 10].

4.3 Expert Comments

Yingjiang Ye

The major advantages of STER for esophageal GIST include avoiding damage to surrounding tissues and organs and preventing serious complications by applying tunnel endoscopic technology and resecting muscularis propria lesions under direct vision. When performing STER, an incision is made in the mucosa 4–5 cm above the tumor to establish a submucosal tunnel, and as a result, the mucosal layer at the tumor resection site remains intact. Meanwhile, the wound surface is closed at the tunnel entrance instead of tumor resection site, which ensures that the integrity of the digestive tract can be completely restored after suturing the mucosal incision, avoiding postoperative gastrointestinal leakage and secondary infections of the chest and abdominal cavity. Not only is STER different to traditional endoscopic treatment in the esophagus and gastric cavity, but it is also different to conventional endoscopic treatment. Submucosal tunneling endoscopic resection uses the gastrointestinal mucosa and muscularis propria to establish a tunnel as a space for surgery. However, the anatomical position of the esophagus is considered a special location for GIST and the esophageal wall is thin, giving a high risk of perforation and bleeding. Therefore, it is necessary to selectively conduct the relevant treatment while expanding the indications of endoscopic treatment for GIST [7, 11].

During the development of STER, gas-related complications, fever, pain, and pleural effusion were common complications. Gas-related complications included subcutaneous emphysema, pneumothorax or pneumoperitoneum, and the incidence of these was as high as 66.7%. However, gas-related complications often do not require special treatment, and usually can resolve spontaneously. If pneumoperitoneum is severe, a 14G puncture needle can be used to puncture the abdomen at the McBurney's point in the right lower quadrant of the abdomen for deflation. If the blood oxygen saturation is less than 90% or the airway pressure is higher than 30 mmHg due to pneumothorax, closed chest drainage can be performed. Fever and pain can often relieve spontaneously after supportive care. A small amount of pleural effusion after STER usually does not require treatment. If the patient presents with hyperpyrexia or their breathing is affected, ultrasound-guided intubation should be performed for drainage [12].

In recent years, due to the popularization of endoscopy and the development progression of endoscopic ultrasound technology, the detection rate of SMTs has significantly increased. Among these, gastric GIST is the most commonly diagnosed gastric SMT, followed by leiomyoma and ectopic pancreas. Generally, GIST present as hypoechoic on endoscopic ultrasound, with a diameter of <2 cm and with smooth, spherical, uniform boundaries. Malignant tumors can present with irregular boundaries in the cavity. In most cases, GIST originates from the muscularis propria, and laparoscopic resection is often considered. However, endoscopic resection has the advantages of minimally invasive procedures such as faster recovery and small surgical trauma; thus, some surgeons adopt endoscopic methods such as ESD or STER to remove small GIST. However, endoscopic resection has higher requirements for anatomical position, and risks of bleeding and perforation, which is technically demanding for the surgeon and require fine control. Despite these risks, endoscopic resection for GIST attracts more and more attention due to the minimally invasive advantages.

References

1. Li QL, Yao LQ, Zhou PH, Xu MD, Chen SY, Zhong YS, Zhang YQ, Chen WF, Ma LL, Qin WZ. Submucosal tumors of the esophagogastric junction originating from the muscularis propria layer: a large study of endoscopic submucosal dissection (with video). Gastrointest Endosc. 2012;75(6):1153–8. https://doi.org/10.1016/j.gie.2012.01.037.
2. Zhang Y, Ye LP, Zhu LH, Zhou XB, Mao XL, Ding JX. Endoscopic muscularis excavation for subepithelial tumors of the esophagogastric junction originating from the muscularis propria layer. Dig Dis Sci. 2013;58(5):1335–40. https://doi.org/10.1007/s10620-012-2487-7.
3. Chien CH, Chien RN, Yen CL, Fang KM, Liu CJ, Lin CL, Chang JJ, Chen LW, Lee TS, Chen SW, Hu CC, Chang LC. The role of endoscopic ultrasonography examination for evaluation and surveillance of gastric subepithelial masses. Chang Gung Med J. 2010;33(1):73–81. http://cgmj.cgu.edu.tw/3301/330109.pdf
4. Zhou P, Zhong Y, Li Q. Chinese consensus on endoscopic diagnosis and management of gastrointestinal submucosal tumor (Version 2018). Zhonghua Wei Chang Wai Ke Za Zhi. 2018;21(8):841–52. https://doi.org/10.3760/cma.j.issn.1671-0274.2018.08.001.
5. Kim JW, Kim HS, Park DH, Park YS, Jee MG, Baik SK, Kwon SO, Lee DK. Risk factors for delayed postendoscopic mucosal resection hemorrhage in patients with gastric tumor. Eur J Gastroenterol Hepatol. 2007;19(5):409–15. https://doi.org/10.1097/MEG.0b013e32801015be.
6. Zhou DJ, Dai ZB, Wells MM, Yu DL, Zhang J, Zhang L. Submucosal tunneling and endoscopic resection of submucosal tumors at the esophagogastric junction. World J Gastroenterol. 2015;21(2):578–83. https://doi.org/10.3748/wjg.v21.i2.578.
7. Wang L, Ren W, Zhang Z, Yu J, Li Y, Song Y. Retrospective study of endoscopic submucosal tunnel dissection (ESTD) for surgical resection of esophageal leiomyoma. Surg Endosc. 2013;27(11):4259–66. https://doi.org/10.1007/s00464-013-3035-z.
8. Robb WB, Bruyere E, Amielh D, Vinatier E, Mabrut JY, Perniceni T, Piessen G, Mariette C, FREGAT Working Group--FRENCH. Esophageal gastrointestinal stromal tumor: is tumoral enucleation a viable therapeutic option? Ann Surg. 2015;261(1):117–24. https://doi.org/10.1097/SLA.0000000000000505.
9. Technology Committee ASGE, Aslanian HR, Sethi A, Bhutani MS, Goodman AJ, Krishnan K, Lichtenstein DR, Melson J, Navaneethan U, Pannala R, Parsi MA, Schulman AR, Sullivan SA, Thosani N, Trikudanathan G, Trindade AJ, Watson RR, Maple JT. ASGE guideline for endoscopic full-thickness resection and submucosal tunnel endoscopic resection. VideoGIE. 2019;4(8):343–50. https://doi.org/10.1016/j.vgie.2019.03.010.
10. Deprez PH, Moons LMG, O'Toole D, Gincul R, Seicean A, Pimentel-Nunes P, Fernández-Esparrach G, Polkowski M, Vieth M, Borbath I, Moreels TG, Nieveen van Dijkum E, Blay JY, van Hooft JE. Endoscopic management of subepithelial lesions including neuroendocrine neoplasms: European Society of Gastrointestinal Endoscopy (ESGE) Guideline. Endoscopy. 2022;54(4):412–29. https://doi.org/10.1055/a-1751-5742.
11. Peng W, Tan S, Huang S, Ren Y, Li H, Peng Y, Fu X, Tang X. Efficacy and safety of submucosal tunneling endoscopic resection for upper gastrointestinal submucosal tumors with more than 1-year' follow-up: a systematic review and meta-analysis. Scand J Gastroenterol. 2019;54(4):397–406. https://doi.org/10.1080/00365521.2019.1591500.
12. Liu BR, Song JT, Kong LJ, Pei FH, Wang XH, Du YJ. Tunneling endoscopic muscularis dissection for subepithelial tumors originating from the muscularis propria of the esophagus and gastric cardia. Surg Endosc. 2013;27(11):4354–9. https://doi.org/10.1007/s00464-013-3023-3.

Part II

Preoperative Treatment of Gastrointestinal Stromal Tumors

Rectal Gastrointestinal Stromal Tumors with Preoperative Treatment

5

Yao Lin, Youwei Kou, Chengguo Li, Xing Liu, and Jiren Yu

Keywords

Rectum · Gastrointestinal stromal tumor · Targeted therapy · Preoperative treatment

5.1 Case 8 A 65-Year-Old Man with Rectal GIST Who Underwent Preoperative Treatment

Yao Lin and Youwei Kou

5.1.1 Introduction

Generally, GIST occurs in the stomach and small intestine, accounting for 50–60%, and 20–30% of cases, respectively. Primary rectal GIST are relatively rare [1]. When considering treatment for rectal GIST, especially low rectal GIST, whether the anus can be preserved during surgery determines the patient's postoperative quality of life. Preoperative treatment can reduce the size of the tumor, reduce the clinical stage, and increase the distance between the tumor and the anus. Subsequently, this can allow some patients with low rectal GIST to retain the anus without affecting their overall survival time and improve the postoperative quality of life.

5.1.2 Case Background

A 65-year-old man was admitted to the hospital to investigate a 1-year history of frequent urination and difficulty defecating. He had no fever, nausea, vomiting, abdominal pain, or bloating. Since the onset of illness, the diet and sleep have been good, the patient has been in good spirits, and there was no significant weight loss.

5.1.2.1 Past History and Family History

The patient was diagnosed with diabetes 3 years previously, but had good blood sugar control. The patient did not have coronary heart disease, hypertension, or previous infection with hepatitis or tuberculosis. The patient had undergone internal hemorrhoidectomy 10 years previously, but had no history of trauma or blood transfusion.

5.1.2.2 Physical Examination

The patient had a flat abdomen, no observable gastrointestinal or peristaltic waves, no abdominal wall varicose veins, no tenderness, and no rebound pain or muscle tension. The liver and spleen were not palpable under the ribs, and the Murphy's sign was negative. The bowel sounds occurred 4 times/min, and there were no high-pitched bowel sounds. Digital rectal examination (DRE) revealed a hemispherical mass protruding into the intestinal cavity on the anterior wall of the rectum at a distance of 3 cm. The upper boundary of the mass could not be felt. The mass was hard, with smooth surface mucosa and poor movement. The intestinal cavity was slightly narrowed.

Y. Lin · C. Li
Department of Gastrointestinal Surgery, Union Hospital, Tongji Medical College, Huazhong University of Science and Technology, Wuhan, China
e-mail: lichengguo@hust.edu.cn

Y. Kou (✉)
Department of Gastrointestinal Surgery, Shengjing Hospital of China Medical University, Shenyang, China
e-mail: kouyw@sj-hospital.org

X. Liu (✉)
Department of Colorectal Surgery, Fujian Medical University Union Hospital, Fuzhou, China

J. Yu
Department of Gastrointestinal Surgery, The First Affiliated Hospital of Zhejiang University School of Medicine, Hangzhou, China

K. Tao, H. Cao (eds.), *Clinical Management of Gastrointestinal Stromal Tumor*, https://doi.org/10.1007/978-981-99-9392-5_5

Fig. 5.1 PET-CT revealed a rectal tumor approximately 5.5 cm in size

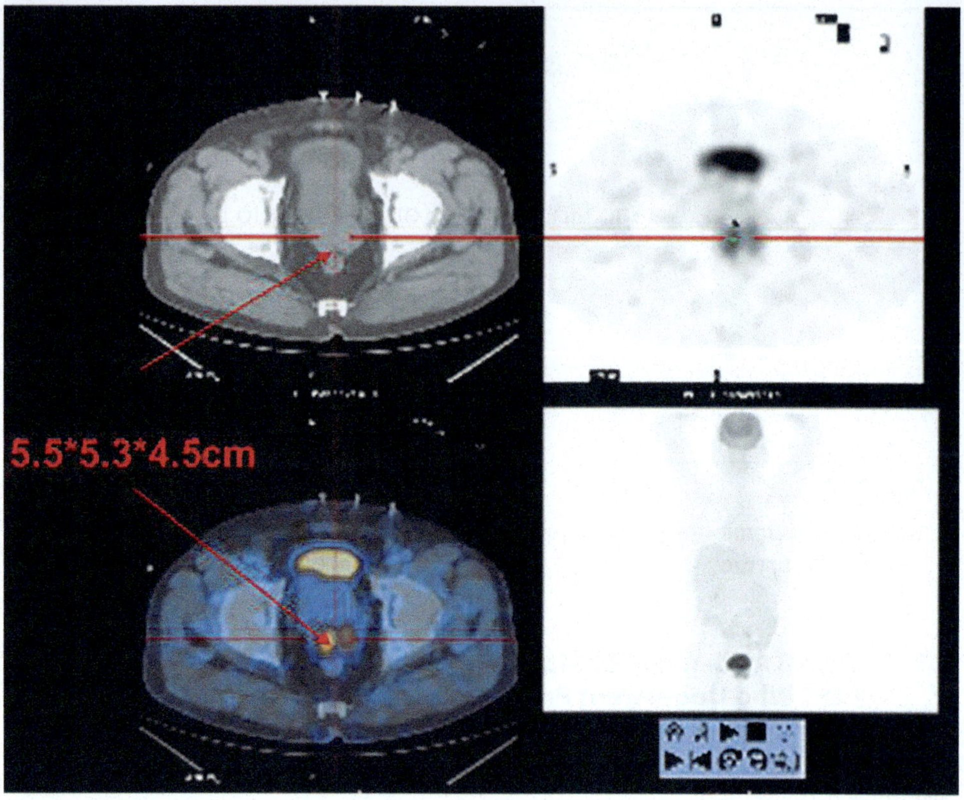

5.1.2.3 Auxiliary Examination

PET-CT Rectal tumor, approximately 5.5 cm in size (Fig. 5.1).

5.1.3 Therapy

5.1.3.1 Case Analysis

Considering that the tumor was close to the anus, a combined abdominal and perineal rectal tumor resection procedure was considered, where the anus would not be preserved. The patient refused surgery in order to preserve the anus. Subsequently, the patient underwent a needle biopsy, the tumor was pathologically diagnosed as GIST, and he was treated with oral imatinib with regular follow-up. The patient was treated with oral imatinib for 40 months, and continuous reexamination of the tumor using CT, MRI, and ultrasound showed that the mass was increasing in size (the results of CT, MRI, and ultrasound examinations at 40 months are shown in Figs. 5.2 and 5.3). Following this, the patient chose to undergo surgery.

5.1.3.2 Treatment

The patient underwent laparoscopic resection of the rectal mass in April 2013. A 2 cm × 2 cm mass was seen outside the left anterior wall of the rectum. The mass was freed along the periphery of the tumor and was completely resected.

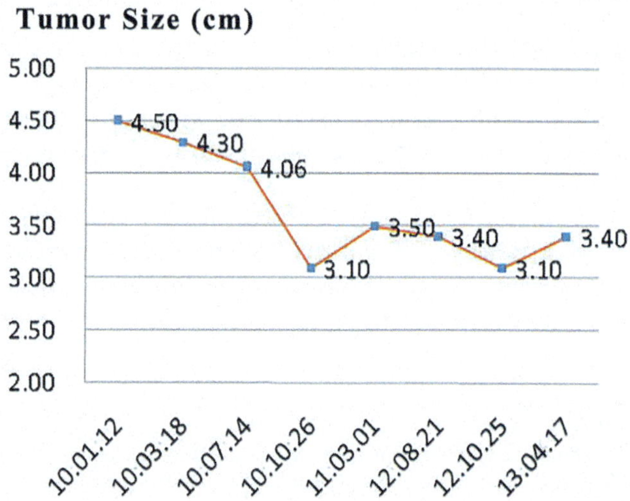

Fig. 5.2 Reexamination of CT and MRI

5.1.3.3 Postoperative Pathology and Genetic Testing

Pathological Diagnosis Rectal GIST, with no obvious mitotic figures, in line with the preoperative treatment.

Immunohistochemistry CD117 (+), CD34 (+), DOG-1 (+), SMA (−), S-100 (−), Ki-67 (Li: 6%).

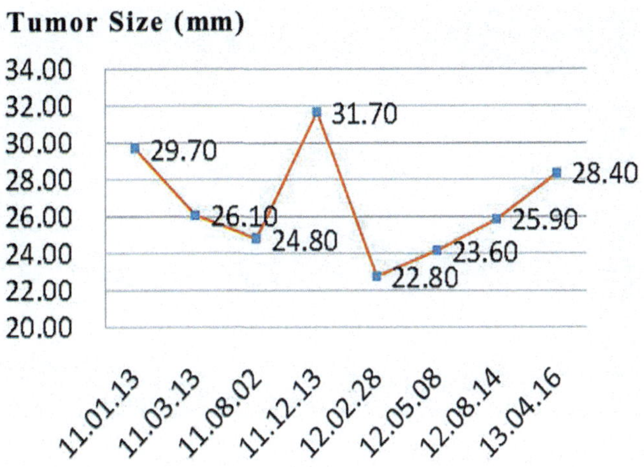

Fig. 5.3 Reexamination of ultrasound

Genetic Testing A mutation in *KIT* exon 11 was found. The mutation was p.W557_K558del. Exons 9, 13, and 17 of the *KIT* and exons 12 and 18 of *PDGFRA* were wild-type.

5.1.4 Prognosis

The patient continued to take imatinib for 3 years after the operation. During regular review, no tumor recurrence or metastasis was found.

5.1.5 Experience of Diagnosis and Therapy

Rectal GIST accounts for 5–10% of all GIST. The main clinical symptoms are bleeding, obstruction, and pain. About 10% of rectal GIST demonstrate infiltration, without lymph node metastasis [2]. For tumors in important parts of the gastrointestinal tract, such as the rectum, cardia, or duodenum, if the tumor is large, the function may be lost following tumor resection; thus, preoperative treatment may be considered before surgery. Preoperative treatment is mainly undertaken to reduce the tumor volume, downstage the tumor, and reduce the scope of surgery in order to avoid unnecessary combined organ resection, reduce the risks associated with surgery, and increase the chance of radical resection. For tumors in significant areas, preoperative treatment can protect the structure and function of important organs. For patients with huge tumors and a greater risk of intraoperative rupture and bleeding, preoperative treatment can reduce the possibility of iatrogenic dissemination [3]. The indications for preoperative treatment are that R0 resection will be difficult to achieve; the tumor is huge (>10 cm) and could easily bleed or rupture during surgery, which may cause iatrogenic dissemination; tumors in special locations (such as at the EGJ, or in the duodenum, or lower rectum); where surgery is likely to damage the function of important organs; when the tumor can be removed, but the estimated risk of surgery and the postoperative recurrence rate and mortality are high; and where it is estimated that multiple organ resection will be required.

Pathological examination must be performed before treatment for GIST is commenced. Needle biopsy is the preferred method to obtain pathological tissues, and intracavitary needle biopsy is recommended. The European Society for Medical Oncology (ESMO) guidelines also suggest that if performed properly, the risk of tumor dissemination caused by needle biopsy is negligible [4]. Drug therapy should be stopped for about 1 week before surgery, which can be considered after the basic conditions of the patient meet the requirements for the procedure. The patient took medicine for about 10 months and the maximum therapeutic effect was achieved. Due to the difficulty of defecation and a noticeable increasement in urination frequency the patient refused surgical treatment and continued to take the medication. During the 40 months of preoperative medication, the CT and MRI tumor diameter fluctuated within a certain range, but the results of the last two ultrasounds before resection showed that the diameter of the tumor continued to increase, and the patient finally chose surgery. The pathological results showed that the tumor had been completely degenerated and was necrotic, and no normal tumor cells were seen.

Post-surgery, in principle, as long as the patient's gastrointestinal function recovers and the patient can tolerate drug treatment, drug treatment should be commenced as soon as possible. For patients with R0 resection, the postoperative drug maintenance time can be determined based on the standard of adjuvant treatment; for patients with palliative resection, metastasis, or recurrence (regardless of whether R0 resection is achieved), the postoperative treatment is similar to that for GIST patients with recurrence or metastasis without surgery. For rectal GIST, due to the high cost of CT and MRI, transanal ultrasound is an economical and convenient means of review which also has a certain reference value.

5.2 Case 9 A 70-Year-Old Man with Rectal GIST

Chengguo Li and Xing Liu

5.2.1 Case Background

The patient, a 70-year-old man, was admitted to the Department of Colorectal Surgery, Union Hospital Affiliated to Fujian Medical University in June 2013 to investigate a 1-year history of tenesmus. One year ago, the patient had tenesmus without obvious inducement with defecation five to eight times a day, and occasional episodes of paroxysmal abdominal pain. The patient reported no mucus or bloody stools. A colonoscopy performed at the local hospital 1 week earlier revealed submucosal lesions in the anal area of the lower rectum (possible GIST) occupying the rectal cavity, and the colonoscope could not be passed beyond that point. To clarify the diagnosis and treatment, he was admitted to Union Hospital of Fujian Medical University. Since the onset of the disease, the patient's food intake was normal, with no significant weight loss.

5.2.1.1 Past History and Family History

He had a 5-year history of hypertension and controlled well with amlodipine. The patient reported no drug allergies. Both parents were deceased, the causes of death were unknown, and there was no similar medical history in the family.

5.2.1.2 Physical Examination

The vital signs were stable, and the skin and mucous membranes were not yellowish or pale. The abdomen was flat, and no gastrointestinal and peristaltic waves were observed. The abdominal muscles were soft, and there was no obvious tenderness, rebound pain, or palpable mass anywhere in the abdomen. The Murphy's sign was negative, there was no mobile dullness, and the bowel sounds were normal. Digital rectal examination revealed normal anal sphincter tension, and a huge submucosal mass was palpable at 3–9 points in the lithotomy position. The tumor was 4 cm from the anal verge. The mass boundary was clear, the surface was smooth, the texture was hard, and the mass was in a fixed position, resulting in obvious narrowing of the rectal cavity. No blood stains were seen when the finger was removed.

5.2.1.3 Auxiliary Examination

Blood Routine and Biochemistry No obvious abnormalities.

Coagulation Function Fibrinogen 4.63 g/L, D-dimer 5.21 ug/mL.

Tumor Markers Carcinoembryonic antigen (CEA): 1.3 ng/mL, CA19-9: 2.37 U/mL.

Enhanced CT of the Whole Abdomen Lower rectal mass, 7.1 cm × 6.3 cm in size, with a high possibility of GIST (Fig. 5.4).

Trans-anorectal Ultrasound A hypoechoic mass in the muscular layer of the posterior rectum wall was identified approximately 5 cm from the anal margin, approximately 6.8 cm × 6.2 cm in size (Fig. 5.5).

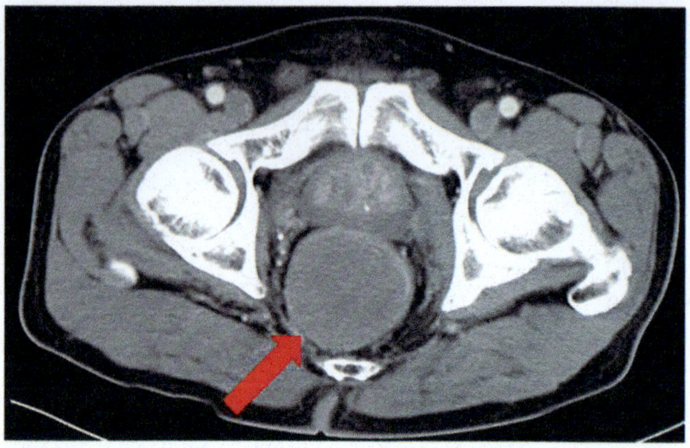

Fig. 5.4 The enhanced CT showed a lower rectal mass, 7.1 cm × 6.3 cm in size

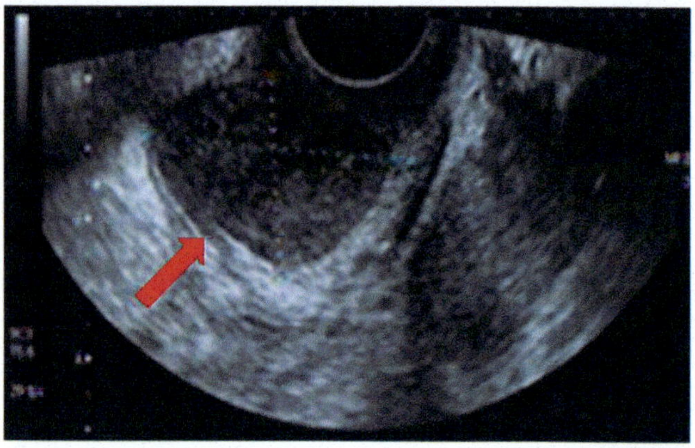

Fig. 5.5 Ultrasound enteroscopy showed a hypoechoic mass in the posterior rectal wall

Trans-anorectal Mass Biopsy Pathology Rectal mass puncture biopsy specimens showed spindle cells with nuclear atypia and visible mitotic figures. The mass was considered to be a rectal GIST.

Immunohistochemistry CD117 (+), CD34 (+), DOG- 1 (+), SMA (−), desmin (−).

Genetic Testing A mutation in *KIT* exon 11 was identified. The mutation type was K550_P551delinsF. Exons 9, 13, and 17 of *KIT* and exons 12 and 18 of *PDGFRA* were wild type.

5.2.2 Therapy

5.2.2.1 Case Analysis

The MDT discussion opinion was that the current diagnosis was clear: the mass was a rectal GIST (*KIT* Exon 11 mutant). Because the tumor was large and located in the lower rectum, it was a special GIST. If surgical treatment was performed

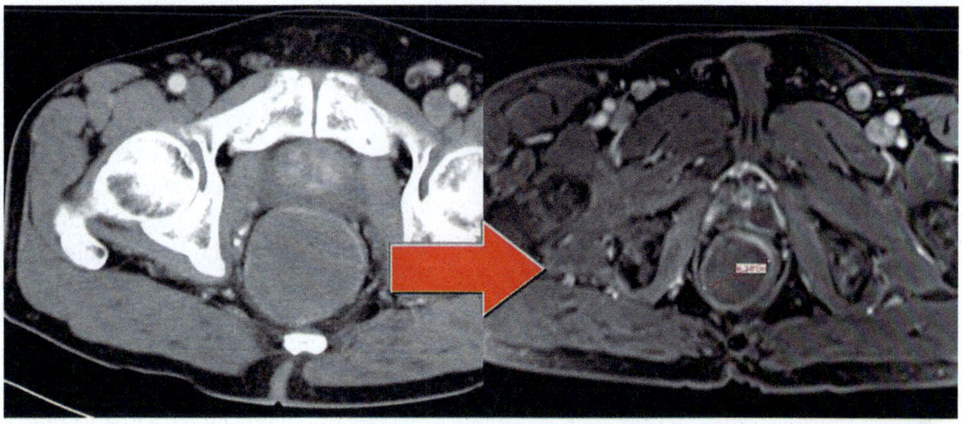

Fig. 5.6 Enhanced MRI after 8 months of imatinib therapy

directly, the anus may not have been preserved, there may have been a greater impact on postoperative anal function, and there was a risk of tumor rupture during the procedure. Therefore, imatinib was recommended for preoperative treatment. Subsequently, the tumor changes were monitored and evaluated every 2–3 months, with the aim to perform surgical treatment when the treatment had achieved the maximal effect.

5.2.2.2 Treatment

The patient started oral imatinib, 400 mg/d, on July 3, 2013. Enhanced MRI revealed that after 6 months of treatment the rectal tumor had reduced to an estimated 4.2 cm × 3.8 cm (Partial response, PR), and after 8 months of treatment, it had further reduced in size to 4.2 cm × 3.6 cm (Stable disease, SD). No metastatic lesions were found in the liver, abdomen, or pelvis (Fig. 5.6). While taking regular oral imatinib, the main adverse reaction experienced by the patient was second-degree lower extremity edema. The second MDT discussion was held on March 26, 2014. After 6 months of neoadjuvant treatment with imatinib, the patient's rectal tumor had significantly regressed, and the best curative effect had reached PR. Experts recommend surgery for the patient.

The patient underwent laparoscopic ultra-low anterior rectal resection and preventive loop ileostomy on April 1, 2014. Intraoperative exploration revealed no obvious ascites, and no metastases in the liver, peritoneum, or pelvis. The tumor was located in the lower rectum, approximately 6 cm from the anal margin and was approximately 4.5 cm × 3.5 cm in size, with soft texture and clear boundaries. There were no obvious enlarged lymph nodes near the rectum or mesenteric vessels. The operation process went smoothly, R0 resection was achieved, and there were no intraoperative complications such as tumor rupture (Fig. 5.7).

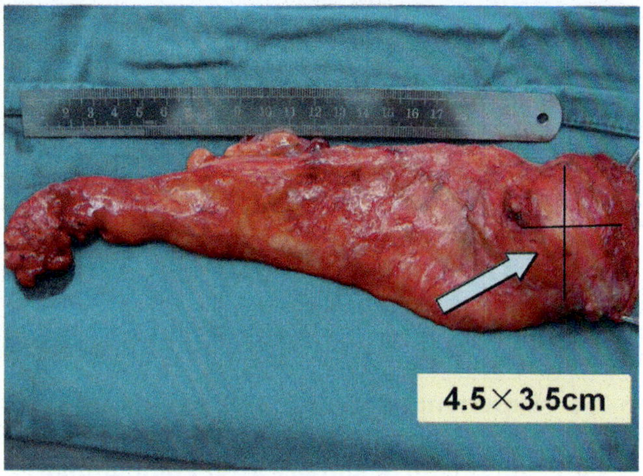

Fig. 5.7 Postoperative rectal and tumor gross specimens

5.2.2.3 Postoperative Pathology and Genetic Testing

Pathological Diagnosis After rectal GIST targeted therapy, the excised mass was 4.4 cm × 3.3 cm × 2.8 cm in size, most of the tumor exhibited necrosis, and a small amount of lymphocytic cell infiltration with calcification was seen in the interstitium. Combined with the results of needle biopsy and the clinical history, the characteristics were consistent with the changes in GIST after treatment. The upper and lower cut ends were clean, and no tumor metastasis was found (Fig. 5.8).

Immunohistochemistry CD117 (+), CD34 (−), DOG-1 (+), SMA (−), S-100 (−), desmin (−).

Genetic Testing *KIT* exon 11 mutation.

5.2.3 Prognosis

The patient recovered smoothly after the operation. Gas was passed through the ileostomy 2 days after the operation, he was started on a semi-liquid diet 4 days after surgery, and oral imatinib 400 mg/d treatment was recommenced 1 week after the operation. Ileostomy closure was performed 3 months after the initial operation. The Wexner scores for

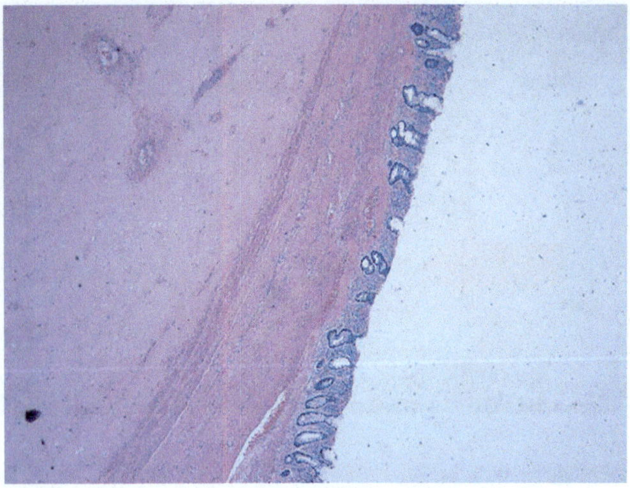

Fig. 5.8 Postoperative pathological H&E staining

anal function assessment were 8 and 5 points, at 6 and 12 months after stoma closure, respectively. Imatinib was taken orally for 3 years after the operation, and lung and whole abdominal CT images were reviewed every 3–6 months. The patient was followed-up until August 2022, and no tumor recurrence or metastasis was found.

5.2.4 Experience of Diagnosis and Therapy

5.2.4.1 The Timing of Surgery After Preoperative Treatment

The purpose of preoperative treatment for GIST should be to reduce tumor size and stage, reduce the required scope of surgery, protect the structure and function of organs, and reduce the possibility of iatrogenic dissemination, rather than pursuing complete tumor remission. Therefore, it is generally believed that surgery should be performed when the best effect of preoperative treatment has been observed, which may be 6–12 months after preoperative therapy [5]. Excessive prolongation of the preoperative treatment time may lead to secondary drug resistance and the best opportunity for surgery may be missed. Significant tumor shrinkage usually starts 2–3 months after initiation of treatment, so the target lesions should be evaluated every 2–3 months [5–7]. After 6 months of treatment, the rate of tumor shrinkage often slows down significantly. At this time, the review cycle should be appropriately shortened, such as by conducting a monthly review, to confirm that the best efficacy has been achieved in a timely manner. It is sufficient to cease imatinib administration 1 week before the operation [7], and preoperative hematological examination should be conducted to determine whether there are any abnormalities.

5.2.4.2 Common Surgical Methods and Indications for Rectal GIST

Common surgical methods for rectal GIST include low anterior resection, abdominal perineal resection, trans-sacral or trans-anal resection, and trans-anal endoscopic microsurgery. Low anterior resection is mostly suitable for mid-to-high rectal GIST, or GIST that is still large after preoperative treatment. Because abdominal perineal resection leads to the complete sacrifice of anal function, the technique is rarely used for GIST treatment in the era of targeted drugs and is only suitable for cases where the anal sphincter is still affected after preoperative treatment. Trans-sacral and trans-anorectal GIST resection can reduce the scope of rectal resection. For low rectal GIST, especially in men with pelvic stenosis, trans-sacral or trans-anorectal resection can reduce the difficulty of surgery, but there are risks of tumor crushing and rupture, anal sphincter injury, and higher local wound infection rate. Trans-anal endoscopic microsurgery has emerged in recent years and is a fast-developing surgical method which can preserve the function of the rectum and anus to the greatest extent [8]. However, due to the particular characteristics of the surgical instruments, this technique is mainly used to treat upper and middle rectal GIST with small diameters. It should be emphasized that no matter which surgical method is selected, the tumor should be completely removed with the aim of "non-contact, less squeezing, and no rupture," to protect the rectal and anal function and reduce trauma as much as possible as the principle aims [7].

5.3 Expert Comments

Jiren Yu

At present, there is still widespread controversy regarding the duration of preoperative treatment of GIST and the timing of surgery. The sensitivity to imatinib varies greatly because of the diverse types of GIST gene mutations, and secondary mutations may occur during treatment [6, 7, 9]. Therefore, the CSCO and NCCN guidelines point out that the duration of preoperative treatment should be based on the maximum response to drug therapy [6, 7]. Blindly prolonging the preoperative treatment time of imatinib is very likely to lead to drug resistance and the best opportunity for surgery will be missed. During the preoperative treatment period, the imaging changes should be closely observed to prevent instances of being unable to perform salvage surgery for marginal resectable lesions due to progress during the treatment period. Appropriately shortening the imaging review time during the preoperative treatment period (2–3-month interval between review) will help confirm the best timing for surgery.

References

1. Qu H, Xu Z, Ren Y, Gong Z, Ju RH, Zhang F, Kang H, Xu Y, Chen X. Recent advancements in the treatment of rectal gastrointestinal stromal tumor: in era of imatinib. Cancer Manag Res. 2022;14:1141–52. https://doi.org/10.2147/CMAR.S352860.
2. Baik SH, Kim NK, Lee CH, Lee KY, Sohn SK, Cho CH, Kim H, Pyo HR, Rha SY, Chung HC. Gastrointestinal stromal tumor of the rectum: an analysis of seven cases. Surg Today. 2007;37(6):455–9. https://doi.org/10.1007/s00595-006-3424-1.
3. Li W, Li X, Yu K, Xiao B, Peng J, Zhang R, Zhang L, Wang K, Pan Z, Li C, Wu X. Efficacy and safety of neoadjuvant imatinib therapy for patients with locally advanced rectal gastrointestinal stromal tumors: a multi-center cohort study. Front Pharmacol. 2022;13:950101. https://doi.org/10.3389/fphar.2022.950101.
4. Landi B, Blay JY, Bonvalot S, Brasseur M, Coindre JM, Emile JF, Hautefeuille V, Honore C, Lartigau E, Mantion G, Pracht M, Le Cesne A, Ducreux M, Bouche O, Thésaurus National de Cancérologie Digestive (TNCD), Fédération Francophone de Cancérologie Digestive (FFCD), Fédération Nationale de Centres de Lutte Contre les Cancers (UNICANCER), Groupe Coopérateur Multidisciplinaire en Oncologie (GERCOR), Société Française de Chirurgie Digestive (SFCD), Société Française de Radiothérapie Oncologique (SFRO), Société Française d'Endoscopie Digestive (SFED), Société Nationale Française de Gastroentérologie (SNFGE). Gastrointestinal stromal tumours (GISTs): French Intergroup Clinical Practice Guidelines for diagnosis, treatments and follow-up (SNFGE, FFCD, GERCOR, UNICANCER, SFCD, SFED, SFRO). Dig Liver Dis. 2019;51(9):1223–31. https://doi.org/10.1016/j.dld.2019.07.006.
5. Tang S, Yin Y, Shen C, Chen J, Yin X, Zhang B, Yao Y, Yang J, Chen Z. Preoperative imatinib mesylate (IM) for huge gastrointestinal stromal tumors (GIST). World J Surg Oncol. 2017;15(1):79–86. https://doi.org/10.1186/s12957-017-1143-2.
6. von Mehren M, Randall RL, Benjamin RS, Boles S, Bui MM, Ganjoo KN, George S, Gonzalez RJ, Heslin MJ, Kane JM, Keedy V, Kim E, Koon H, Mayerson J, McCarter M, McGarry SV, Meyer C, Morris ZS, O'Donnell RJ, Pappo AS, Paz IB, Petersen IA, Pfeifer JD, Riedel RF, Ruo B, Schuetze S, Tap WD, Wayne JD, Bergman MA, Scavone JL. Soft tissue sarcoma, version 2.2018, NCCN clinical practice guidelines in oncology. J Natl Compr Cancer Netw. 2018;16(5):536–63. https://doi.org/10.6004/jnccn.2018.0025.
7. Li J, Ye Y, Wang J, Zhang B, Qin S, Shi Y, He Y, Liang X, Liu X, Zhou Y, Wu X, Zhang X, Wang M, Gao Z, Lin T, Cao H, Shen L, Chinese Society of Clinical Oncology CSCO Expert Committee on Gastrointestinal Stromal Tumor. Chinese consensus guidelines for diagnosis and management of gastrointestinal stromal tumor. Chin J Cancer Res. 2017;29(4):281–93. https://doi.org/10.21147/j.issn.1000-9604.2017.04.01.
8. Wu X, Lin G, Qiu H, Zhou J, Xu J. Transanal endoscopic microsurgery for local excision of rectal gastrointestinal stromal tumors. Zhonghua Wei Chang Wai Ke Za Zhi. 2018;21(11):1296–300. https://doi.org/10.3760/cma.j.issn.1671-0274.2018.11.017.
9. Gounder MM, Maki RG. Molecular basis for primary and secondary tyrosine kinase inhibitor resistance in gastrointestinal stromal tumor. Cancer Chemother Pharmacol. 2011;67(Suppl 1(Suppl 1)):S25–43. https://doi.org/10.1007/s00280-010-1526-3.

Giant Abdominal Gastrointestinal Stromal Tumors with Preoperative Treatment

6

Lei Yang, Xiaodong Gao, and Kuntang Shen

Keywords

Gastrointestinal stromal tumor · Abdominal · Giant Surgery

6.1 Case 10 A 68-Year-Old Man with a Giant Abdominal GIST

Lei Yang and Xiaodong Gao

6.1.1 Introduction

GIST is the most common gastrointestinal mesenchymal tumor and is most commonly found in the stomach (50–60%) and small intestine (20–30%) [1]. It is currently believed that the possible origin of GIST is the interstitial cells of Cajal, which controls gastrointestinal peristalsis [2]. Extra-gastrointestinal stromal tumor (EGIST) refers to GIST that occurs outside the gastrointestinal tract, and is common in the omentum, mesentery, and retroperitoneum [3]. Both EGIST and GIST have similar cell morphology, immunohistochemical expression, and gene mutation types. Since EGIST often lacks early symptoms, it is usually large when diagnosed. This report describes a typical huge EGIST case.

L. Yang
Department of Gastrointestinal Surgery, Union Hospital, Tongji Medical College, Huazhong University of Science and Technology, Wuhan, China

X. Gao (✉)
Department of General Surgery, Zhongshan Hospital, Fudan University, Shanghai, China

K. Shen
Department of Gastrointestinal Surgery, Zhongshan Hospital, Fudan University, Shanghai, China
e-mail: shen.kuntang@zs-hospital.sh.cn

6.1.2 Case Background

The patient, a 68-year-old man, presented to the Zhongshan Hospital of Fudan University on April 8, 2014, for investigation of middle and lower abdominal pain. A CT scan of the abdomen showed a huge, cystic, solid mass in the abdomen and pelvis. Blood tests revealed Hb 76 g/L, and WBC 10.3×10^9/L. The abdominal and pelvic enhanced CT showed the following: (1) A huge mass in the abdomen and pelvic space, measuring 19.4 cm × 9.6 cm in size, which was considered to be a mesenchymal malignant tumor with a high chance of hemorrhage; (2) A chronic hematoma under the liver capsule (Fig. 6.1).

An ultrasound-guided pathological biopsy of the abdominal mass on April 18, 2014, revealed spindle cells, abundant cell numbers, and mild to moderate atypia. Tumor cells were seen growing in clusters around blood vessels in focal areas, but mitotic count was difficult to discern.

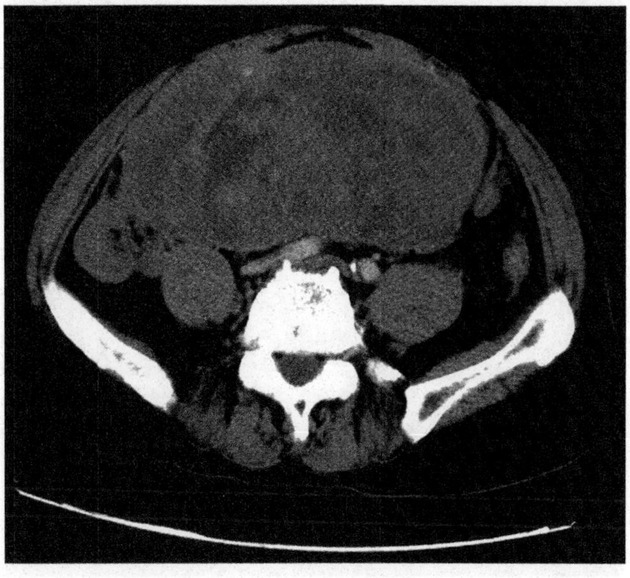

Fig. 6.1 Enhanced CT showed a huge mass in the abdominal and pelvic cavity

K. Tao, H. Cao (eds.), *Clinical Management of Gastrointestinal Stromal Tumor*, https://doi.org/10.1007/978-981-99-9392-5_6

Immunohistochemistry and genetic testing revealed a GTT/GTA mutation at codon 559 in exon 11 of *KIT*, consistent with an abdominal GIST diagnosis. On April 27, 2014, treatment with oral imatinib, 400 mg/d, was initiated.

The enhanced CT scan of the abdominal and pelvic cavities on May 23, 2014, showed that the abdominal and pelvic cavity measured 13.9 cm × 6.6 cm, which was markedly smaller than observed in the images from April 10, 2014 (Fig. 6.2). Enhanced CT of the abdomen and pelvic cavity on August 20, 2014, showed that the lesion had further reduced to 11 cm × 7.7 cm, and the center of the lesion was liquefied and necrotic (Fig. 6.3). Enhanced CT of the abdominal and pelvic cavity on October 27, 2014, showed an abdominal GIST measuring 11 cm × 6.6 cm, which was slightly smaller than the observed dimensions on August 20, 2014 (Fig. 6.4).

After 6 months of oral imatinib therapy, the patient came to our hospital's Gastrointestinal Stromal Tumor Specialty Outpatient Clinic and was admitted to the hospital with "abdominal GIST following 6 months of targeted therapy."

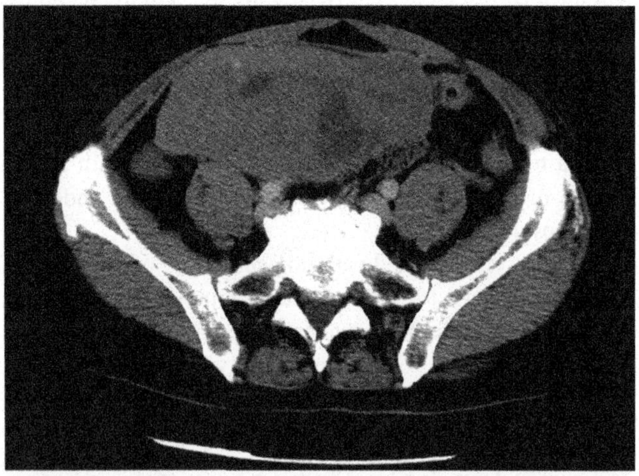

Fig. 6.2 Abdominal and pelvic enhanced CT after 1 month of oral imatinib therapy

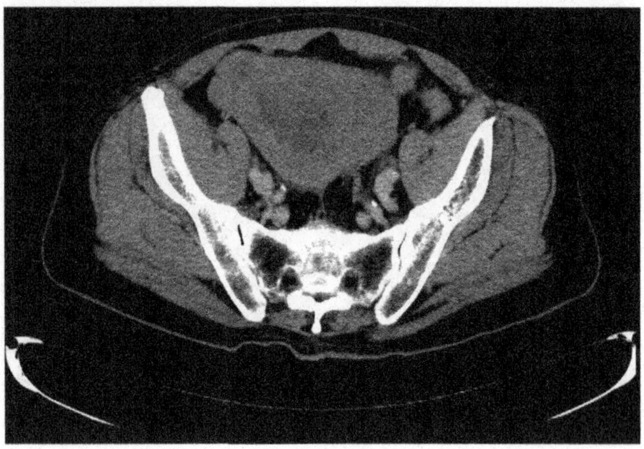

Fig. 6.3 Abdominal and pelvic enhanced CT after 4 months of oral imatinib therapy

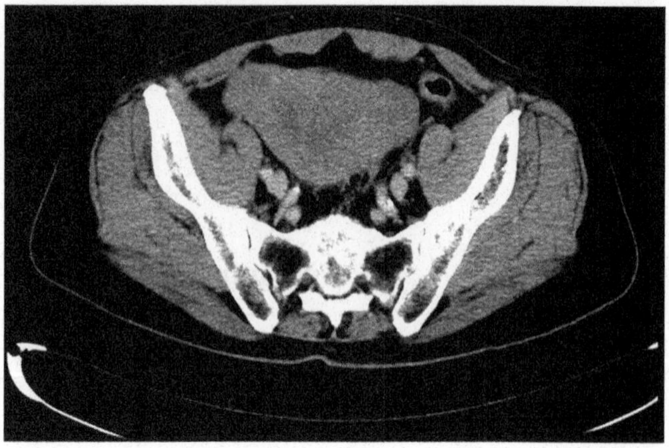

Fig. 6.4 Abdominal and pelvic enhanced CT after 6 months of oral imatinib therapy

6.1.2.1 Past History and Family History

The patient was previously physically fit and reported no drug allergies. The patient's parents were alive, and there was no similar medical history within the family.

6.1.2.2 Physical Examination

The vital signs were stable, and the skin and mucous membranes were not yellowish or pale. The abdomen was flat, and no gastrointestinal and peristaltic wave was seen. The abdomen was soft, with no tenderness, guarding, rebound tenderness, or obvious masses. There was no shifting dullness and the bowel sounds were normal. A digital rectal examination revealed that the intestinal wall was smooth and there were no obvious masses.

6.1.2.3 Auxiliary Examination

Blood Routine RBC 4.15×10^{12}/L; HCT% 39.4%; NEUT% 37.0%; neutrophil count 1.40×10^{9}/L.

Enhanced CT of the Abdomen and Pelvis (1) There was a huge mixed-density soft tissue mass in the lower abdomen-pelvic cavity, with a sheet-like low-density area. The mass was approximately 11.0 cm × 6.6 cm in size, and the margins were not clearly distinguishable from the adjacent intestine. There was no enhancement in the low-density area, and there was no obvious expansion of the intestinal lumen; (2) There was a round, cystic low-density shadow in the liver, with a clear boundary, and a diameter of approximately 2.0 cm. Additionally, a nodular dense area was visible on the edge of the right lobe of the liver. No enlargement or abnormalities were detected in the gallbladder, spleen, or pancreas; (3) There was nodular dense area in the right renal pelvis, but no obvious abnormality in the left kidney. The bladder was not well filled, and there were no abnormalities in the prostate and seminal vesicle glands; (4) No obvious enlarged lymph nodes were observed in the posterior peritoneum, and there was no fluid accumulation in the abdomen or pelvis.

6.1.3 Therapy

6.1.3.1 Case Analysis

The patient was a middle-aged man who presented with a 2-month history of middle and lower abdominal pain. An abdominal and pelvic CT scan revealed a huge mass in the abdominal and pelvic cavity. The pathology was consistent with GIST. After 6 months of imatinib targeted therapy, the lesion was smaller than at the time of diagnosis. At the time of admission to our center, the size of the tumor was significantly relieved, and the tumor had not significantly decreased further in size in the final 2 months. The patient was generally in a good health, and the tumor was considered to be resectable. It was decided that surgical treatment should be performed, followed with postoperative targeted therapy.

6.1.3.2 Treatment

Retroperitoneal tumor resection was performed on November 6, 2014. During the operation, it was seen that the abdominal tumor was located behind the bladder on the front wall of the rectum, extended to the right abdominal wall and was approximately 12 cm in size. The adhesion between the mass and the bladder, along the edge of the mass, was excised, the posterior wall of the mass on the anterior wall of the rectum was separated, the ureter and vas deferens on the side wall of the tumor were dissected and freed, and finally, the mass was separated and the tumor blood vessels were cut and ligated one by one (Figs. 6.5 and 6.6). The operation was completed smoothly.

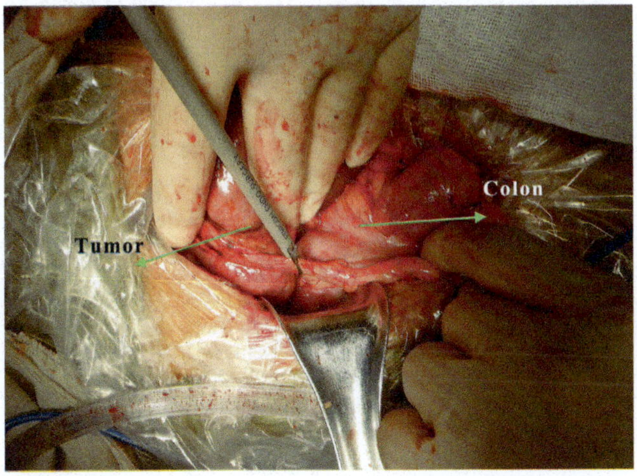

Fig. 6.5 Intraoperative separation of tumor and colon

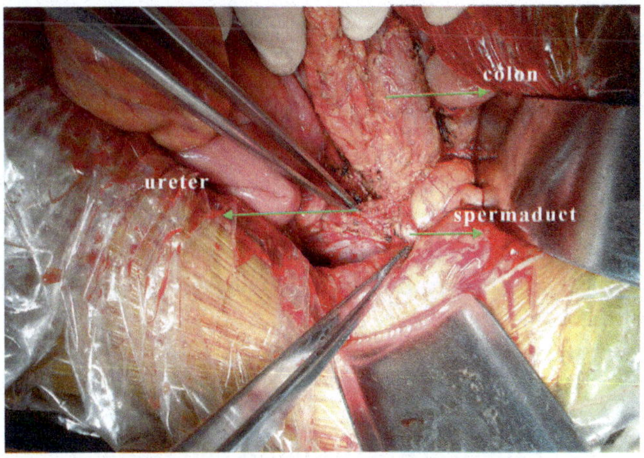

Fig. 6.6 Abdominal cavity after tumor removal

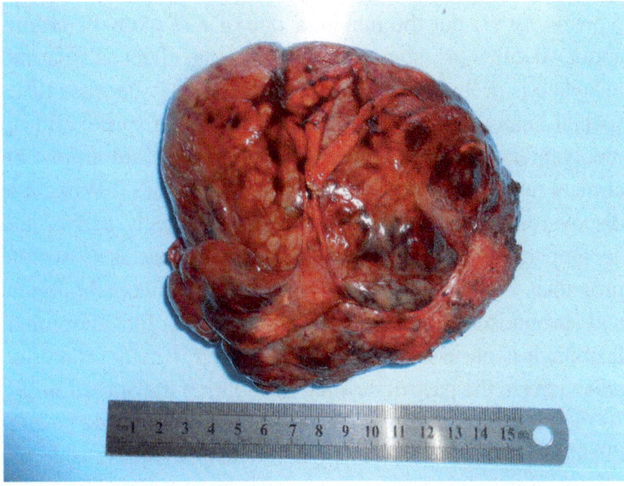

Fig. 6.7 The gross specimen

6.1.3.3 Postoperative Pathology and Genetic Testing

Pathological Diagnosis After preoperative treatment of GIST was densely packed and obviously abnormal, some cells were degenerated, tumors could be seen in clusters around blood vessels, and focal necrosis was observed. Cholesterol crystals were observed in the necrotic area, foam tissue cells were present, the necrotic area was less than 5% of the total mass, and mitotic count was hard to find. Morphologically, the drug response area was less than 5% (images suggested that the tumor had shrunk from 19.4 to 11 cm) (Fig. 6.7).

Immunohistochemistry CD117 (+), DOG-1 (+), CD34 (−), DES (−), Ki-67 (Li: <1%), NES (+), S-100 (+), SMA (+).

Genetic Testing There was a mutation of GTT (Val) at codon 559 in exon 11 of *KIT* to GAT (Asp). There were no mutations in *KIT* exons 9, 13, and 17 or *PDGFRA* exons 12 and 18.

6.1.4 Prognosis

The patient was discharged from the hospital on the seventh day postoperatively, and imatinib 400 mg/d targeted therapy was resumed on the 14th day after the operation. In the first postoperative year, the abdominal and pelvic cavity enhanced CT was reviewed every 3 months. In the second year after the operation, the abdominal and pelvic cavity enhanced CT was reviewed every 6 months. No obvious signs of recurrence or metastasis were detected. As of the last follow-up, the patient survived without recurrence.

6.1.5 Experience of Diagnosis and Therapy

Extra-gastrointestinal stromal tumor has similar cell morphology, immunohistochemical expression, and gene mutation types to GIST, but the mutation rate of *KIT* exon 11 is low, about 40–50% [4], suggesting the curative effect of imatinib mesylate is probably lower than that for GIST. Because of its special anatomical location, sufficient growth space, and no involvement of the gastrointestinal tract, there are almost no clinical manifestation in the early stages of EGIST. When it is discovered, the tumor is often huge, mitotically active, and accompanied by lymphatic or distant metastasis, so the prognosis is poor. In view of the special clinicopathological and prognostic characteristics of EGIST, for abdominal lesions, it is necessary to carefully explore whether there are adhesions to the gastrointestinal tract during the operation [5]. At the same time, postoperative pathology tests should be conducted to determine whether gastrointestinal wall muscle tissue remains on the tumor pseudocapsule.

For GIST patients who intend to undergo preoperative targeted therapy, biopsy should be performed to clarify the diagnosis and the type of gene mutation. Fine-needle aspiration biopsy via endoscopic ultrasonography is preferred [6], but is limited to accessible areas within the digestive tract lumen. This patient presented to the emergency department due to acute lower abdominal pain. Plain scan CT showed that the tumor had ruptured and was not suitable for endoscopic ultrasonography. Therefore, percutaneous biopsy was performed. After biopsy, a *KIT* exon 11 mutation was identified, and 400 mg/d imatinib treatment was commenced [7]. While imatinib therapy was being administered, the abdominal and pelvic cavity enhanced CT was reviewed every 2–3 months, and the treatment effect was evaluated according to Choi's standard [8]. Regarding the preoperative treatment time for imatinib, it is generally considered that 6–12 months is appropriate. After 6 months of targeted therapy with imatinib, the size of the patient's lesion was significantly lessened compared to the time of the first diagnosis, with little change in the final 2 months, so the lesion was surgically removed. Considering that the patient's tumor was larger than 10 cm before targeted therapy, and the tumor had ruptured, the patient continued to receive imatinib 400 mg/d after the operation.

6.2 Expert Comments

Kuntang Shen

At diagnosis, EGIST tumors are generally large (often >10 cm) and have a higher likelihood of local organ infiltration or metastasis compared to gastric GIST. Many studies have shown that EGIST has a higher degree of malignancy. At present, the main treatment method is surgical resection, and the tumor should be removed as completely as possible. If there is invasion of adjacent tissue, surgery should also be considered for the affected organs. Therefore, surgery for EGIST is often more difficult and traumatic. With the advent of targeted drugs, more and more scholars have found that preoperative imatinib treatment can significantly reduce the tumor volume of EGIST, reduce the risk of surgery, and increase the rate of complete surgical resection. In this case, the patient's tumor body was reduced from 19 to 11 cm, which greatly reduced the difficulty of the operation, increased the R0 resection rate, and the patient achieved a significant improvement in curative effect.

References

1. Greenson JK. Gastrointestinal stromal tumors and other mesenchymal lesions of the gut. Mod Pathol. 2003;16(4):366–75. https://doi.org/10.1097/01.mp.0000062860.60390.c7.
2. Robinson TL, Sircar K, Hewlett BR, Chorneyko K, Riddell RH, Huizinga JD. Gastrointestinal stromal tumors may originate from a subset of CD34-positiveinterstitial cells of Cajal. Am J Pathol. 2000;156(4):1157–63. https://doi.org/10.1016/s0002-9440(10)64984-x.
3. Reith JD, Goldblum JR, Lyles RH, Weiss SW. Extragastrointestinal (soft tissue) stromal tumors: an analysis of 48 cases with emphasis on histologic predictors of outcome. Mod Pathol. 2000;13(5):577–85. https://doi.org/10.1038/modpathol.3880099.
4. Yi JH, Park BB, Kang JH, Hwang IG, Shin DB, Sym SJ, Ahn HK, Lee SI, Lim DH, Park KW, Won YW, Lim SH, Park SH. Retrospective analysis of extra-gastrointestinal stromal tumors. World J Gastroenterol. 2015;21(6):1845–50. https://doi.org/10.3748/wjg.v21.i6.1845.
5. Agaimy A, Wünsch PH. Gastrointestinal stromal tumours: a regular origin in the muscularis propria, but an extremely diverse gross presentation. A review of 200 cases to critically re-evaluate the concept of so-called extra-gastrointestinal stromal tumours. Langenbeck's Arch Surg. 2006;391(4):322–9. https://doi.org/10.1007/s00423-005-0005-5.
6. Sepe PS, Brugge WR. A guide for the diagnosis and management of gastrointestinal stromal cell tumors. Nat Rev Gastroenterol Hepatol. 2009;6(6):363–71. https://doi.org/10.1038/nrgastro.2009.43.
7. Gronchi A, Blay JY, Trent JC. The role of high-dose imatinib in the management of patients with gastrointestinal stromal tumor. Cancer. 2010;116(8):1847–58. https://doi.org/10.1002/cncr.24944.
8. Choi H. Response evaluation of gastrointestinal stromal tumors. Oncologist. 2008;13(Suppl 2):4–7. https://doi.org/10.1634/theoncologist.13-s2-4.

Preoperative Treatment of Duodenal Gastrointestinal Stromal Tumors

7

Yongzhou Huang, Yuan Yin, and Zhiqiang Ma

Keywords

Gastrointestinal stromal tumor · Preoperative treatment Duodenal · Surgical treatment

7.1 Case 11 Duodenal GIST with Preoperative Treatment

Yongzhou Huang and Yuan Yin

7.1.1 Introduction

Duodenal GIST account for 12–18% of small intestinal GIST and 1–3% of all GIST. Surgical treatment is still the primary treatment for localized GIST. Because of the special anatomical location of duodenal GIST, immediately adjacent to the pancreatic head and biliary tract, complex surgical methods are required, and surgeons must consider surgical methods according to specific anatomical sites, tumor size, and other factors. The preoperative treatment of GIST has an important role, as some unresectable tumors shrink after targeted therapy, reducing the possibility of multi-organ resection, such as pancreaticoduodenectomy, increasing the resection rate, and reducing surgical trauma.

Y. Huang
Department of Gastrointestinal Surgery, Union Hospital, Tongji Medical College, Huazhong University of Science and Technology, Wuhan, China

Y. Yin (✉)
Department of Gastrointestinal Surgery, West China Hospital, Sichuan University, Chengdu, China
e-mail: yinyuan10@wchscu.cn

Z. Ma
Department of Gastrointestinal Cancer, Arion Cancer Center, Beijing, China

7.1.2 Case Background

A 67-year-old man presented with abdominal discomfort for 1 week. He underwent an abdominal ultrasound in West China Hospital, Sichuan University in August 2016, which revealed a large cystic and solid mass in the right retroperitoneum, approximately 10.8 cm × 5.3 cm in size. The mass pushed against the right side of the liver, squeezed the right ureter, and was located immediately adjacent to the inferior vena cava and abdominal aorta, with a less clear boundary. The abdominal enhanced CT showed a cystic and solid mass in front of the right anterior pararenal space (Fig. 7.1), and the parenchyma showed significant heterogeneous enhancement in which many large vessels were observed. The larger cross-sectional area of the mass was approximately 11.3 cm × 5.9 cm, the super-inferior diameter was 13.2 cm, the upper edge was close to the lower wall of the gallbladder neck, and the gallbladder wall showed no significant thickening. The medial edge of the mass was indistinct from the uncinate process of the pancreas, the horizontal, and descending part of the duodenum, the local duodenum was indistinct, and the anterior vessels of the mass were indistinct from the duodenal wall. The ascending colon, duodenum, and pancreatic head were displaced anteriorly. Right abdominal paracentesis showed a pike cell tumor, which revealed GIST when combined with immunohistochemistry results. The primary diagnosis was duodenal GIST.

7.1.2.1 Past History and Family History

Previously healthy, the patient reported no drug allergies. The patient's parents were alive, and there was no similar medical history within the family.

7.1.2.2 Physical Examination

The abdomen was flat, and no gastrointestinal or peristaltic waves were seen. The abdomen was soft, with no rebound tenderness. A large, firm, well-defined mass of approximately 10.0 cm × 10.0 cm was palpable in the right upper abdominal quadrant. The bowel sounds were normal.

K. Tao, H. Cao (eds.), *Clinical Management of Gastrointestinal Stromal Tumor*, https://doi.org/10.1007/978-981-99-9392-5_7

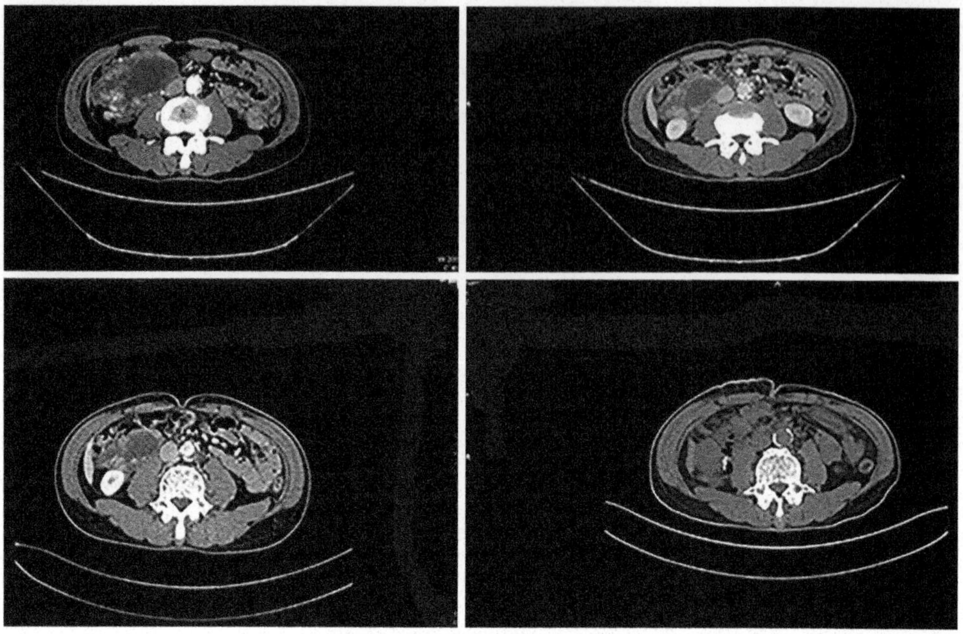

Fig. 7.1 Abdominal CT before preoperative treatment

7.1.2.3 Auxiliary Examination

The blood routine and biochemistry and tumor marker examinations revealed no significant abnormalities.

7.1.2.4 Primary Diagnosis

Duodenal GIST.

7.1.3 Therapy

7.1.3.1 Case Analysis

The patient was an elderly man with duodenal GIST. Abdominal CT showed a large retroperitoneal space occupying lesion, approximately 11.3 cm × 5.9 cm in size, close to the adjacent tissues. The MDT considered that surgical resection would be difficult, the possibility of complete resection was low, and combined organ resection was required. A definitive diagnosis was made based on the results of tumor biopsy. Therefore, the team recommended preoperative treatment with imatinib 400 mg/d and a close evaluation of the tumor changes.

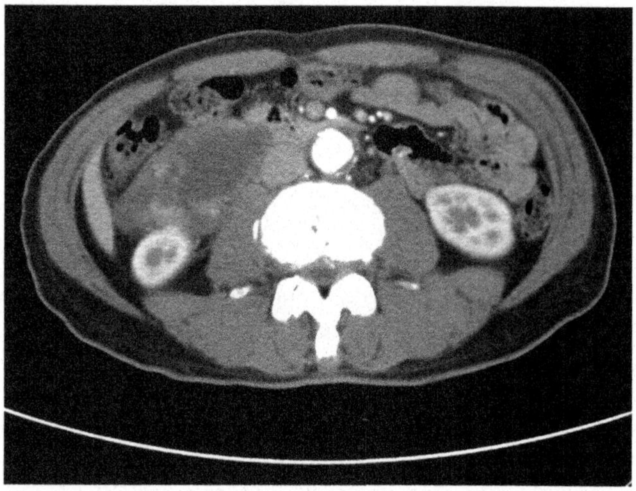

Fig. 7.2 Abdominal enhanced CT after 4 months of imatinib therapy

7.1.3.2 Treatment

The patient started preoperative treatment with imatinib at a dose of 400 mg/d without serious adverse effects. After 4 months of imatinib therapy, abdominal enhanced CT showed that the cross-sectional area of the mass had reduced to 8.2 cm × 4.5 cm (Fig. 7.2). After 8 months of imatinib therapy, the maximum cross-sectional area of the mass was 7.9 cm × 3.6 cm (Fig. 7.3). After re-evaluation of the mass, the patient was scheduled for surgical resection.

One week after preoperative drug withdrawal, the patient underwent exploratory laparotomy under general anesthesia. Intraoperative exploration showed no intraperitoneal effu-

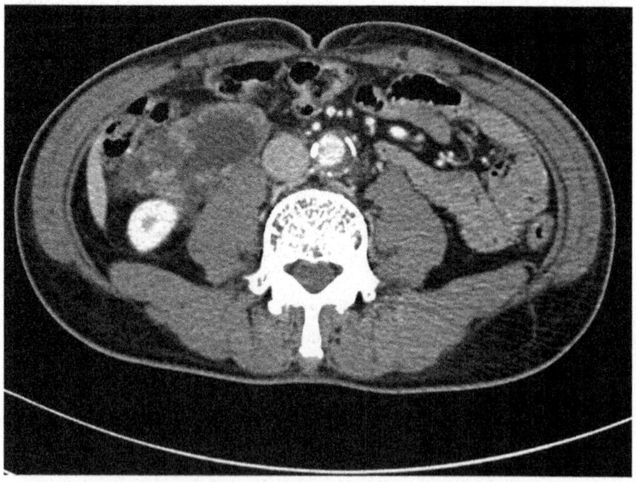

Fig. 7.3 Abdominal enhanced CT after 8 months of imatinib therapy

sion, significant adhesion in the right upper quadrant, and a mass in the right pararenal space, approximately 8.0 cm × 4.0 cm in size, closely adhered to the duodenum. The mass was irregular with an intact capsule, and the profile was fish-like. No retroperitoneal lymphadenopathy was detected, and other intra-abdominal organs showed no abnormalities. The intraoperative diagnosis was duodenal GIST. Therefore, partial duodenectomy and duodenal-jejunal side-to-side anastomosis were performed. The total operation time was 3 hours. Intraoperative blood loss was approximately 200 mL, and no intraoperative blood transfusion was performed.

7.1.3.3 Postoperative Pathology and Genetic Testing

Pathological Diagnosis Duodenal GIST, 9.5 cm × 8.0 cm × 3.9 cm in size, mitotic count 2/50 HPF.

Immunohistochemistry CD117 (+), CD34 (−), DOG-1 (+), SDHB (+), MIB-1 (positive rate < 2%), SMA (+), Desmin (−), and S-100 (−).

Genetic Testing A 557–558 deletion mutation was identified in exon 11 of *KIT*. Exons 9, 13, and 17 of *KIT* and exons 12 and 18 of *PDGFRA* were wild type.

7.1.4 Prognosis

The patient recovered uneventfully after surgery.

After discharge, the patient continued to receive imatinib 400 mg/d, and no recurrence was observed during the 30 months of follow-up.

7.1.5 Experience of Diagnosis and Therapy

Surgical resection is the primary treatment for patients with localized GIST more than 2 cm in diameter without surgical contraindications, who are expected to achieve R0 resection without combined organ resection or seriously affected organ function. For patients with giant tumors or tumors at special sites, owing to surgical difficulties, the current standard treatment includes preoperative treatment with imatinib which increases the tumor R0 resection rate and reduces the tumor volume, surgical risk, and the scope of surgery [1]. According to the Chinese Consensus on the Diagnosis and Treatment of Gastrointestinal Stromal Tumors (2017 Edition), the indications for preoperative treatment are where surgery will be difficult; GIST diameter greater than or equal to 10 cm, as these are susceptible to intraoperative rupture, bleeding, and iatrogenic transmission; where the tumor is located in a special anatomical site, such as EGJ, duodenum, or lower rectum, as in these locations there will be inevitable damage to the main organ function; where the tumor may be removed, but the surgical risk is high, the recurrence rate is high, or the mortality rate is high; where combined multiple organ resection is required; and where there is recurrence and metastasis of GIST [2]. The duration of preoperative treatment is generally 6–12 months, and Choi criteria can be used to determine the effect of preoperative treatment. The requirement for postoperative adjuvant targeted drug therapy is based on the modified 2008 NIH postoperative risk classification of GIST, and the time limit of postoperative adjuvant therapy is selected according to the grade and genetic test results.

Surgical resection of duodenal GIST commonly includes duodenal wedge resection, duodenectomy, distal partial gastrectomy, pancreatic-preserving duodenectomy, or pancreaticoduodenectomy [3]. From the perspective of protecting organ function and reducing trauma, local surgical resection of the tumor should be pursued. On the basis of ensuring complete resection of the tumor, Vater and pancreatic function should be protected as much as possible with physiological digestive tract reconstruction, and the implementation of extended surgery such as pancreaticoduodenectomy should be minimized.

Given the patient's large tumor volume at the initial diagnosis and its location in the duodenum, performing surgery at that time would have involved a combined organ resection, which would have been highly traumatic and posed significant risks. Therefore, preoperative treatment with imatinib was administered. After 8 months of treatment, as the tumor volume reduction plateaued and maximum efficacy was reached, a partial pancreatic-sparing duodenectomy was performed.

Duodenal GIST has the particularity of anatomical location and biology, so preoperative treatment is necessary, but the proportion of preoperative treatment is still low. A multicenter retrospective study of duodenal GIST found that only 13.1% of patients received preoperative treatment [4]. We believe that the concept of preoperative treatment still needs to be continuously promoted, and hope that the report of this case, can provide some reference for the standardized treatment of duodenal GIST.

7.2 Expert Comments

Zhiqiang Ma

Primary duodenal GIST is rare in clinical practice and account for approximately 1–3% of GIST [5]. However, the duodenum is an abdominal organ with the most complex anatomical relationship, and duodenal GIST surgery should try to protect Vater and pancreatic function and physiological digestive tract reconstruction should be performed. From the perspective of protecting organ function, local surgical resection of the tumor is pursued, and extended surgery such as pancreaticoduodenectomy was minimized on the basis of ensuring complete resection of the tumor [6]. Our retrospective study summarized the selection of surgical approach based on the size of duodenal GIST: (1) GIST less than 3 cm in size: partial resection of duodenal intestinal wall (wedge resection) is usually feasible; (2) GIST 3–5 cm in size: if tumor is not adjacent to the duodenal papilla, duodenal resection can be considered. (3) GIST greater than or equal to 5 cm in size: mostly requires pancreatic preserving duodenectomy, or pancreaticoduodenectomy (Whipple operation). However, the location of the tumor (medial or lateral), whether there is inward or outward growth, and whether the duodenal papilla can be avoided should be considered more in clinical practice, and even the texture of the tumor will affect the treatment choice. In the selection of non-Whipple operation, duodenoplasty and reconstruction of digestive tract are still a critical issue for patient prognosis, and the outflow of bile and pancreatic juice and anastomotic blood supply should be fully considered.

In above mentioned case, the longest diameter of the tumor was more than 5 cm, the demarcation from the surrounding organs was unclear, direct surgical R0 resection was difficult and combined organ resection was unavoidable, so preoperative treatment was performed after a diagnosis of duodenal GIST was confirmed by biopsy. In this case, the tumor shrank after 8 months of treatment with imatinib. Although the tumor was still 9.5 cm × 8.0 cm × 3.9 cm in size, partial duodenectomy was possible because the tumor grew outwardly (retroperitoneally) and was distant from the duodenal papilla.

Preoperative treatment of GIST can usually achieve tumor shrinkage, reduction of tumor density, and a clearer definition of the relationship between the tumor and adjacent organs. These are the key factors to improve the resection rate, avoid combined organ resection, narrow the scope of surgery, reduce surgical trauma, and reduce surgical complications. However, some GIST (about 10%) still have primary drug resistance during first-line targeted therapy. Therefore, it is very important to perform timely and reasonable imaging follow-up examinations during the initial preoperative targeted drug therapy period. In recent years, it has become clear that, while preoperative drug therapy for partial GIST may be initially effective, this can be followed by stagnation of the effect, or secondary drug resistance, such that R0 resection is still unfeasible. Some research has reported that further tumor shrinkage using second-line targeted therapy or the combination of first-line and second-line therapies can be explored to obtain successful surgery [7].

The data from 10 European centers showed that a total of 161 locally advanced but non-metastatic GIST (duodenal GIST accounted for 10%) received an average of 40 months of preoperative treatment, 83% achieved R0 resection, and the postoperative 5-year disease-free survival for locally advanced duodenal GIST was 65% [8]. These results suggest that preoperative treatment of duodenal GIST is a safe and effective method for increasing the surgical R0 resection rate and reducing the surgical risk.

References

1. Renberg S, Zhang Y, Karlsson F, Bränström R, Åhlen J, Jalmsell L, Linder-Stragliotto C, Haglund de Flon F, Papakonstantinou A. The role of neoadjuvant imatinib in gastrointestinal stromal tumor patients: 20 years of experience from a tertial referral center. Int J Cancer. 2022;151(6):906–13. https://doi.org/10.1002/ijc.34052.
2. Li J, Ye Y, Wang J, Zhang B, Qin S, Shi Y, He Y, Liang X, Liu X, Zhou Y, Wu X, Zhang X, Wang M, Gao Z, Lin T, Cao H, Shen L, Chinese Society of Clinical Oncology Csco Expert Committee on Gastrointestinal Stromal Tumor. Chinese consensus guidelines for diagnosis and management of gastrointestinal stromal tumor. Chin J Cancer Res. 2017;29(4):281–93. https://doi.org/10.21147/j.issn.1000-9604.2017.04.01.
3. Vassos N, Perrakis A, Hohenberger W, Croner RS. Surgical approaches and oncological outcomes in the management of duodenal gastrointestinal stromal tumors (GIST). J Clin Med. 2021;10(19):4459. https://doi.org/10.3390/jcm10194459.
4. Colombo C, Ronellenfitsch U, Yuxin Z, Rutkowski P, Miceli R, Bylina E, Hohenberger P, Raut CP, Gronchi A. Clinical, pathological and surgical characteristics of duodenal gastrointestinal stromal tumor and their influence on survival: a multi-center study. Ann Surg Oncol. 2012;19(11):3361–7. https://doi.org/10.1245/s10434-012-2559-0.
5. Sugase T, Takahashi T, Nakajima K, Hirota S, Masuzawa T, Nishida T, Kimura Y, Miyazaki Y, Makino T, Kurokawa Y, Yamasaki M, Takiguchi S, Mori M, Doki Y. Clinicopathological characteristics, surgery and survival outcomes of patients with duodenal gastrointestinal stromal tumors. Digestion. 2016;94(1):30–6. https://doi.org/10.1159/000447665.
6. Tien YW, Lee CY, Huang CC, Hu RH, Lee PH. Surgery for gastrointestinal stromal tumors of the duodenum. Ann Surg Oncol. 2010;17(1):109–14. https://doi.org/10.1245/s10434-009-0761-5.
7. Serrano C, Leal A, Kuang Y, Morgan JA, Barysauskas CM, Phallen J, Triplett O, Mariño-Enríquez A, Wagner AJ, Demetri GD, Velculescu VE, Paweletz CP, Fletcher JA, George S. Phase I study of rapid alternation of sunitinib and regorafenib for the treatment of tyrosine kinase inhibitor refractory gastrointestinal stromal tumors. Clin Cancer Res. 2019;25(24):7287–93. https://doi.org/10.1158/1078-0432.CCR-19-2150.
8. Rutkowski P, Gronchi A, Hohenberger P, Bonvalot S, Schöffski P, Bauer S, Fumagalli E, Nyckowski P, Nguyen BP, Kerst JM, Fiore M, Bylina E, Hoiczyk M, Cats A, Casali PG, Le Cesne A, Treckmann J, Stoeckle E, de Wilt JH, Sleijfer S, Tielen R, van der Graaf W, Verhoef C, van Coevorden F. Neoadjuvant imatinib in locally advanced gastrointestinal stromal tumors (GIST): the EORTC STBSG experience. Ann Surg Oncol. 2013;20(9):2937–43. https://doi.org/10.1245/s10434-013-3013-7.

8 Avapritinib Therapy for Preoperative Treatment of Gastrointestinal Stromal Tumors with *PDGFRA* Mutation

Bo Ni, Linxi Yang, and Kaixiong Tao

Keywords

Avapritinib · Advanced GIST · Preoperative treatment

8.1 Case 12 A 67-Year-Old Man with Metastatic GIST with *PDGFRA* D842V Mutation Who Received Preoperative Avapritinib Therapy

Bo Ni and Linxi Yang

8.1.1 Introduction

Imatinib is still the first-line therapy for unresectable or recurrent/metastatic GIST [1, 2]. However, the number of cases that achieve complete remission has been unsatisfactory and a large number of patients who receive imatinib therapy suffer from primary or secondary resistance [3]. Approximately 5–10% of GIST harbor oncogenic mutations in the juxtamembrane domain or activation loop of platelet-derived growth factor receptor alpha (*PDGFRA*), a receptor tyrosine kinase that is highly homologous to *KIT* [4]. Most patients with *PDGFRA* gene mutation on exon 18, including the D842V subtypes, are highly resistant to imatinib (primary resistance), which is a major clinical difficulty for prescribing individual therapy [5–7]. Hence, it is necessary to discover novel targeted therapies for refractory GIST to improve patient prognosis and create better surgical opportunities [8].

B. Ni · L. Yang (✉)
Department of Gastrointestinal Surgery, Renji Hospital, Shanghai Jiaotong University School of Medicine, Shanghai, China

K. Tao
Department of Gastrointestinal Surgery, Union Hospital, Tongji Medical College, Huazhong University of Science and Technology, Wuhan, China
e-mail: kaixiongtao@hust.edu.cn

8.1.2 Case Background

In December 2019, the patient, a 67-year-old man, presented to Renji Hospital Affiliated to Shanghai Jiao Tong University School of Medicine with recurrent abdominal distension over the course of one month. The previous abdominal CT showed a huge soft tissue mass in the lesser curvature of the stomach (possible GIST) and multiple annular low-density enhanced shadows in the liver (considered metastasis, Fig. 8.1). A previous biopsy of the mass indicated a possible diagnosis of GIST with strongly positive expression of DOG-1 and negative expression of CD117 and CD34. Moreover, Sanger sequencing of the biopsy specimen revealed the D842V mutation of *PDGFRA* on exon 18.

The patient was prescribed 300 mg/d avapritinib from February 2020 to February 2021. In which CT scans showed regression of the primary and liver-metastatic lesions (Figs. 8.2, 8.3, and 8.4 show the findings of abdomen CT after 2 months, 6 months, and 12 months, respectively). Specifically, the size of the primary tumor had decreased by 27.2%, 33.6%, and 38.9% after 2, 6, and 12 months, respectively, compared to the initial images.

In February 2021, the patient suffered sudden abdominal pain and continuous weakness, and blood tests revealed a hemoglobin level of 50 g/L. Emergency abdominal CT images revealed a huge mass in the abdominal and pelvic cavities with partially unclear margins with the gastrointestinal tract, accompanied by thickening of peritoneal blood vessels and central ischemic necrosis of the gastric lesion. The pelvic ascites progressed significantly (Fig. 8.5). An abdominal puncture was performed, which revealed the fluid was noncoagulating blood, considered to represent tumor rupture and hemorrhage.

The patient was admitted to the emergency department and hospitalized for treatment of rupture and hemorrhage of GIST previously treated with avapritinib.

K. Tao, H. Cao (eds.), *Clinical Management of Gastrointestinal Stromal Tumor*, https://doi.org/10.1007/978-981-99-9392-5_8

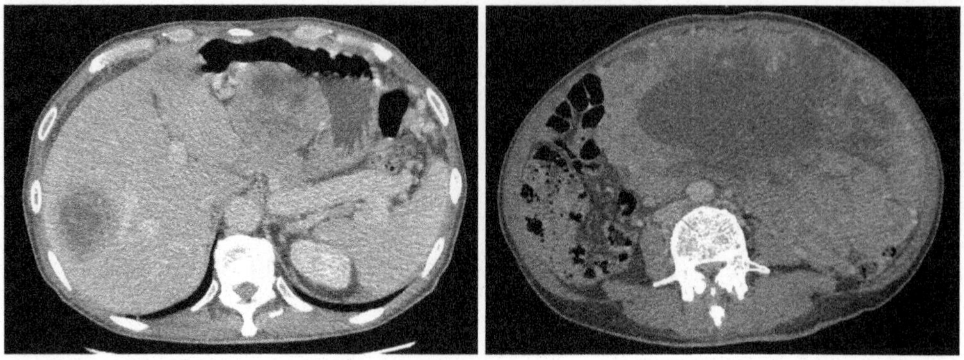

Fig. 8.1 Abdominal CT before avapritinib therapy

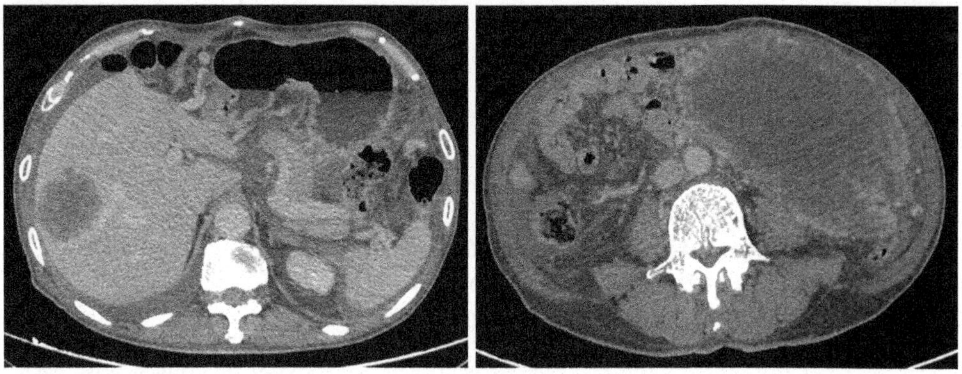

Fig. 8.2 Abdominal enhanced CT after 2 months of avapritinib therapy

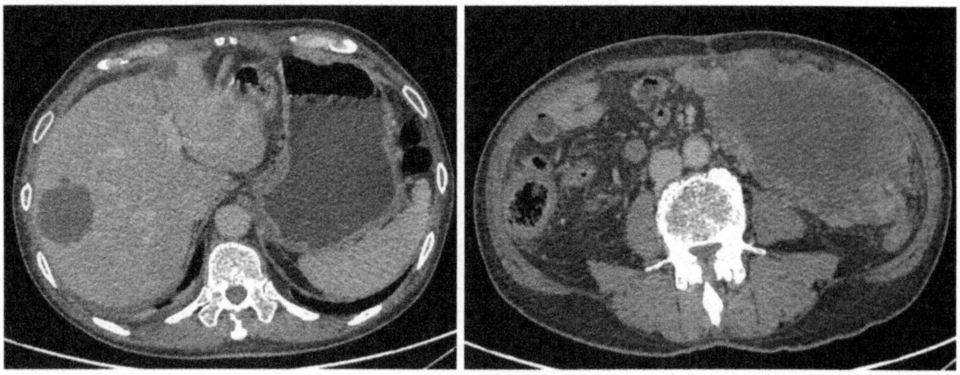

Fig. 8.3 Abdominal enhanced CT after 6 months of avapritinib therapy

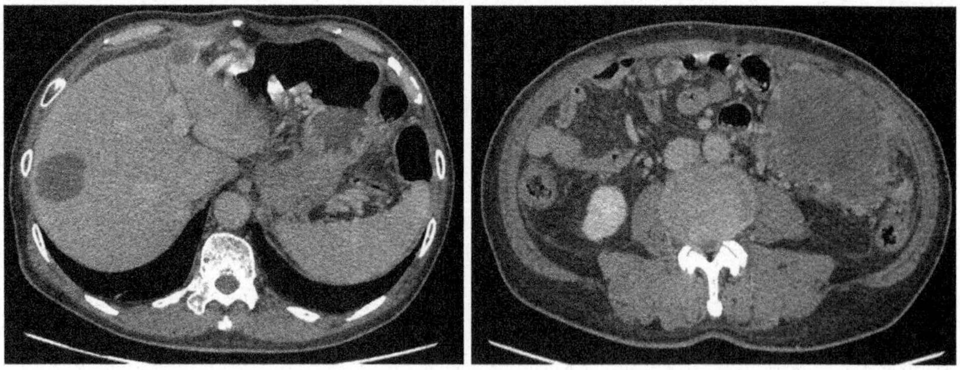

Fig. 8.4 Abdominal enhanced CT after 12 months of avapritinib therapy

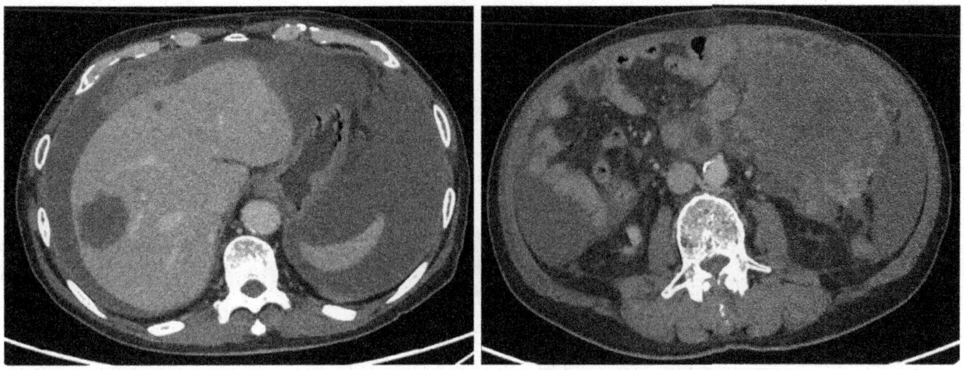

Fig. 8.5 Preoperative abdominal CT showed the increased pelvic ascites with several new nodular lesions

8.1.2.1 Past History and Family History

The patient had a history of coronary heart disease with stent implantation and previous surgery for an inguinal hernia. The patient reported no drug allergies or relevant family history.

8.1.2.2 Physical Examination

The patient had an increased heart rate and slightly low blood pressure, with pale conjunctivae. He reported tenderness in his entire abdomen and a tight mass was palpated in the left upper quadrant.

8.1.2.3 Auxiliary Examination

Blood Routine Examination Hb 50 g/L.

Abdominal CT A huge mass was identified in the abdominal and pelvic cavities with partially unclear margins with the gastrointestinal tract, accompanied by thickening of peritoneal blood vessels and central ischemic necrosis of the lesion and the pelvic scan revealed ascites and several nodular lesions.

8.1.2.4 Preliminary Diagnosis

1. Metastatic GIST (after preoperative avapritinib targeted therapy)
2. Intra-abdominal hemorrhage
3. Severe anemia
4. Coronary heart disease (CHD)

8.1.3 Therapy

8.1.3.1 Case Analysis

The patient was an elderly man with advanced GIST who had received a 12-month course of preoperative avapritinib therapy. Although the drug effect was promising, a sudden emergency occurred and indicated tumor rupture and hemorrhage. Considering the slowly tumor remission, tumor rupture, and severe anemia of the patient, it was determined that surgical treatment should be performed immediately. The postoperative targeted therapy was subsequently determined by the results of pathological examination and genetic testing.

8.1.3.2 Therapy

On February 19, 2021, partial gastrectomy, partial transverse colectomy, and palliative liver tumor enucleation were simultaneously performed under general anesthesia. During the operation, the bloody ascites in abdominal cavity was found to be approximately 5000 mL, and the primary tumor was 20 cm × 10 cm in size and originated from the posterior wall of the gastric body. The tumor exhibited signs of rupture and hemorrhage. The mass had invaded the transverse mesocolon, surrounded the left branch of the middle colonic blood vessels, and also invaded the left lower abdominal parietal peritoneum. Moreover, multiple, soft-textured metastatic nodules were found in the liver (Fig. 8.6).

8.1.3.3 Postoperative Pathology and Genetic Testing

Pathology Gastric tumor: the tumor was 20.0 cm × 13.0 cm × 6.0 cm in size, the tumor cells had obviously decreased in size, and appeared as mostly fibrotic stroma with abundant focal tumor cells, and a high mitotic count of >10/50 HPF. Left and right liver tumor: most metastatic GIST tumor cells had decreased in size and demonstrated stromal fibrosis with a few tumor cells left. The maximum diameter of both tumors was 0.1 cm.

Immunohistochemistry Ki-67 (LI: 60%), VIM (+), CD117 (+), CD34 (+), DOG-1 (+), SMA (−), Desmin (−), S-100 (−), SDHB (+), BRAF (−).

Genetic Testing There was a mutation in *PDGFRA*, and the mutation type was 842GAC > GTC (homozygous) on exon 18, resulting in the change of the encoded amino acid D842V, without any further mutations in *KIT* or *PDGFRA*.

Pathological Diagnosis Metastatic GIST with D842V mutation on exon 18 of *PDGFRA*.

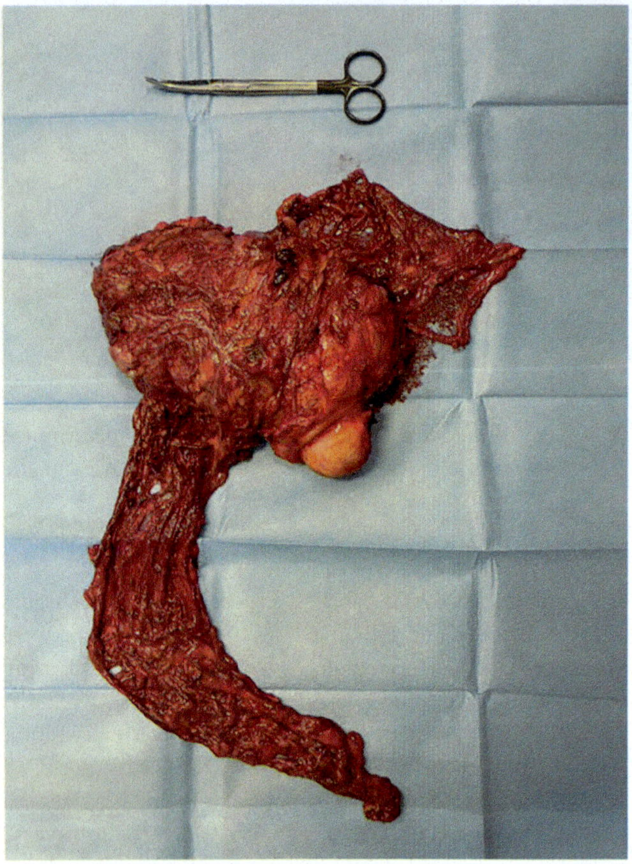

Fig. 8.6 Picture of the primary huge GIST originating from stomach and invading transverse mesocolon

8.1.4 Prognosis

The patient recovered smoothly and received 200 mg/d avapritinib after the surgery. However, the disease had shown marked progression and several novel lesions appeared during the course of avapritinib therapy. The patient ultimately died in July 2021 as a result of disease progression.

8.1.5 Experience of Diagnosis and Therapy

8.1.5.1 Advanced GIST with *PDGFRA* Mutation on Exon 18 is Potential Candidates to Benefit from Preoperative Avapritinib

From this case, we observed that patients with GIST caused by *PDGFRA* mutation on exon 18 could obtain partial benefits from avapritinib, especially regarding tumor remission. The patient had reached the maximal response of partial remission and received a surgical resection in emergency state. The progression-free survival time was 12 months and overall survival time was around 17 months. Compared to imatinib, avapritinib seems to have promising effects on GIST with specific mutation types during the preoperative targeted therapy. This also indicates the importance of biopsy and genetic testing, which could guide individual therapy and precision medicine.

8.1.5.2 Close Assessment Is Key during Preoperative Therapy

Although the patient had obtained remarkable tumor remission while receiving avapritinib therapy, the emergency of tumor rupture and hemorrhage occurred, which led to avapritinib discontinuation and emergency surgery. Because the rupture, the swift growth of the tumor should be taken into account when considering the progression in this case. Mainstream guidelines state that the duration of preoperative treatment is dependent on when the maximal response to therapy is achieved [9]. Nevertheless, few reports of preoperative avapritinib administration have been published, and more cases should be reported to explore ways to achieve the best surgical outcomes. During preoperative therapy courses, changes in imagining studies should be closely recorded to avoid losing opportunities for surgery due to progression of unresectable lesions. Appropriately shortening the imaging examination interval during preoperative treatment can be of benefit to patients and help to guide surgical timing.

8.1.5.3 Mechanism Exploration of Avapritinib Resistance Should Be Concerned

The prognosis of this patient was not satisfactory, because the tumor progressed quickly after palliative surgery. Moreover, mechanism of GIST resistance to avapritinib should be taken into consideration, as this could provide more effective targeted strategies for refractory GIST.

8.2 Expert Comments

Kaixiong Tao

Gastrointestinal stromal tumors are not sensitive to radiotherapy or chemotherapy, but the administration of imatinib created the era of targeted therapy for GIST [3, 4]. However, patients with certain primary mutations, such as exon 18 mutations in *PDGFRA*, are resistant to standard imatinib therapy, especially patients with D842V mutations with intermediate to high risk of recurrence. In the first-, second-, or third-line targeted therapy, secondary mutations always occur, which lead to drug resistance. Therefore, exploration of resistance mechanisms and development of novel TKIs has been a recent study focus. In 2020, the FDA approved avapritinib for the treatment of adult patients with inoperable or metastatic GIST with exon 18 mutations in *PDGFRA*, providing treatment opportunities for those refractory patients [10, 11].

From the perspective of a surgeon, accomplishment of surgery is important for GIST prognosis, but more effective targeted therapy is equally important. The first-, second-, and third-line TKIs, imatinib sunitinib, and regorafenib, respectively, all provide survival benefits for patients with advanced GIST to varying degree. We hope that patients with special genotypes could receive more effective and precise treatment. Surgeons and physicians are both looking forward to the development of novel drugs for this purpose. In addition, during the administration of drugs with latter-lines, patient management is the key, and it is necessary to understand the indications, administration methods and control of adverse reactions. This is a problem that needs to be solved through series of study.

The clinicians are looking forward to the continuous promotion of novel TKIs for clinical application, because patients with advanced or unresectable *PDGFRA* mutation (exon 18) are clearly recommended for first-line treatment with avapritinib [5, 6, 11–13]. At present, avapritinib is also considered as neoadjuvant or adjuvant therapy for genotyped patients with *PDGFRA* mutations, which may maximize the effect of this drug and survival benefit.

References

1. Kelly CM, Gutierrez Sainz L, Chi P. The management of metastatic GIST: current standard and investigational therapeutics. J Hematol Oncol. 2021;14(2):1–12. https://doi.org/10.1186/s13045-020-01026-6.
2. McAuliffe JC, Hunt KK, Lazar AJ, Choi H, Qiao W, Thall P, Pollock RE, Benjamin RS, Trent JC. A randomized, phase II study of preoperative plus postoperative imatinib in GIST: evidence of rapid radiographic response and temporal induction of tumor cell apoptosis. Ann Surg Oncol. 2009;16(4):910–9. https://doi.org/10.1245/s10434-008-0177-7.
3. Serrano C, George S. Gastrointestinal stromal tumor: challenges and opportunities for a new decade. Clin Cancer Res. 2020;26(19):5078–85. https://doi.org/10.1158/1078-0432.CCR-20-1706.
4. Blay JY, Kang YK, Nishida T, von Mehren M. Gastrointestinal stromal tumours. Nat Rev Dis Primers. 2021;7(1):22. https://doi.org/10.1038/s41572-021-00254-5.
5. Henriques-Abreu M, Serrano C. Avapritinib in unresectable or metastatic gastrointestinal stromal tumor with PDGFRA exon 18 mutation: safety and efficacy. Expert Rev Anticancer Ther. 2021;21(10):1081–8. https://doi.org/10.1080/14737140.2021.1963235.
6. Jones RL, Serrano C, von Mehren M, George S, Heinrich MC, Kang YK, Schoffski P, Cassier PA, Mir O, Chawla SP, Eskens F, Rutkowski P, Tap WD, Zhou T, Roche M, Bauer S. Avapritinib in unresectable or metastatic PDGFRA D842V-mutant gastrointestinal stromal tumours: long-term efficacy and safety data from the NAVIGATOR phase I trial. Eur J Cancer. 2021;145:132–42. https://doi.org/10.1016/j.ejca.2020.12.008.
7. von Mehren M, Heinrich MC, Shi H, Iannazzo S, Mankoski R, Dimitrijevic S, Hoehn G, Chiroli S, George S. Clinical efficacy comparison of avapritinib with other tyrosine kinase inhibitors in gastrointestinal stromal tumors with PDGFRA D842V mutation: a retrospective analysis of clinical trial and real-world data. BMC Cancer. 2021;21(1):291. https://doi.org/10.1186/s12885-021-08013-1.
8. BLU-285, DCC-2618 show activity against GIST. Cancer Discov. 2017;7(2):121–2. https://doi.org/10.1158/2159-8290.CD-NB2016-165.
9. Qi J, Liu HL, Ren F, Liu S, Shi W, Liu WH, Cai GQ, Liao GQ. Preoperative adjuvant therapy for locally advanced and recurrent/metastatic gastrointestinal stromal tumors: a retrospective study. World J Surg Oncol. 2020;18(1):70. https://doi.org/10.1186/s12957-020-01840-9.
10. Dhillon S. Avapritinib: first approval. Drugs. 2020;80(4):433–9. https://doi.org/10.1007/s40265-020-01275-2.
11. Gebreyohannes YK, Wozniak A, Zhai ME, Wellens J, Cornillie J, Vanleeuw U, Evans E, Gardino AK, Lengauer C, Debiec-Rychter M, Sciot R, Schoffski P. Robust activity of avapritinib, potent and highly selective inhibitor of mutated KIT, in patient-derived xenograft models of gastrointestinal stromal tumors. Clin Cancer Res. 2019;25(2):609–18. https://doi.org/10.1158/1078-0432.CCR-18-1858.
12. George S, Jones RL, Bauer S, Kang YK, Schoffski P, Eskens F, Mir O, Cassier PA, Serrano C, Tap WD, Trent J, Rutkowski P, Patel S, Chawla SP, Meiri E, Gordon M, Zhou T, Roche M, Heinrich MC, von Mehren M. Avapritinib in patients with advanced gastrointestinal stromal tumors following at least three prior lines of therapy. Oncologist. 2021;26(4):e639–e49. https://doi.org/10.1002/onco.13674.
13. Kang YK, George S, Jones RL, Rutkowski P, Shen L, Mir O, Patel S, Zhou Y, von Mehren M, Hohenberger P, Villalobos V, Brahmi M, Tap WD, Trent J, Pantaleo MA, Schoffski P, He K, Hew P, Newberry K, Roche M, Heinrich MC, Bauer S. Avapritinib versus regorafenib in locally advanced unresectable or metastatic GI stromal tumor: a randomized, open-label phase III study. J Clin Oncol. 2021;39(28):3128–39. https://doi.org/10.1200/JCO.21.00217.

Preoperative Treatment of Rectal-Vaginal Septum Gastrointestinal Stromal Tumors

9

Wenchang Yang, Zhidong Gao, and Yingjiang Ye

Keywords

Gastrointestinal stromal tumors · Rectovaginal septum
Targeted therapy · Surgery

9.1 Case 13 Preoperative Treatment of Rectal-Vaginal Septum GIST

Wenchang Yang and Zhidong Gao

9.1.1 Introduction

The most common site of GIST is the digestive tract, but a few originate from other soft tissues in the abdominal cavity, such as the greater omentum, mesentery, or retroperitoneum. These tumors are called extra-gastrointestinal stromal tumors (EGIST). Due to the special location, the treatment of EGIST which occur in the pelvic floor region (including the rectum, rectovaginal septum, posterior vaginal wall, anterior and posterior bladder regions, anterior and posterior prostate regions, and presacral region) requires the protection of pelvic floor organs, so clinicians need to pay more attention to it.

W. Yang
Department of Gastrointestinal Surgery, Union Hospital, Tongji Medical College, Huazhong University of Science and Technology, Wuhan, China
e-mail: yangwenchang@hust.edu.cn

Z. Gao (✉) · Y. Ye
Department of Gastrointestinal Surgery, Peking University People's Hospital, Beijing, China
e-mail: gaozhidong@pkuph.edu.cn; yeyingjiang@pkuph.edu.cn

9.1.2 Case Background

The patient, a 33-year-old woman, presented to the hospital on 8 April, 2016, for investigation of a mass in the perineum which had been present for one and a half years. The patient was found to have a "left vaginal wall cyst" during physical examination in October 2014. There was no pain, no contact bleeding, and no treatment was performed. In October 2015, the patient felt that the left side of the vagina was swollen during menstruation, and an ultrasound at that time showed a "left Bartholin gland cyst" which was treated with traditional Chinese medicine, with little effect. In November 2015, the patient felt that the mass was enlarged and bulged outward, and this was accompanied by thin urine and incomplete urination, with no abnormal secretions. Gynecological ultrasound examination showed a cystic and solid structure on the left side of the external orifice of the vaginal wall, approximately 2.3 cm × 2.1 cm × 2.3 cm in size, with a clear boundary, poor internal sound transmission, and dense punctate echo. In February 2016, she felt that the tumor was enlarged with pain and swelling in the perineal area. She was admitted to hospital for treatment of "Bartholin's cyst with infection." She received antibiotic treatment, and the symptoms were slightly relieved. In March 2016, the patient was scheduled for Bartholin's gland cyst resection, and a cystic and solid mass was found which was mainly composed of solid components during the operation. As the nature of the mass was not clear, the surgery was suspended. The cystic component was punctured and 3 mL of bloody fluid was aspirated. The bacterial culture was negative. After the operation, the patient continued to have bloody exudation, and felt that the tumor became larger, but the pain was slightly relieved after the antibiotic treatment. Ultrasound-guided transperineal biopsy was performed, and the pathology showed spindle cell tumor with moderate cell atypia and mitotic count (18/50 HPF). Immunohistochemistry showed CD117 (+), CD34 (+), S-100 (−), Ki-67 (Li: 10–20%), ER (−) and PR (−), and the tumor was considered to be high risk GIST. Genetic testing showed

K. Tao, H. Cao (eds.), *Clinical Management of Gastrointestinal Stromal Tumor*, https://doi.org/10.1007/978-981-99-9392-5_9

a deletion mutation in exon 11 of *KIT* (c.1670-1675 del GGAAGG). After the biopsy, the patient felt that the mass was obviously enlarged, and the pain was aggravated. Subsequently, a pelvic MRI was performed (Fig. 9.1), which revealed an oval-shaped, mixed soft tissue signal between the lower rectum and the vagina, with the maximum section of approximately 5.7 cm × 3.7 cm, and uneven enhancement in the enhanced scan. The boundary between the lesion and the anterior wall of the rectum and the posterior wall of the vagina was not clear, and the adjacent tissue was compressed and displaced. There was upper vaginal obstruction with effusion.

Transrectal ultrasound showed that the lower part of the rectum and the anterior wall of the anal canal, 1 cm above the anus, had uneven low echo, the size was approximately 4.3 cm × 3.7 cm, the internal blood flow was rich and disordered, and the arterial spectrum could be derived. The tumor was located below the peritoneal reflection and the puborectalis and external anal sphincter were intact. Transabdominal ultrasound showed that the pelvic cavity was inhomogeneous and hypoechoic, approximately 5.9 cm × 4.8 cm in size, and the boundary with the vagina was not clear. Transperineal ultrasound showed that the pelvic cavity was inhomogeneous and hypoechoic, approximately 5.2 cm × 5.5 cm in size, the front of the mass was approximately 0.2 cm from the skin, the boundary was not clear, the shape was irregular, the blood flow signal was rich, and the arterial spectrum could be derived. A PET-CT scan showed a round mass in the lower part of the vagina and the anterior wall of the rectum, approximately 5.0 cm × 3.5 cm × 5.9 cm in size, with a slightly inhomogeneous density, unclear boundary between the mass and the vagina and anterior wall of the rectum, and local protrusion to the vulva. Preoperatively, it was assessed as a potentially resectable rectal GIST. Considering that the tumor was large and closely related to the surrounding tissues and organs, direct resection had the possibility of combined organ resection, and it would have been difficult to preserve the function of vagina and anus; therefore, preoperative therapy was administered. The patient started to take imatinib mesylate 400 mg/d from April 15, 2016. After that, she was reviewed regularly.

Enhanced CT was performed 1 month after initiation of imatinib treatment and revealed a round-like mixed density shadow between the lower rectum and the vagina, approximately 4.2 cm × 2.5 cm × 2.6 cm in size (Fig. 9.2). The density of the lesion was uneven, and a liquid density area was observed. The solid component was obviously enhanced, and the boundary between the lesion and the anterior wall of the rectum and the posterior wall of the vagina was not clear. Compared to the first pelvic MRI, the lesion was smaller (Choi criteria: PR status). Enhanced CT was repeated 4 months after initiation of imatinib treatment which revealed

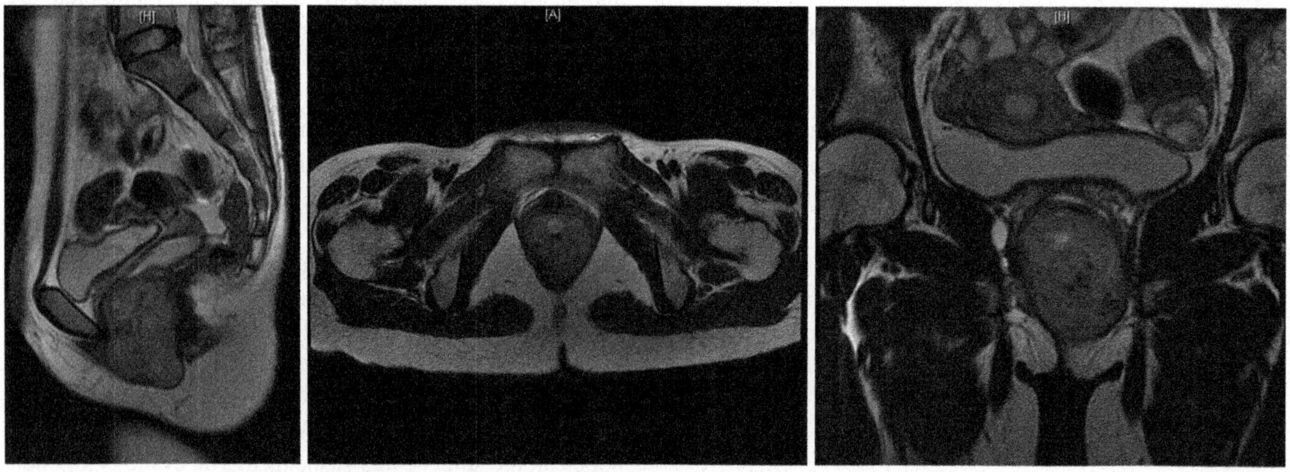

Fig. 9.1 The initial pelvic MRI examination showed an oval-shaped, mixed soft tissue signal shadow between the lower rectum and the vagina

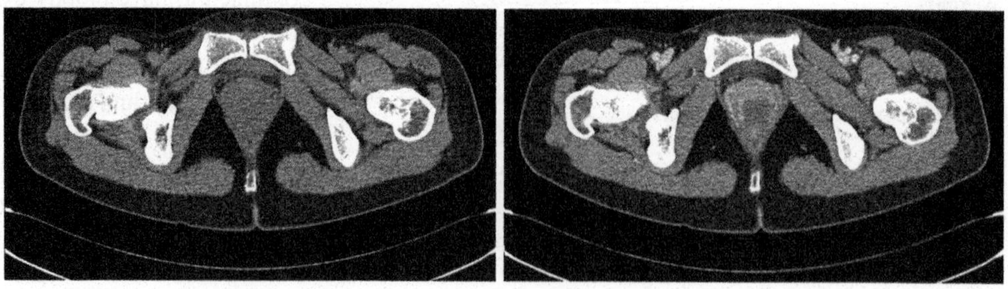

Fig. 9.2 Enhanced CT after 1 month of imatinib therapy

a round low-density lesion between the lower rectum and the vagina, approximately 3.5 cm × 2.3 cm × 1.8 cm in size, with slight enhancement (Fig. 9.3). The boundary between the lesion and the anterior wall of the rectum and the posterior wall of the vagina was not clear. Compared to the previous results, the lesion was slightly smaller (Choi criteria: PR status). Enhanced CT was again performed 6 months after initiation of imatinib treatment, and this scan revealed a round low-density lesion between the lower part of the rectum and the vagina, approximately 3.9 cm × 2.1 cm × 1.9 cm in size, and the local boundary between the lesion and the anterior wall of the rectum and the posterior wall of the vagina was still not clear (Fig. 9.4). Compared to the previous scan, there was no significant change in the lesion (Choi criteria: maintaining PR status). Considering that the preoperative targeted therapy had been carried out for more than 6 months, and the effect of drug therapy had been maximized, the patient could undergo surgical treatment. On November 1, 2016, she was admitted to the Department of Gastrointestinal Surgery of Peking University People's Hospital for treatment of GIST following preoperative therapy.

9.1.2.1 Past and Family History

The patient was previously healthy, and reported no drug allergies. Her parents were alive, and there was no similar medical history in the family.

9.1.2.2 Physical Examination

The abdomen was flat, and no gastrointestinal pattern or peristaltic waves were seen. There was no tenderness, rebound tenderness, or guarding in the whole abdomen, the liver and spleen were not palpable, and there was no palpable abdominal mass. There was no shifting dullness and the bowel sounds were normal.

Gynecological examination showed an incision biopsy scar on the skin of the left vulva, which had healed well. There was a palpable mass under the skin of the left vulva, approximately 4 cm × 3 cm in size, with hard texture and poor mobility. The left vaginal mucosa was everted due to the swelling of the mass, and the vaginal orifice was narrow, making it difficult to insert the fingers. Lithotomy position: The mass was palpable at 4–9 o'clock by the vaginal entrance, especially at 9 o'clock. There was contact bleeding, but the upper boundary was not touched.

Digital examination of the anus in the KC position showed no obvious abnormality in anal shape and skin. When the finger was inserted about 2 cm from the anus, a hard mass could be palpated at 7 o'clock, the upper edge of the mass could not be reached and there was tenderness. There was no blood stain.

9.1.2.3 Auxiliary Inspection

Routine Blood Test White blood cells 4.20 × 10^9/L, red blood cells 4.74 × 10^{12}/L, hemoglobin 138 g/L, platelets 175 × 10^9/L, neutrophils (%) 56.6%, lymphocytes (%) 30.7%.

Blood Biochemistry No abnormality was found.

Pelvic MRI A GIST between the lower rectum and the vagina was identified, with an unclear boundary with the posterior wall of the vagina and the anterior wall of the rec-

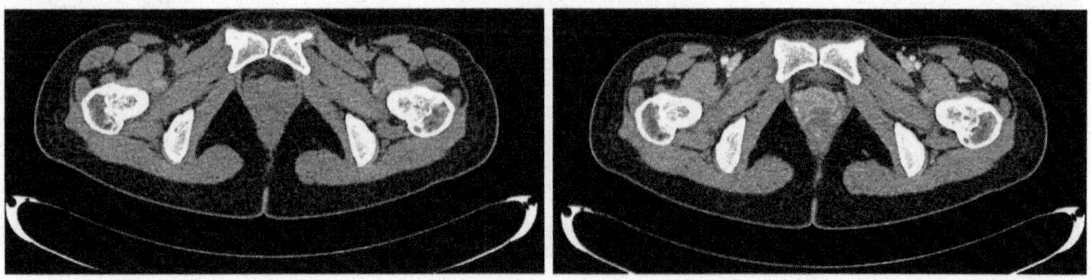

Fig. 9.3 Enhanced CT after 4 months of imatinib therapy

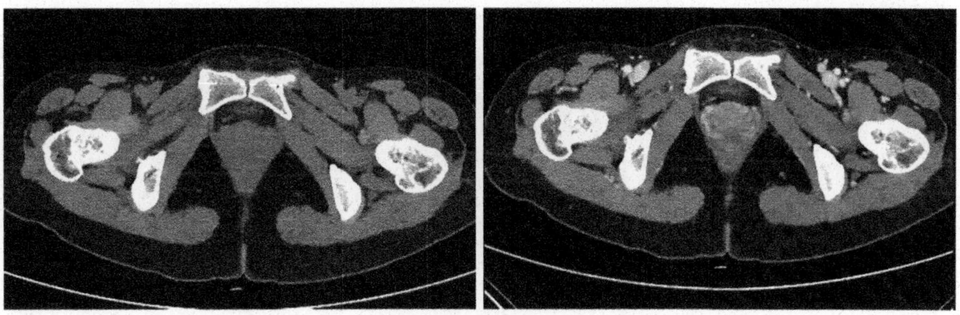

Fig. 9.4 Enhanced CT after 6 months of imatinib therapy

tum. The tumor was approximately 3.3 cm × 2.1 cm × 1.7 cm in size, and there was no significant change in size compared to the previous images. There was no obvious high signal on DWI, and no obvious enhancement. A small amount of fluid was observed in the pelvic cavity (Fig. 9.5).

9.1.3 Therapy

9.1.3.1 Case Analysis

The patient was a young woman, diagnosed with GIST. Because the tumor was large and located in the pelvic floor rectovaginal septum, involving the vagina and low rectum, it was difficult to preserve the anal and vaginal structures when performing direct resection; therefore, surgery would inevitably affect defecation and sexual function. To avoid this, imatinib pretreatment was administered. After 6 months of 400 mg/d imatinib treatment, two consecutive efficacy evaluations showed PR status, indicating the tumor had stopped shrinking and the maximum effect of preoperative therapy had been achieved. At that time, the patient's general condition was good, there was no distant metastasis, and surgical intervention was planned. Although the tumor had reduced in size, it formed strong adhesion with the surrounding tissue and the boundary was not clear. Local excision was determined to be the appropriate method to ensure R0 excision while preserving anal and vaginal function. Pathology and genetic testing of gross specimens was conducted again after surgery, and the adjuvant targeted therapy was guided by these results.

9.1.3.2 Treatment

After ceasing imatinib therapy for 1 week, surgery for mass resection with vaginal and rectal repair and temporary ileostomy was performed on November 7, 2016. In the lithotomy position, the intraoperative findings were of a solid mass in the pelvic cavity, with a clear boundary and a pseudocapsule, approximately 3.5 cm × 2.5 cm in size, which invaded part of the posterior vaginal wall upward and adhered to part of the anterior rectal wall. A portion of the involved posterior vaginal wall was resected along the border of the mass. Sharp dissection was performed along the space behind the tumor, part of the anterior rectal wall muscle layer tissue was resected, the integrity of the rectal mucosa was preserved without damage, and the tumor was completely resected. The operation went smoothly.

The mass was located in the rectovaginal septum, invaded the posterior wall of the vagina anteriorly and the anterior wall of the rectum posteriorly. It was hard with approximately 3.5 cm × 2.5 cm in size (Fig. 9.6).

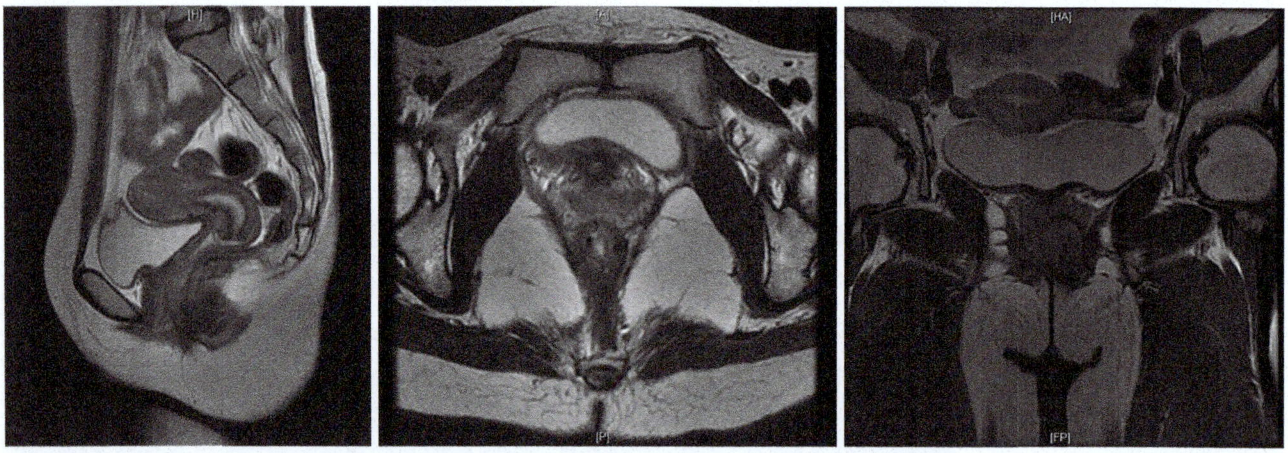

Fig. 9.5 Preoperative pelvic MRI

Fig. 9.6 The gross specimen

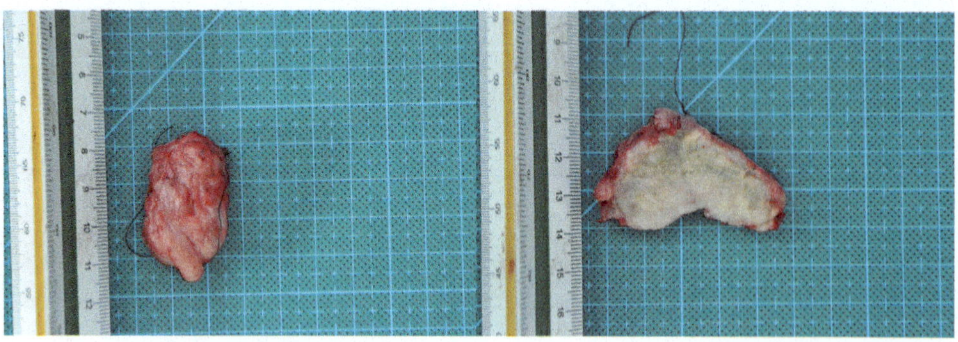

9.1.3.3 Postoperative Pathology and Genetic Testing

Pathological Diagnosis Postoperative pathology showed a spindle cell tumor with extensive degeneration and necrosis, focal cell abundance, moderate atypia, and mitotic count >10/50 HPF. The size was approximately 3.5 cm × 2.5 cm × 1.5 cm, which was consistent with the changes after targeted therapy for GIST. Vaginal mucosa sample: a small piece of mucosal tissue with a few neoplastic elements. Rectal resection margin: no tumor component was found.

Immunohistochemistry CD117 (+), CD34 (+), DOG-1 (+), S-100 (−), SMA (−), CK (−), Vimentin (+), Desmin (−) Ki-67 (Li: 40%).

Genetic Testing A deletion mutation in exon 11 of *KIT* (c.1670-1675delGGAAGG) was identified. Exons 9, 13, and 17 of *KIT* and exons 12 and 18 of *PDGFRA* were wild type.

9.1.3.4 Prognosis

Intestinal function recovered well after the operation and the patient was discharged 10 days after the operation without other serious complications. Ileostomy resection was performed 3 months postoperatively. Oral imatinib 400 mg/d adjuvant therapy was continued after the first operation, and no signs of recurrence were found in follow-up in March 2019.

9.1.4 Experience of Diagnosis and Therapy

9.1.4.1 General Description of EGIST at Rectovaginal Septum

The incidence of extra-gastrointestinal stromal tumors is reported to be approximately 10% of all GIST [1]. Most EGIST occur in the lesser or greater omentum, mesentery, and retroperitoneum, and rarely occur in areas of the women genital tract such as the vulva and vagina and are especially rare in the rectovaginal septum. There are few reports of EGIST in the women genital tract at home and abroad (Table 9.1). There are several possibilities for the histological origin of EGIST. The earliest type of tumor was thought to originate from the outward growth of GIST in the gastrointestinal tract. Under the action of external forces and other factors, the mass eventually breaks away from the digestive tract to form the so-called EGIST, which is not a real EGIST. Later, some scholars speculated that EGIST might originate from extra-gastrointestinal stromal cells, which acquired the phenotype of Cajal stromal cells during tumorigenesis. It has been confirmed that interstitial cells of Cajal also exist in extra-gastrointestinal organs such as the uterus, fallopian tubes, bladder, breasts, gallbladder, and pancreas. Therefore, many scholars believe that EGIST originates from the neoplastic transformation of interstitial cells of Cajal outside the gastrointestinal tract. To support this theory, some literatures have reported that Cajal cells with the same cell morphology, phenotype and function as gastrointestinal pacemaker cells also exist in the vaginal wall of women in normal physiological conditions.

9.1.4.2 Diagnosis and Differential Diagnosis of EGIST

Vaginal EGIST have been reported on MRI as lobulated oval masses with long T1 and slightly longer T2 signal intensity, which are relatively homogeneous. The mass showed obvious homogeneous enhancement, and the degree of enhancement was basically consistent with the vaginal wall. However, in this case, the MRI showed a nodular mass with low signal intensity on T1WI, slightly low signal intensity on T2WI, and progressive enhancement on enhanced scan. The slight signal intensity on T2WI in this case is inconsistent with the above and may be due to coagulative necrosis of the tumor.

The pathological features of EGIST are similar to other GIST. Grossly, it is usually a poorly defined nodule with a diameter of 2.0–10.0 cm. The cut surface of the tumor is gray-white or gray-red. It is solid, smooth, and fish-like in texture. Often, EGIST lacks the hard and woven structure of leiomyoma. Sometimes there may be obvious necrosis, hemorrhage, or cystic degeneration. The tumor tissue often invades the surrounding tissues. Microscopically, most of the tumor cells were fusiform. Tumor cells are arranged in bundles and swirls, and some are composed of epithelioid cells, which are arranged in diffuse patches or trabeculae, or in palisades, which are common in schwannomas.

Gastrointestinal stromal tumors can differentiate into smooth muscle cells and are often misdiagnosed as smooth muscle-derived tumors. For tumors in the women genital tract, EGIST should be differentiated from leiomyoma and leiomyosarcoma. Histologically, the cytoplasm of smooth muscle cells is often strongly eosinophilic, while the cytoplasm of EGIST cells is only slightly eosinophilic. Leiomyosarcoma cells are more pleomorphic. Immunohistochemistry showed that 95% of GIST expressed CD117 (KIT protein), 90% expressed DOG-1, and 60–70% expressed CD34. Additionally, DOG-1 was expressed in KIT negative GIST and PDGFRA mutated GIST. Recently, it has been reported that immunohistochemical detection of PKC-θ expression is of great significance in the diagnosis of CD117 and DOG-1 double-negative GIST. In addition, 30–40% of GIST express SMA, 1–2% express desmin, and 5% express S-100. In contrast, smooth muscle tumors express desmin, SMA, and H-Caldesmon almost exclusively and CD117, CD34, and DOG-1 are generally not expressed. Approximately 80% of GIST also express H-Caldesmon, although H-Caldesmon expression is very specific for differentiation toward smooth muscle. Schwannomas generally express S-100 diffusely but not CD117 and CD34. It

Table 9.1 Case data of EGIST occurring in vagina or recto-vagina

References	Age (y)	Tumor site	Tumor size (cm)	Treatment	Mitotic count (/50 HPF)	CD117	CD34	*KIT* mutation	Follow-up time
Nasu et al. [2]	54	Recto-vagina	8.5	Surgery	1 ~ 2	+	+	ND	13 months
Ceballos et al. [3]	75	Vagina	4.5	Surgery	12 ~ 15	+	+	ND	7.5 years
Weppler et al. [4]	66	Recto-vagina	8	Imatinib	>5	+	+	ND	ND
Takano et al. [5]	38	Vagina	7	Surgery	1–2	+	+	ND	1 year
Lam et al. [6]	36	Vagina	4	ND	15	+	+	9	2 years
Lam et al. [6]	48	Vagina	6	ND	12	+	+	11	10 years
Lam et al. [6]	61	Vagina	8	ND	16	+	+	11	ND
Nagase et al. [7]	42	Recto-vagina	3.5	Surgery	<1	+	+	ND	4 years
Nagase et al. [7]	66	Vagina	5	Surgery+ Imatinib	2–3	+	+	ND	6 months
Zhang et al. [8]	42	Recto-vagina	8	Surgery	10	+	+	ND	11 months
Molina et al. (2009) [9]	56	Recto-vagina	5	Surgery+ radiotherapy	>25	+	+	ND	ND
Vazquez et al. [10]	29	Recto-vagina	7	Surgery+ Imatinib	10	+	+	11	2 years
Melendez et al. [11]	80	Recto-vagina	6	Surgery+ Imatinib	5	+	+	ND	22 months

HPF high powered field, *ND* no description

should also be noted that soft tissue tumors with positive immunohistochemical markers for CD34, CD117, and DOG-1 are not necessarily GIST. Microarray analysis of 775 soft tissue specimens showed that a few leiomyosarcomas, synovial sarcomas, and melanomas also expressed CD117, DOG-1, and CD34. It has been reported that leiomyosarcomas and endometrial stromal sarcomas of the women reproductive system can diffusely express CD117, but these tumors do not have *KIT* mutations. Therefore, the detection of *KIT* molecular mutations has important differential significance in the pathological diagnosis of GIST or EGIST. Mutations in *KIT* or *PDGFRA* are key mechanisms in the morbidity of GIST. Approximately 80% of GIST had mutations in *KIT*, with 80% and 15% occurring in exons 11 and 9, respectively, and less than 2% in exons 13 and 17. Only about 30% of GIST with *PDGFRA* mutations had no *KIT* mutations. About 44% of EGIST have mutations in the *KIT*, and most of them are in exon 11.

9.1.4.3 Biological Behavior of EGIST

Because EGIST is rare, there is no clear and unified standard to evaluate its biological behavior. The biological behavior of GIST varies according to the site of occurrence, and generally the closer the mass is to the distal gastrointestinal tract, the higher the malignant potential. Additionally, EGIST are considered to be similar to GIST occurring in the distal gastrointestinal tract and generally have a higher malignant potential than GIST occurring in the gastrointestinal tract. In addition, some studies have shown that, contrary to GIST, the biological behavior of EGIST is not related to tumor size, which may be related to the fact that most EGIST are large at the time of discovery. Reith et al. showed that the risk factors for the malignant potential of EGIST included high cell density, a mitotic count >2/50 HPF, and necrosis. For patients with fewer than 2 risk factors, only 5% of which have a poor prognosis. On the contrary, 95% of those having 2 or more risk factors have a poor prognosis. Although most EGIST in this study were located in the mesentery and retroperitoneal space, the histological features (high cell density and mitotic count) of this patient were classified as having poor biological behavior based on the criteria of Reith et al.

9.1.4.4 Treatment Strategy for EGIST

A radical resection is the treatment of choice for EGIST. Lymph node metastasis is rare in GIST, and routine lymph node dissection is usually not required, but an extended resection could be necessary. The effect of radiotherapy and chemotherapy is minimal, but adjuvant therapy with tyrosine kinase inhibitors is effective. The thoroughness of surgical treatment for EGIST is closely related to the prognosis of the disease, and en bloc resection of the lesion is recommended. In some patients, because of extensive adhesion or dissemination of surrounding tissues, only palliative surgery is performed to achieve the purpose of definite diagnosis or to reduce tumors and alleviate symptoms. If necessary, molecular targeted drug therapy can be carried out before operation to reduce the tumor volume and the risk of operation, which can also reduce the possibility of iatrogenic dissemination of tumors with high risk of rupture and bleeding during operation. Because EGIST are rare, there is no unified standard for the malignant risk assessment of EGIST, so the malignant risk assessment of EGIST is compared with that of GIST. In this case, the tumor was approximately 10 cm in diameter, and the microscopic mitotic count was 4–6/50 HPF. The tumor occurred in the vagino-rectal septum and was classified as a high-risk case according to Joensuu's risk classification after GIST resection. Patients with moderate and high risk of recurrence need adjuvant therapy after operation. Imatinib is currently recommended as first-line adjuvant therapy. It is generally recommended that the initial recommended dose be 400 mg/d for 1 year, with follow-up.

9.1.4.5 How to Follow Up After EGIST?

Because peritoneal and hepatic metastases can occur after EGIST, patients at moderate and high risk should have CT or MRI scans conducted every 3 months for 3 years, then every 6 months until 5 years postoperative. Then patients should have a follow-up every year after 5 years. Low-risk patients should have CT or MRI every 6 months for 5 years. Because of the relatively low incidence of lung and bone metastases, chest X-ray examination is recommended at least once a year. Enhanced CT bone scans and, if necessary, PET/CT are recommended in the presence of relevant symptoms.

9.2 Expert Comments

Yingjiang Ye

An EGIST is a primary GIST that occurs outside the gastrointestinal tract, with a low incidence and relative rarity in the clinical setting; therefore, there is a lack of relevant research and unified norms and standards for treatment. Extra-gastrointestinal stromal tumors, especially those located in the pelvic floor area (such as the rectovaginal septum, posterior vaginal wall, anterior and posterior bladder areas), are often larger than 5 cm in diameter at the first diagnosis because of their insidious symptoms and difficult diagnosis. The anatomical structure of the pelvic floor region is complex, and GIST in this region may originate from multiple organs and tissues, so it is difficult to determine the origin of the tumor, which has been a clinical problem to be solved. A study of GIST in this region in our center showed that GIST from the rectum were the most common (68.0%), followed by those from the prostate, the posterior vaginal wall, rectovaginal septum, presacral region, and bladder. Preoperative imaging examination is helpful to detect the tumor, in which MRI has the highest coincidence rate in judging the primary site of the tumor. CT is also an appropriate imaging modality. Surgery remains the treatment of choice for EGIST. The thoroughness of surgical treatment is closely related to the prognosis of the disease, and en bloc and complete resection of the lesion is recommended. However, for GIST in the pelvic floor region, because it requires organ preservation and functional protection, the patient's condition needs to be fully discussed by a multidisciplinary expert collaboration group to develop a multidisciplinary comprehensive treatment based on surgery.

Through the diagnosis and treatment of this case, the following points are worth learning.

1. The incidence of EGIST is low, the onset is usually insidious, and the clinical symptoms are different from those of gastrointestinal GIST, which requires a certain degree of clinical diagnostic vigilance.
2. For some cases of EGIST, it is difficult to diagnose the source of the tumor before surgery, and it is helpful to select appropriate examination methods for diagnosis.
3. For EGIST requiring multiple organ resection or functional protection, imatinib should be used before surgery, biopsy is helpful to confirm the diagnosis, and genetic testing should be carried out to guide treatment.
4. EGIST are considered to be more aggressive biologically and usually require imatinib therapy.
5. During preoperative treatment, the therapeutic effect should be evaluated regularly (every 2–3 months), and assessment using Choi criteria should be performed. When the effect of drug treatment is maximized (generally after no more than 6 months of treatment, or when the tumor does not recede after two consecutive evaluations), timely surgical intervention should be carried out to avoid delaying the best time for surgical treatment.
6. Pathological examination and genetic testing should be repeated postoperatively to evaluate whether there are secondary mutations or other rare conditions, and to guide the implementation of adjuvant therapy.

References

1. Cho M-Y, Sohn JH, Kim JM, Kim K-M, Park YS, Kim WH, Jung JS, Jung ES, Jin S-Y, Kang DY, Park JB, Park HS, Choi YD, Sung SH, Kim Y-B, Kim H, Bae Y-K, Kang M, Chang HJ, Chae YS, Lee HE, Park DY, Lee YS, Kang YK, Kim HK, Chang H-K, Hong SW, Choi YH, Shin O, MiJin G, Kim YW, Kim GI, Sei Jin Chang. Current Trends in the Epidemiological and Pathological Characteristics of Gastrointestinal Stromal Tumors in Korea. 2003-2004. J Korean Med Sci. 2010;25(6):853–62. https://doi.org/10.3346/jkms.2010.25.6.853.
2. Nasu K, Ueda T, Kai S, Anai H, Kimura Y, Yokoyama S, Miyakawa I. Gastrointestinal stromal tumor arising in the rectovaginal septum. Int J Gynecol Cancer. 2004;14(2):373–7. https://doi.org/10.1111/j.1048-891x.2004.014230.x.
3. Ceballos KM, Francis JA, Mazurka JL. Gastrointestinal stromal tumor presenting as a recurrent vaginal mass. Arch Pathol Lab Med. 2004;128(12):1442–4. https://doi.org/10.5858/2004-128-1442-GSTPAA.
4. Weppler EH, Gaertner EM. Malignant extragastrointestinal stromal tumor presenting as a vaginal mass: report of an unusual case with literature review. International journal of gynecological cancer. Int J Gynecol Cancer. 2005;15(6):1169–72. https://doi.org/10.1111/j.1525-1438.2005.00269.x.
5. Takano M, Saito K, Kita T, Furuya K, Aida S, Kikuchi Y. Preoperative needle biopsy and immunohistochemical analysis for gastrointestinal stromal tumor of the rectum mimicking vaginal leiomyoma. Int J Gynecol Cancer. 2006;16(2):927–30. https://doi.org/10.1111/j.1525-1438.2006.00217.x.
6. Lam MM, Corless CL, Goldblum JR, Heinrich MC, Downs-Kelly E, Rubin BP. Extragastrointestinal stromal tumors presenting as vulvovaginal/rectovaginal septal masses: a diagnostic pitfall. Int J Gynecol Pathol. 2006;25(3):288–92. https://doi.org/10.1097/01.pgp.0000215291.22867.18.
7. Nagase S, Mikami Y, Moriya T, Niikura H, Yoshinaga K, Takano T, Ito K, Akahira J, Sasano H, Yaegashi N. Vaginal tumors with histologic and immunocytochemical feature of gastrointestinal stromal tumor: two cases and review of the literature. Int J Gynecol Cancer. 2007;17(4):928–33. https://doi.org/10.1111/j.1525-1438.2007.00892.x.
8. Zhang WJ, Peng ZL, Xu L. Extragastrointestinal stromal tumor arising in the rectovaginal septum: report of an unusual case with literature review. Gynecol Oncol. 2009;113(3):399–401. https://doi.org/10.1016/j.ygyno.2009.02.019.
9. Molina I, Seamon LG, Copeland LJ, Suarez A. Reclassification of leiomyosarcoma as an extra-gastrointestinal stromal tumor of the gynecologic tract. Int J Gynecol Pathol. 2009;28(5):458–63. https://doi.org/10.1097/PGP.0b013e31819c7fc1.
10. Vázquez J, Pérez-Peña M, González B, Sánchez A. Gastrointestinal stromal tumor arising in the rectovaginal septum. J Low Genit Tract Dis. 2012;16(2):158–61. https://doi.org/10.1097/LGT.0b013e31823b52af.
11. Meléndez MN, Revello R, Cuerva MJ, De Santiago J, Zapardiel I. Misdiagnosis of an extragastrointestinal stromal tumor in the rectovaginal septum. J Low Genit Tract Dis. 2014;18:e66–70. https://doi.org/10.1097/LGT.0b013e3182a72156.

Part III

Uncommon Pathological Types of Gastrointestinal Stromal Tumors

Small Hypermitotic Gastrointestinal Stromal Tumors

10

Jianbo Lyu, Xin Chen, and Yong Li

Keywords

Gastrointestinal stromal tumor · Hypermitotic
Prognosis

10.1 Case 14 A 49-Year-Old Man with Small Hypermitotic GIST

Jianbo Lyu and Xin Chen

10.1.1 Introduction

The origin and pathogenesis of GIST has been basically clarified. However, the high recurrence and metastasis rates of GIST still present difficulties for clinicians. Most GIST classification criteria are based on tumor size, mitotic count, and tumor location, but these criteria cannot accurately predict the recurrence of GIST. It is widely believed that the size of the primary tumor and mitotic count are important indicators to judge the degree of malignancy and determine the operation method, in which mitotic count should be more heavily weighted. Clinically, during the diagnosis and treatment of GIST, it is not uncommon to find that the tumor volume is small, but the number of mitotic images is high. The Union Hospital, Tongji Medical College of Huazhong University of Science and Technology conducted a single center investigation of this kind of patient. Among 269 cases of GIST, with a maximum tumor diameter < 2 cm, 14 cases (about 5%) were accompanied by a high mitotic count. The diagnosis and treatment of such patients should pay more attention to genetic testing and adjuvant therapy, and comprehensive evaluation should be conducted.

J. Lyu · X. Chen (✉)
Department of Gastrointestinal Surgery, Union Hospital, Tongji Medical College, Huazhong University of Science and Technology, Wuhan, China
e-mail: u201610420@hust.edu.cn; chenxinzju@zju.edu.cn

Y. Li
Department of Gastrointestinal Surgery, Guangdong Provincial People's Hospital, Guangzhou, China
e-mail: liyong@gdph.org.cn

10.1.2 Case Background

The patient, a 49-year-old man, presented to the local hospital in December 2016 for investigation of intermittent hiccups for more than 3 years which had been aggravated for 6 months. Electronic gastroscopy showed chronic erosive gastritis with ulceration and a bulge in the gastric body. Gastroscopic ultrasound showed suspected hypoechoic eminence of muscularis propria in the gastric body. After gastric protection and antacid treatment, the patient's hiccup symptom was improved. In order to clarify the nature of the gastric protuberant lesion, the patient visited the Outpatient Department of the Union Hospital, Tongji Medical College of Huazhong University of Science and Technology. The patient was subsequently admitted to the hospital with a gastric body bulge, suspected to be a GIST.

10.1.2.1 Past History and Family History

The patient had a 3-year history of hypertension, and the highest recorded blood pressure was 180/100 mmHg. He took medicine regularly, and usually had good blood pressure control. The patient was previously healthy, and reported no drug allergies. The parents were deceased, and there was no similar medical history in the family.

10.1.2.2 Physical Examination

The vital signs were stable, and the skin and mucous membranes were not yellowish or pale. The abdomen was flat, and no gastrointestinal or peristaltic waves were seen. The abdomen was normal in shape, and the whole abdomen was soft, with no tenderness, rebound pain, muscle tension, or

K. Tao, H. Cao (eds.), *Clinical Management of Gastrointestinal Stromal Tumor*, https://doi.org/10.1007/978-981-99-9392-5_10

palpable mass in the abdomen. The liver, spleen and ribs were not reached, and the bowel sounds were normal.

10.1.2.3 Auxiliary Examination

Blood Routine No obvious abnormalities.

Blood Biochemistry TBil 23.2 μmol/L ↑, DBil 9.4 μmol/L ↑, TP 49.5 g/L ↓, GLO 12.7 g/L ↓, Na^+ 139 mmol/L, K^+ 3.37 mmol/L ↓, Ca^{2+} 1.97 mmol/L ↓, P 0.83 mmol/L ↓.

Tumor Markers No abnormalities were detected.

Abdominal CT (1) The gastric cavity was generally filled, and a soft tissue density nodule shadow was seen on the greater curvature of the gastric fundus, protruding outside the cavity, with a diameter of approximately 1.5 cm. This was considered to be possible GIST; (2) The size and shape of the liver were normal, and no obvious metastasis was found; (3) No obvious metastasis was found in the remaining abdominal cavity (Fig. 10.1).

Electronic Ultrasonic Gastroscopy There was a flat bulge on the posterior wall of the gastric body with a smooth surface. A class of circular hypoechoic lesions was seen at the lesion in the gastric body, protruding out of the cavity, with clear boundary and homogeneous internal echo. The maximum section was 1.5 cm × 1.6 cm, the mass originated from the deep layer of muscularis propria, no enlarged lymph nodes were found in the surrounding area, and the quality of ultrasonic elastic imaging was hard (Fig. 10.2).

10.1.3 Therapy

10.1.3.1 Case Analysis

The patient was a middle-aged man who was treated for the discovery of a gastric bulge. The preoperative examination was perfect. At the time of consultation and assessment, the bulge was diagnosed as a gastric body GIST. Imaging examination showed that the size of the tumor was approximately 1.5 cm, the boundary was clear, and no obvious metastasis

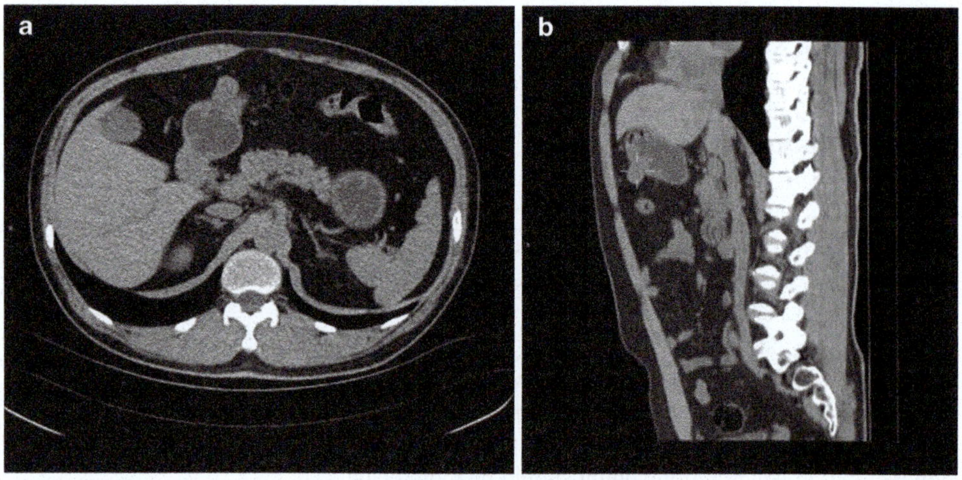

Fig. 10.1 Abdominal CT revealed a soft tissue density nodule shadow. **a** Transverse position. **b** Vector position

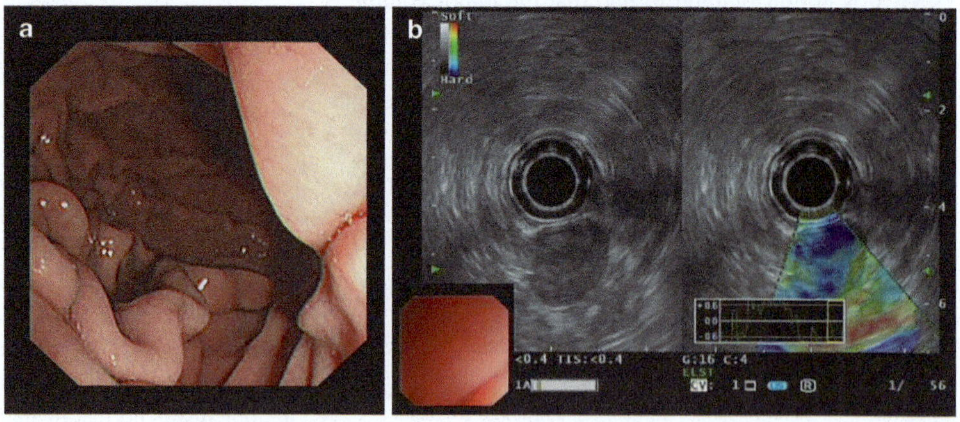

Fig. 10.2 Electronic ultrasonic Gastroscopy revealed a flat bulge on the posterior wall of gastric body with smooth surface. **a** Gastroscope. **b** Ultrasonic endoscope

was found. According to The Consensus of Experts on Standardized Surgical Treatment of Gastrointestinal Stromal Tumors (2015 Edition), because the patient had a localized gastric GIST with a size of less than 2 cm and no adverse factors in imaging examination, regular endoscopic or imaging follow-up and close observation could be conducted. After communicating the treatment plan with the patients and their family, the patient and their family requested surgical treatment.

10.1.3.2 Treatment

In December 2016, the patient underwent combined laparoscopic and gastroscopic local resection of gastric mass. During the operation, gastroscopic positioning was first performed, followed by laparoscopic preparation. A 1 cm diameter protuberant lesion could be seen near the gastric antrum on the rear wall of the gastric body, and there were no obvious abnormalities in the liver and other organs. Local resection of the gastric mass was performed, and the operation process was smooth.

10.1.3.3 Postoperative Pathology and Genetic Testing

Pathological Diagnosis (1) Gastric GIST, 2.0 cm × 1.0 cm in size, mitotic count >10/50 HPF. The modified NIH risk grade was high risk. (2) No tumor involvement was found on the cut edge of the specimen from the gastric body, and no tumor tissue metastasis was found on the sections of lesser curvature lymph nodes (5) and greater curvature lymph nodes (6) (Fig. 10.3).

Immunohistochemistry CD117 (+), CD34 (+), DOG-1 (+), SMA (−), S-100 (−), Ki-67 (Li: >10%), SDHB (+).

Genetic Testing Mutation in exon 9 of *KIT*, the mutation was c.1509_1510 ins GCCTAT. The 11, 13 and 17 exons of *KIT* and the 12 and 18 exons of *PDGFRA* were all wild type.

10.1.4 Prognosis

The patient was discharged 11 days after surgery. Imatinib 400 mg/d targeted therapy was started 27 days after the operation. As of January 2022, the patients had been followed up for 61 months, and there were no obvious adverse reactions or signs of tumor recurrence or metastasis.

10.1.5 Experience of Diagnosis and Therapy

10.1.5.1 Is Surgical Treatment Better for (Gastric) Small GIST?

Surgical resection is the most important and effective treatment for GIST, but not all small gastric GIST are suitable for surgical treatment. At present, there is controversy about the tumor cut-off size for the surgical treatment of gastric GIST. Some scholars support that small gastric GIST (less than 2 cm) do not need to be treated with surgery, but only require regular follow-up. Great results can be also achieved by surgery when the disease is found to be progressing [1]. According to The Chinese Consensus on Endoscopic Diagnosis and Management of Gastrointestinal Submucosal Tumors (Version 2018), gastric GIST less than 2 cm in size, with clinical symptoms, may be considered for surgical treatment, and treatment of asymptomatic suspected GIST should be based on endoscopy and endoscopic ultrasound findings to determine whether there is a risk of progression. The unfavorable factors under endoscopic ultrasound are irregular borders, ulceration, strong internal echoes, and heterogeneity. For patients without adverse factors, endoscopic or imaging follow-up can be performed regularly.

In this case, the patient went to the doctor because of the discovery of a gastric bulge. The possibility of gastric GIST considered to be high, given that the tumor originated in the gastric body and was small in size, and there were no adverse factors found under gastroscopy ultrasound. According to

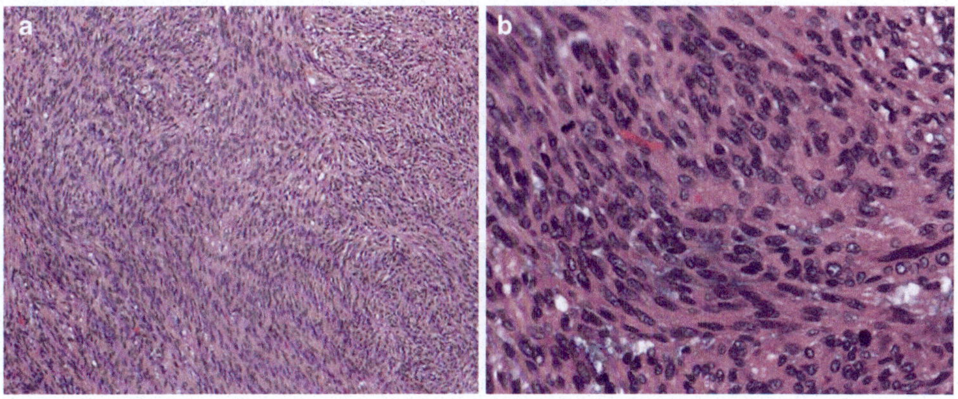

Fig. 10.3 Postoperative pathological H&E staining: **a** 100X, **b** 400X

the guidelines, surgical resection may be temporarily delayed, but regular imaging follow-ups are required. After communicating with the patient and family members, the patient indicated his willingness to undergo surgery. However, postoperative pathology found that the patient's mitotic count was >10/50 HPF, and he was classified as a patient with high risk of recurrence according to the modified NIH risk classification. Therefore, for this patient, surgical treatment had a great benefit. Based on this, it is necessary to refer to various guidelines for small gastric GIST, comprehensively analyze various examination indicators, and carefully decide whether surgical treatment should be performed. How to identify small GIST with different recurrence risks is worthy of our further discussion.

10.1.5.2 Is Endoscopic Resection Suitable for Small GIST?

The choice of surgical methods for GIST has been a hot topic in academic circles. The treatment of GIST using various endoscopic techniques and dual-lens combined techniques has only been proposed in recent years. There is still controversy about how to choose a suitable treatment for patients. Although different centers have reported on the treatment of GIST using endoscopy or endoscopy combined with laparoscopy technology, they all have the problem of small sample size and short follow-up time. Therefore, when formulating a treatment plan, it is necessary to fully consider the size of the tumor, the growth direction of the invasion, and the functional impact after resection. Endoscopic resection and dual-lens combined technology should be performed in an experienced endoscopy center [2, 3].

According to The Chinese Consensus on Endoscopic Diagnosis and Management of Gastrointestinal Submucosal Tumors (Version 2018), GIST located at the distal end of the esophagus can be treated using endoscopic enucleation and transmucosal resection in an experienced unit according to its size, location, and nature. Different surgical methods such as tunnel endoscopic resection and left thoracotomy can be used for tumor resection.

10.1.5.3 Is the Prognosis Better for GIST with a Smaller Gastric Volume?

At present, it is considered that size and mitotic count of the primary tumor are important indices to judge the malignant degree of the tumor and select the surgical method, but no single factor can reliably evaluate the risk of recurrence. Additionally, the existing guidelines cannot accurately predict the prognosis of GIST with a small tumor volume but a high mitotic count. In 2016, the National Comprehensive Cancer Network (NCCN) pointed out that metastasis or tumor-related mortality of GIST with a diameter less than 2 cm is less than 4% even with a high number of mitotic images [4]. Fourteen cases in the metastasis center had small volume and high number of mitotic images. It was found that the prognosis of the cases assessed in a 13-year follow-up study of Union Medical College Affiliated to Tongji Medical College was relatively poor, although there was no recurrence even in high-risk patients. However, a few reports have referred to a relatively poor prognosis, and their recurrence risk is even similar to that of the high-risk group. Therefore, it is important to evaluate the prognosis and therapeutic effect of this kind of GIST.

In 2022, the National Comprehensive Cancer Network (NCCN) pointed out that metastasis or tumor-related mortality of GIST with a diameter less than 2 cm is about 0% even with a high number of mitotic images [4].

10.2 Expert Comments

Yong Li

The NCCN guidelines define GIST with a gastric origin which are less than 2 cm in diameter as "small GIST." This type of GIST as a special category is mainly derived from its unique biological behavior [5]. With the improvement of people's health awareness, as well as the development of imaging and endoscopy technology, the incidence of small GIST has gradually increased in recent years. In view of this, this type of tumor deserves everyone's attention.

In the NCCN guidelines and Chinese guidelines, the treatment recommendations for small GIST are if there are no high-risk features (such as irregular borders, cystic cavity, ulceration, hyperechoic lesions, and heterogeneity) under endoscopic ultrasound, the patient will only require endoscopic ultrasound follow-up every 6–12 months, without surgery. However, there are certain factors in the clinical practice which interfere with this recommendation, including (1) endoscopy is subjective, and the diagnostic accuracy is greatly affected by the operating doctor; (2) the patient's anxiety about the disease seriously affects the quality of life, and the follow-up time, and economic costs and patient compliance can lead to failure to follow up in the manner recommended by the guidelines; (3) With the development of minimally invasive techniques, some surgeons believe that minimally invasive surgery can be used to completely remove the lesions at a relatively low cost. The more important reason is that not all small GIST exhibit benign biological behaviors. The author retrospectively analyzed China Gastrointestinal Stromal Tumor Study Group (Guangdong Provincial People's Hospital, Union Hospital of Tongji Medical College of Huazhong University of Science and Technology, and Tumor Affiliated to Sun Yat-Sen University Hospital, Southern Hospital of Southern Medical University).

A total of 273 patients with small GIST who underwent surgical treatment (endoscopy or surgery) between 1998 and 2015 were assessed based on the modified NIH risk classification diagnostic criteria. In total, seven patients were assessed as intermediate risk (2.5%), and ten patients were assessed as high risk (3.6%).

At present, endoscopic treatment is not recommended for small GIST, but it is undeniable that the technology is minimally invasive, especially when the tumor is located in a special part such as the gastric outlet and the technology can retain the organ function to the greatest extent. Qualified units can use endoscopic treatment for clinical research projects. Laparoscopy is undoubtedly the mainstream treatment option for small GIST. The traditional abdominal German technique for peach-shaped resection can be used for the treatment of small GIST. For GIST near the cardia or in a specific site, the author team carried out laparoscopic transgastric cardia tumor resection and achieved good results. It is recommended that an experienced medical center carry out this technique for tumors at a specific site.

According to the modified NIH risk classification standard, small GIST patients were given corresponding postoperative adjuvant treatment and follow-up.

References

1. Chien CH, Chien RN, Yen CL, et al. The role of endoscopic ultrasonography examination for evaluation and surveillance of gastric subepithelial masses. Chang Gung Med J. 2010;33(1):73–81. http://cgmj.cgu.edu.tw/3301/330109.pdf
2. Nishida T, Goto O, Raut CP, Yahagi N. Diagnostic and treatment strategy for small gastrointestinal stromal tumors. Cancer. 2016;122(20):3110–8. https://doi.org/10.1002/cncr.30239.
3. Shen K, Gao X. Evaluation and endoscopic treatment of small and micro gastrointestinal stromal tumors. Zhonghua Wei Chang Wai Ke Za Zhi. 2015;18(4):328–31. https://doi.org/10.3760/cma.j.issn.1671-0274.2015.04.008.
4. NCCN Clinical Practice Guidelines in Oncology-Gastrointestinal Stromal Tumors (GISTs) (2022 Version I) [DB/OL]. http://www.nccn.org
5. Sepe PS, Brugge WR. A guide for the diagnosis and management of gastrointestinal stromal cell tumors. Nat Rev Gastroenterol Hepatol. 2009;6(6):363–71. https://doi.org/10.1038/nrgastro.2009.43.

11 Mitotic Extremely High Gastrointestinal Stromal Tumors

Pei Zhou, Zhen Xiong, and Kaixiong Tao

Keywords

Gastrointestinal stromal tumor · Prognostic factors
Mitotic · Extremely high

11.1 Case 15 A Gastric GIST with Super High Mitotic Index

Pei Zhou and Zhen Xiong

11.1.1 Introduction

The grading criteria of a GIST directly affect the selection of treatment strategies, and the current GIST grading criteria were mainly developed based on parameters such as tumor size, number of mitotic count, tumor location, and tumor rupture, but these criteria cannot accurately predict the probability of GIST recurrence. At present, the academic community generally recognizes that mitotic count have a high weight, and the existing NIH risk classification cannot provide an individualized prediction of GIST recurrence and prognosis, especially regarding the prognosis of patients with high mitotic count. From this, it can be seen that it is insufficient to grade the risk of GIST by relying solely on the conventional pathological features of the tumor. The ultimate goal of the evaluation criteria is to reveal the biological behavior of GIST and guide clinical treatment. At present, many evaluation criteria cannot reasonably predict the risk of GIST recurrence, thus making clinical treatment difficult, especially for patients with a certain risk of recurrence.

P. Zhou · Z. Xiong (✉) · K. Tao
Department of Gastrointestinal Surgery, Union Hospital, Tongji Medical College, Huazhong University of Science and Technology, Wuhan, China
e-mail: xiongzhen@hust.edu.cn; kaixiongtao@hust.edu.cn

11.1.2 Case Background

A 64-year-old woman visited a local hospital in September 2015 for investigation of black stool with epigastric discomfort for fortnight. Gastroscopy revealed a large ulcer in the gastric body, considered to be possible gastric cancer, and an elevated lesion in the antrum. The patient visited Union Hospital, Tongji Medical College, Huazhong University of Science and Technology, for further diagnosis and treatment and was admitted for investigation of a gastric space-occupying lesion.

11.1.2.1 Past History and Family History

The patient was previously healthy, and reported no drug allergies. The patient's parents were alive, and there was no similar medical history in the family.

11.1.2.2 Physical Examination

The patient's vital signs were stable, she was anemic in appearance, but the skin and sclera were not yellowish in color. The abdomen was flat, and no gastrointestinal or peristaltic waves were seen. The abdomen was soft, with no tenderness or rebound pain. There was a palpable solid mass under the diaphragm, which was soft and exhibited poor mobility. The bowel sounds were normal.

11.1.2.3 Auxiliary Examination

Blood Routine WBC 9.21×10^9/L, RBC 2.82×10^{12}/L ↓, Hb 77 g/L ↓, PLT 495×10^9/L ↑, NEUT% 78.9% ↑, LY% 15.5% ↓.

Blood Biochemistry Various indicators showed no abnormalities.

Tumor Markers No abnormalities detected.

Endoscopic Ultrasound Endoscopic examination showed a large ulcer on the lesser curvature of the gastric body, with

K. Tao, H. Cao (eds.), *Clinical Management of Gastrointestinal Stromal Tumor*, https://doi.org/10.1007/978-981-99-9392-5_11

a dirty, rough surface. Ultrasound scans showed a large hypoechoic mass on the lesser curvature of the gastric body, most of the lesion protruded outside of the cavity. The mass was approximately 8 cm × 8 cm in size, the boundary with the liver was clear, and no significantly enlarged lymph nodes were observed in the abdominal cavity (Fig. 11.1).

Enhanced CT A soft tissue mass of approximately 11.2 cm × 11.4 cm was found in the hepatogastric space, which had multiple lobes and uneven density. The mass was considered to be a possible mesenchymal tumor (Fig. 11.2).

11.1.2.4 Primary Diagnosis

1. Gastric malignancy: possible GIST
2. Gastrointestinal bleeding
3. Moderate anemia

11.1.3 Therapy

11.1.3.1 Case Analysis

The patient was a middle-aged woman who presented with black stools and epigastric discomfort. The current diagnosis was gastric GIST. Imaging examination showed a large tumor located in the lesser curvature of the gastric body. We summarized the characteristic of this case as follows: (1) The patient had severe melena and moderate anemia. (2) The endoscopy showed tumor surface ulceration. (3) The boundary between the tumor tissue and the surrounding tissue was clear, and no significantly enlarged lymph nodes were observed in the abdominal cavity. Considering factors such as the location and size of the tumor, it is considered appropriate to use open surgery. The patient had moderate anemia, with fair general condition, an Eastern Cooperative

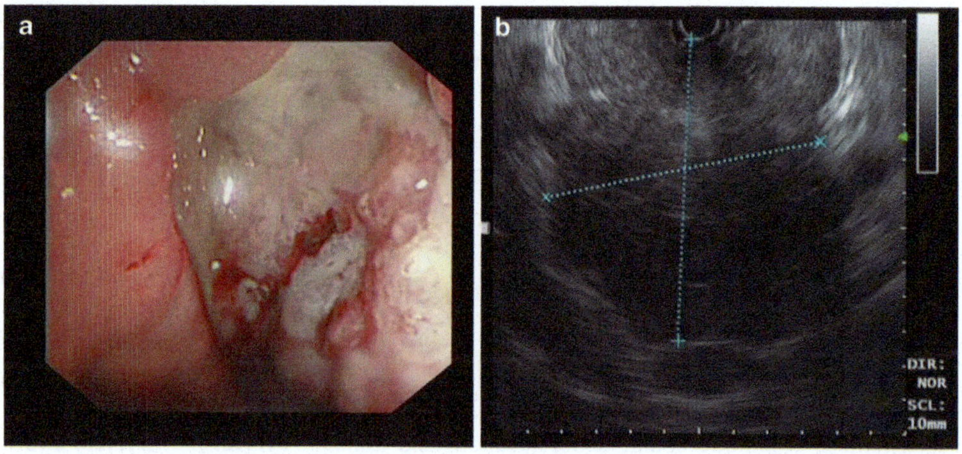

Fig. 11.1 Endoscopic ultrasound revealed a large hypoechoic lesion on the lesser curvature of the gastric body with a section size of approximately 8 × 8 cm. **a** Gastroscope. **b** Ultrasonic endoscope

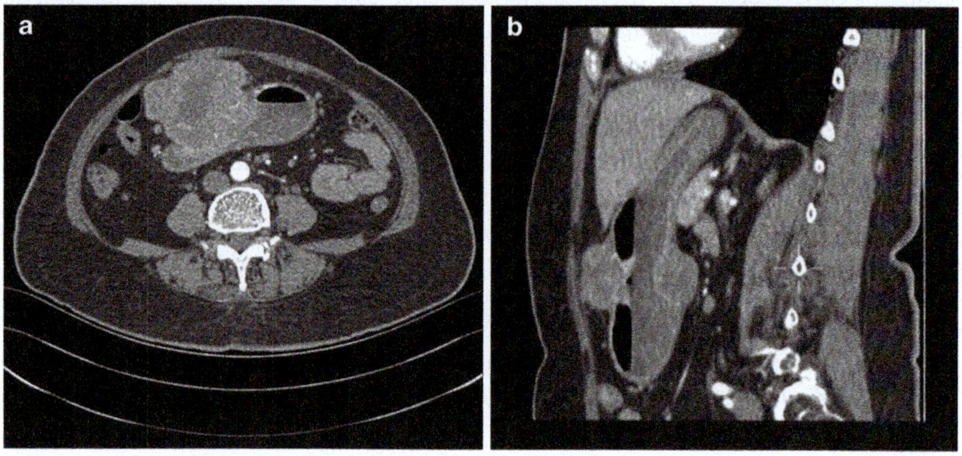

Fig. 11.2 Abdominal CT revealed a large lobulated soft tissue mass in the hepatogastric space. **a** Transverse position. **b** Vector position

Oncology Group (ECOG) score of 2 and NRS (2002) score of 4. Therefore, nutritional support was given, and surgical treatment was performed immediately after correcting anemia.

11.1.3.2 Treatment

Exploratory laparotomy was performed in September 2015, and intraoperative exploration showed a large mass, approximately 13 cm × 12 cm in size, near the pylorus in the greater curvature of the stomach. The mass was irregular in shape and significantly lobulated, without obvious metastases. Distal gastrectomy and regional lymph node dissection were performed, with intraoperative blood loss of approximately 200 mL, and the operation was successful.

11.1.3.3 Postoperative Pathology and Genetic Testing

Pathological Diagnosis (1) Gastric GIST, 13 cm × 9 cm in size, lobulated, with obvious cellular atypia, local hemorrhage and necrosis, mitotic count 85/50 HPF, with a modified NIH risk grade of high risk. (2) No tumor involvement was observed on the resection margin sections of resected gastric body and pylorus tissue, and no tumor tissue metastasis was observed on the sections of lesser curvature lymph nodes and greater curvature lymph nodes (Fig. 11.3).

Immunohistochemistry CD117 (+), CD34 (local +), DOG-1 (+), SMA (−), S-100 (−), Ki-67 (Li: 30%) (Fig. 11.4).

Genetic Testing A mutation in exon 11 of *KIT* was identified, and the mutation type was 17021728del27. Exons 9, 13, and 17 of *KIT* and exons 12 and 18 of *PDGFRA* were wild type.

11.1.4 Prognosis

The patient was discharged from the hospital on postoperative day 13. On the 14th postoperative day, targeted therapy with 400 mg/d imatinib was initiated. As of January 2022, the patient had been followed up for 76 months, and developed edema, leukopenia (grade 2) and other adverse reactions during therapy. The symptoms were relieved without

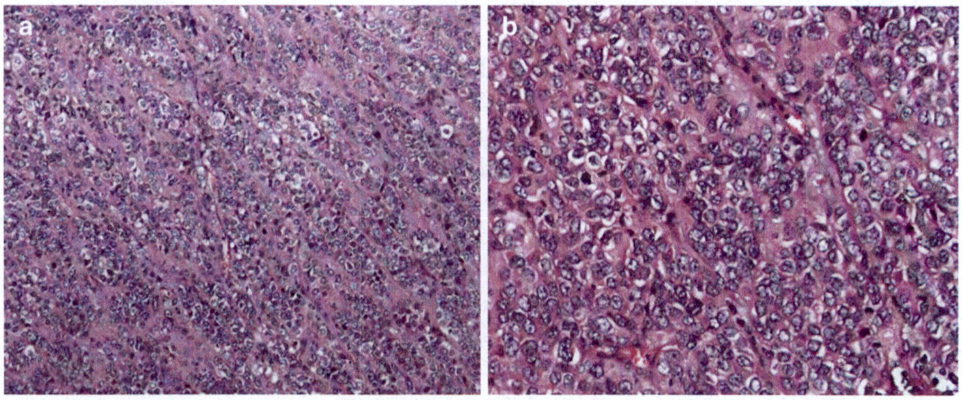

Fig. 11.3 Postoperative pathological H&E staining. **a** HE 100 ×. **b** HE 200 ×

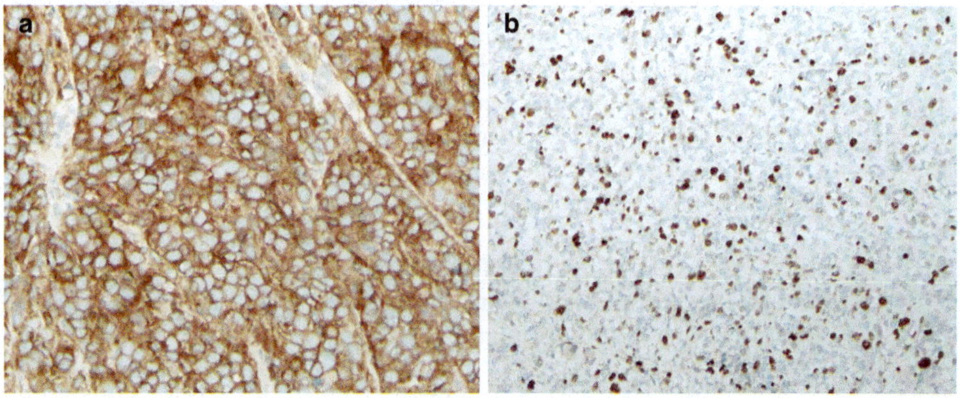

Fig. 11.4 Postoperative pathological immunohistochemistry. **a** CD117 (+) 200 ×. **b** Ki-67 100 ×

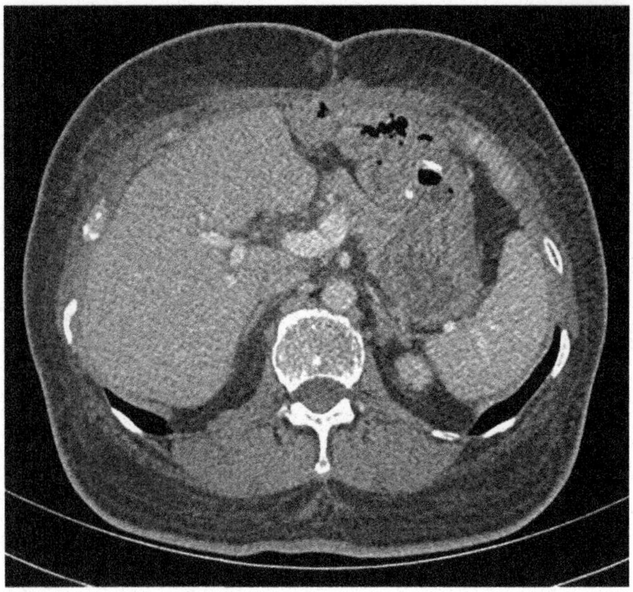

Fig. 11.5 76 months after surgery

special treatment. Reexamination of enhanced CT of the whole abdomen showed no obvious signs of tumor recurrence or metastasis (Fig. 11.5).

11.1.5 Experience of Diagnosis and Therapy

11.1.5.1 Understanding of "Extremely High Risk" Gastrointestinal Stromal Tumors

More and more clinicians are aware that the existing GIST risk grading criteria are flawed and do not guide the clinical implementation of individualized treatment well. Some scholars conducted subgroup analyses for high risk GIST according to mitotic count and found that GIST with high levels of mitotic count had poor prognosis. These findings further expose the shortcomings of the existing grading criteria which are unable to provide individualized guidance for patients.

In recent years, based on the results of previous clinical studies and grading criteria, scholars have defined a class of patients with extremely high risk of GIST recurrence, called extremely high GIST, characterized by high malignancy and a tendency to lead to recurrence or metastasis, and such GIST patients should attract the attention of clinicians [1].

11.1.5.2 How to Select the Course of Treatment for Patients with High Mitotic Count Treated with Imatinib Adjuvant Therapy?

The use of imatinib in the adjuvant treatment of GIST significantly prolongs the postoperative recurrence-free survival of GIST patients. However, 3 years of adjuvant therapy does not guarantee a long-term survival benefit for patients with GIST, and some patients still relapse within 2 years after adjuvant therapy discontinuation [2]. Long-term use of imatinib is currently considered effective in preventing relapse during treatment in patients with sensitive mutations, and randomized controlled trials of imatinib adjuvant therapy at 3 versus 5 years are undergoing. The duration of adjuvant therapy tends to be prolonged. For patients with a high risk of recurrence, the appropriate adjuvant therapy time needs to be based on various characteristics and should pay attention to genotyping to implement an individualized plan.

So far, there is no consensus on the course of adjuvant therapy after GIST surgery, and the optimal course of adjuvant therapy is still being explored. Taking into account the malignant characteristics and genetic subtypes of tumors and implementing more accurate individualized treatment should be the focus of future research.

11.2 Expert Comments

Kaixiong Tao

Tumor size, location, mitotic count, and whether the tumor ruptures are important factors affecting the prognosis of GIST. At present, the common criteria used to determine the risk of postoperative recurrence of GIST include the modified NIH risk classification of recurrence, AFIP criteria, and Joensuu high Hotline Dengjun [3–5]. The modified NIH risk classification of recurrence is the most widely used criteria.

In recent years, with the deepening of the understanding of the condition, GIST has gradually become the focus of attention. In 2015, Maki et al. [6] proposed that the characteristics of extremely high-risk GIST should include at least one of the following criteria: (1) tumor diameter > 10 cm, (2) mitotic bodies >10/50 HPF, (3) tumor diameter > 5 cm and mitotic count >5/50 HPF, (4) tumor rupture during surgery. However, such criteria are not comprehensive, do not include patients with genetic mutations, nor do they include patients with extremely high mitotic count, and their predictive ability is limited. Therefore, it is an urgent problem to establish a more accurate GIST prediction model containing items such as gene mutation type, mitotic count, size, and location.

References

1. Shen C, Zhang B. Preliminary understanding of gastrointestinal stromal tumor with the highest risk. Zhonghua Wei Chang Wai Ke Za Zhi. 2016;19(11):1226–9. https://doi.org/10.3760/cma.j.issn.1671-0274.2016.11.006.

2. Joensuu H, Eriksson M, Sundby Hall K, Hartmann JT, Pink D, Schütte J, Ramadori G, Hohenberger P, Duyster J, Al-Batran SE, Schlemmer M, Bauer S, Wardelmann E, Sarlomo-Rikala M, Nilsson B, Sihto H, Monge OR, Bono P, Kallio R, Vehtari A, Leinonen M, Alvegård T, Reichardt P. One vs three years of adjuvant imatinib for operable gastrointestinal stromal tumor: a randomized trial. JAMA. 2012;307(12):1265–72. https://doi.org/10.1001/jama.2012.347.
3. Joensuu H. Risk stratification of patients diagnosed with gastrointestinal stromal tumor. Hum Pathol. 2008;39(10):1411–9. https://doi.org/10.1016/j.humpath.2008.06.025.
4. Miettinen M, Sobin LH, Lasota J. Gastrointestinal stromal tumors of the stomach: a clinicopathologic, immunohistochemical, and molecular genetic study of 1765 cases with long-term follow-up. Am J Surg Pathol. 2005;29(1):52–68. https://doi.org/10.1097/01.pas.0000146010.92933.de.
5. Joensuu H, Vehtari A, Riihimäki J, Nishida T, Steigen SE, Brabec P, Plank L, Nilsson B, Cirilli C, Braconi C, Bordoni A, Magnusson MK, Linke Z, Sufliarsky J, Federico M, Jonasson JG, Dei Tos AP, Rutkowski P. Risk of recurrence of gastrointestinal stromal tumour after surgery: an analysis of pooled population-based cohorts. Lancet Oncol. 2012;13(3):265–74. https://doi.org/10.1016/S1470-2045(11)70299-6.
6. Maki RG, Blay JY, Demetri GD, Fletcher JA, Joensuu H, Martín-Broto J, Nishida T, Reichardt P, Schöffski P, Trent JC. Key issues in the clinical management of gastrointestinal stromal tumors: an expert discussion. Oncologist. 2015;20(7):823–30. https://doi.org/10.1634/theoncologist.2014-0471.

Neurofibromatosis Type 1 Associated Gastrointestinal Stromal Tumors

12

Yao Lin, Xiangyu Zeng, Chengguo Li, Zhidong Gao, and Jian Li

Keywords

Gastrointestinal stromal tumor · Neurofibromatosis type 1 Wild type · Primary · Genetic testing

12.1 Case 16 A 60-Year-Old Woman with NF1-Related GIST

Yao Lin and Xiangyu Zeng

12.1.1 Introduction

Neurofibromatosis type 1 (NF1), or *von Recklinghausen disease*, is an autosomal dominant genetic disease. Patients with NF1 are prone to develop various types of tumors, including GIST [1]. For patients with NF1, GIST mainly occur in the duodenum and jejunum. Multiple primary tumors and wild-type *KIT* and *PDGFRA* are the most significant features [2].

12.1.2 Case Background

A patient, a 60-year-old woman, was admitted to Union Hospital of Tongji Medical College of Huazhong University of Science and Technology in December 2018 for investigation of abdominal masses and pain in right abdomen. The patient felt a mass in her abdomen 4 months previously but this was not taken seriously. Approximately 10 days ago, the patient suffered pain in the right abdomen without obvious cause, accompanied by difficulty in defecation, and no discomfort such as nausea, vomiting, or diarrhea. The patient went to a secondary hospital and underwent a CT scan of the abdomen. The results showed the retroperitoneal mass with a maximum cross-sectional diameter of approximately 60 mm. The patient came to our hospital for further treatment and was admitted with retroperitoneal space-occupying lesions.

12.1.2.1 Past History and Family History

The patient had a 7-year history of hypertension, the highest blood pressure was 200/150 mmHg, and the condition was well controlled with medication. The patient reported no history of food or drug allergies, and there was no similar medical history in the family.

12.1.2.2 Physical Examination

The body surface was scattered with multiple tumor-like lesions, the largest one was approximately 1.5 cm in diameter, and there were obvious café-au-lait spots on the outer thighs on both sides (Fig. 12.1). A mass was palpated on the right upper abdomen, the boundary was unclear, and the mobility is poor. The patient reported mild abdominal tenderness but no obvious rebound pain.

12.1.2.3 Auxiliary Examination

Blood Routine, Blood Biochemical Examination, Related Tumor Markers Demonstrated no obvious abnormalities.

Enhanced CT Scan of the Abdomen and Pelvis A large mass of approximately 5.4 cm × 5.5 cm × 6.7 cm was seen next to the right lower abdominal aorta with a shadow of slight low density. Stratification with obvious enhancement could be seen in the lesion. The mass was considered to be a duodenal submucosa Tumor: possibly a GIST with cystic change or neurogenic tumor (Fig. 12.2).

Y. Lin · X. Zeng (✉) · C. Li
Department of Gastrointestinal Surgery, Union Hospital, Tongji Medical College, Huazhong University of Science and Technology, Wuhan, China
e-mail: xiangyuzeng@hust.edu.cn; lichengguo@hust.edu.cn

Z. Gao (✉)
Department of Gastrointestinal Surgery, Peking University People's Hospital, Beijing, China
e-mail: gaozhidong@pkuph.edu.cn

J. Li
Department of Gastrointestinal Oncology, Peking University Cancer Hospital & Institute, Beijing, China

K. Tao, H. Cao (eds.), *Clinical Management of Gastrointestinal Stromal Tumor*, https://doi.org/10.1007/978-981-99-9392-5_12

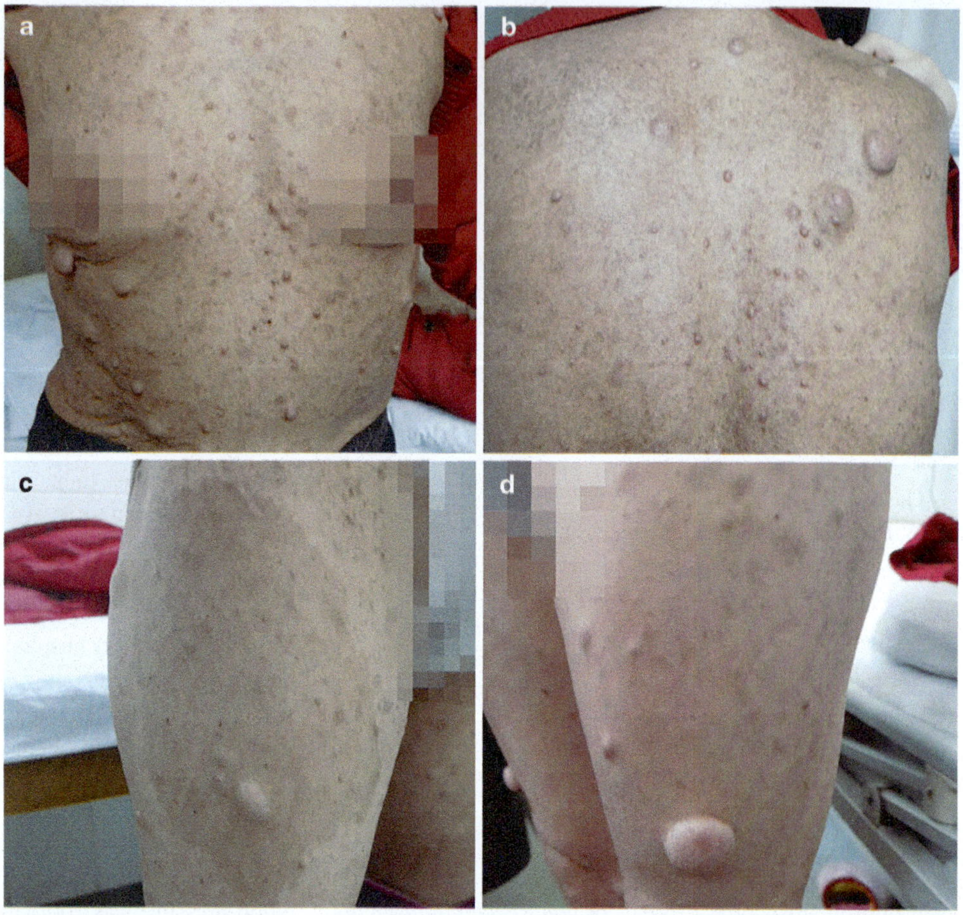

Fig. 12.1 Dermatoma-like lesions and café-au-lait spots: **a** Forebreast and abdomen; **b** Backside; **c** Right thigh; **d** Left thigh

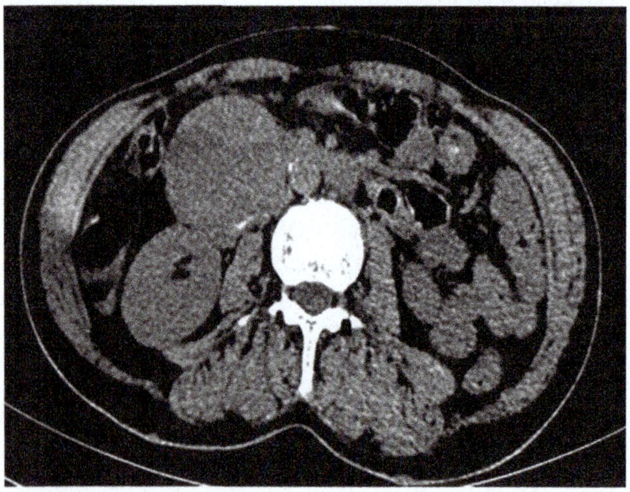

Fig. 12.2 CT of the abdomen

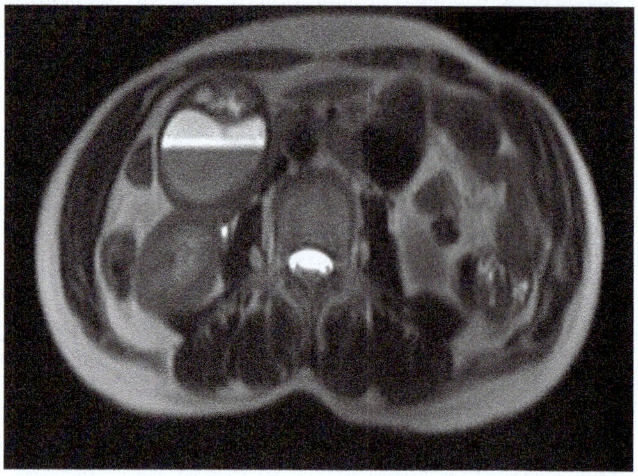

Fig. 12.3 Enhanced MRI of the abdomen

Enhanced MRI Scan of the Abdomen A huge mass of approximately 5.3 cm × 4.9 cm × 7.0 cm was seen next to the right lower abdominal aorta, with iso-intensity on T1WI and stratified signals on T2WI. Inside the mass were shadow nodules with low and short T1 and short T2 signals. The enhancement was not obvious. There was no obvious diffusion limitation on DWI. The tumor was closely related to the duodenum, and the possibility of GIST was considered (Fig. 12.3).

Biopsy of the Abdominal Mass Biopsy the abdomen mass was conducted twice with ultrasound endoscopic puncture and the results were negative. The samples obtained were mainly blood clot when viewed under the microscope.

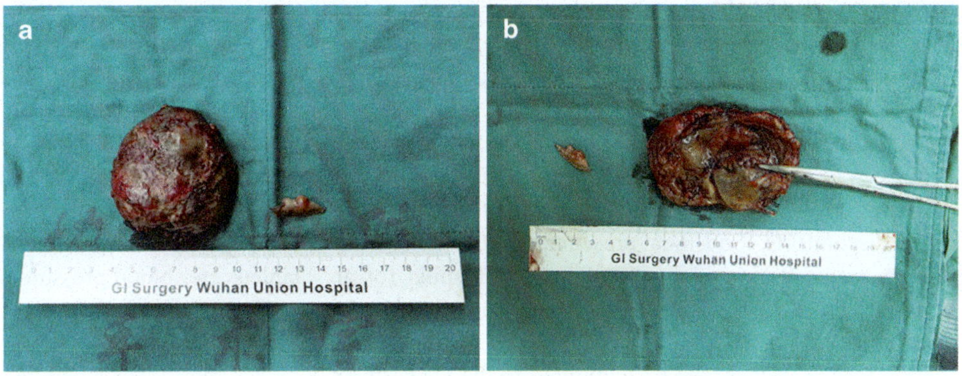

Fig. 12.4 The gross specimen

Biopsy of the Dermatoma-Like Lesions Resection of two tumors on the chest wall and abdominal wall for pathological examination showed that they were neurofibromatosis.

12.1.2.4 Preliminary Diagnosis

1. NF1
2. Duodenal space-occupying lesions, possibly NF1-related GIST
3. Hypertension

12.1.3 Therapy

12.1.3.1 Case Analysis

The patient was an elderly woman with café-au-lait spots and dermatoma-like lesions scattered all over the body, which a biopsy revealed were neurofibromas. Taking the patient's clinical manifestations, imaging examinations, and pathological results into account, it was possible that the patient had NF1-related GIST. However, due to the cystic change of the abdominal mass, the results of the two needle biopsies for the abdomen mass were negative. The patient was generally in good condition and no obvious surgical contraindications were present. It was determined that surgical resection should be performed as soon as possible to remove the abdominal mass, and postoperative adjuvant treatment should be guided according to the postoperative pathological results.

12.1.3.2 Treatment

The patient underwent laparoscopic abdominal exploration in January 2019. A tumor, approximately 8.0 cm × 8.0 cm in size, was seen at the junction of the horizontal part of the descending duodenum, and another tumor approximately 0.5 cm × 0.4 cm was seen protruding from the serosal surface in the middle of jejunum. Laparoscopic duodenal tumor resection and small bowel tumor resection were performed. The operation underwent smoothly.

12.1.3.3 Postoperative Pathology and Genetic Testing

Pathological Diagnosis Figure 12.4

Duodenal GIST, 7 cm × 6 cm × 5 cm in size, with hemorrhagic cystic degeneration, mitotic count >10/50 HPF, and the modified NIH risk classification was high risk.

Jejunum GIST, approximately 0.5 cm in diameter, with mitotic count <5/50 HPF, and the modified NIH risk classification was very low risk.

Genetic Testing *KIT* and *PDGFRA* wild type; *NF1* had somatic and germline mutations (p.C167Qfs*10).

12.1.4 Prognosis

The patient was discharged from hospital 7 days after the operation. The patient did not receive targeted therapy after surgery and was followed up regularly. The last follow-up was conducted on January 2022, there were no signs of recurrence.

12.2 Case 17 A 69-Year-Old Woman with NF1-Related GIST

Chengguo Li and Zhidong Gao

12.2.1 Case Background

The patient, a 69-year-old woman, was admitted to the hospital for examination and treatment of intermittent melena for 2 years and a space-occupying lesion in the fundus of the stomach and descending duodenum identified 1 week earlier in November 2016. Two years previously, the patient had experienced intermittent melena without any obvious cause.

She went to the local hospital and her condition improved after fasting and rehydration therapy. After being discharged from the hospital, she took Yunnan Baiyao regularly and did not have melena while taking the medication. Ten days ago, the patient experienced melena again with no obvious cause and she was accompanied by fatigue, without palpitations, sweating, nausea, vomiting, abdominal pain, diarrhea, or other discomforts. She then presented to the emergency department of Peking University People's Hospital for an urgent check of fecal occult blood (+), hemoglobin 96 g/L, and there were no abnormalities in platelets and blood coagulation factors. Hence, she was admitted to the Department of Gastroenterology for investigation of gastrointestinal bleeding. A CT scan of the abdomen showed the following: (1) Multiple cysts in the liver; (2) space-occupying lesions on the posterior wall of the stomach fundus, and the descending duodenum, the lesions were considered to be GIST. Gastroscopy and endoscopic ultrasonography revealed a duodenal mass with ulcer formation, chronic superficial gastritis, and gastric bulge consistent with GIST or leiomyoma (Fig. 12.5). For further diagnosis and treatment, the patient was transferred to the Department of Gastrointestinal Surgery for continued treatment of gastric and duodenal space-occupying lesions (GIST?).

The patient reported losing about 10 kg in weight in the previous 6 months.

12.2.1.1 Past History and Family History

The patient had a 23-year history of hypertension, and had long-term oral administration of nifedipine sustained-release tablets. Her blood pressure was well controlled.

Twenty-three years ago, the patient underwent a left nephrectomy in other hospital, and the postoperative pathological report was a benign tumor of unknown origin. There was no history of other chronic diseases such as diabetes or coronary heart disease, and no history of drug allergies. There was no family history of gastrointestinal tumors, but the patient's mother had *von Recklinghausen's disease*.

12.2.1.2 Physical Examination

There are scattered café-au-lait spots and neurofibromas on the skin all over the body (Fig. 12.6). The sclera and skin and mucous membranes were not yellowish or pale, and the lymph nodes throughout the body were not swollen. The

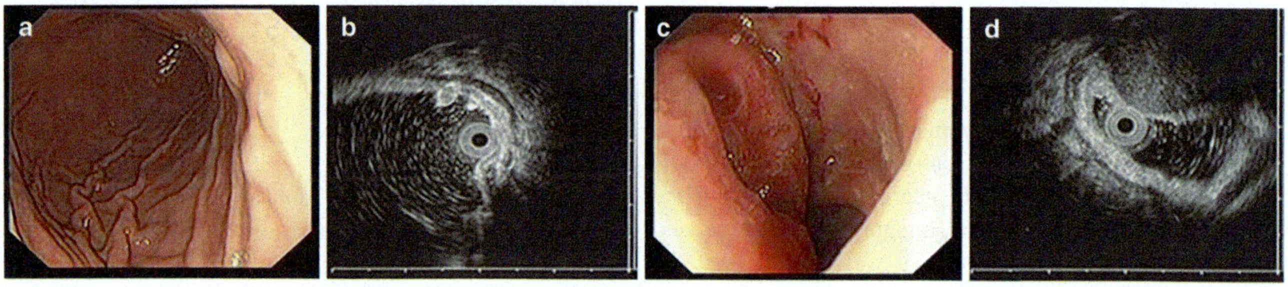

Fig. 12.5 Ultrasound gastroscope. **a**, **b** The gastric body has hypoechoic uplift, the size is approximately 0.6 cm × 0.3 cm; **c**, **d**: Hypoechoic bulge at junction of duodenal bulb and descending segment, approximately 2.0 cm × 2.5 cm in size

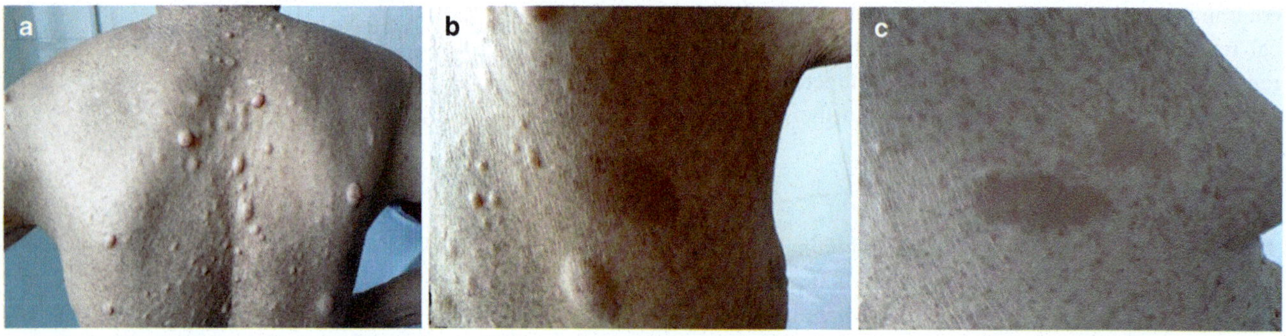

Fig. 12.6 Skin lesions. **a** Multiple neurofibromas were present on the surface of the skin; **b**, **c** café-au-lait spots were scattered in the armpits and all over the body

abdomen was flat, and no gastrointestinal or peristaltic waves were seen. The abdomen was soft with no tenderness, rebound tenderness, or muscle tension. No abdominal masses were palpated, the liver and spleen were not palpable below the costal margin, shifting dullness was negative, and bowel sounds were normal.

12.2.1.3 Auxiliary Examination

Blood Routine WBC 8.61 × 10^9/L, NEUT% 62.2%, LY% 25.8%, RBC 3.08 × 10^{12}/L ↓, Hb 83 g/L ↓, HCT 26.0% ↓, PLT 346 × 10^9/L.

Blood Biochemistry ALB 38.8 g/L ↓, fasting blood glucose 7.31 mmol/L ↑.

Tumor Markers No abnormalities.

Enhanced CT Scan of the Whole Abdomen (1) On the greater curvature of the stomach, a round isodense nodule protruded out of the cavity. The nodule was approximately 1.8 cm × 1.8 cm in size, with clear borders, and obvious enhancement. In the descending segment of the duodenum, a mass of soft tissue density shadow protruding out of the cavity, approximately 3.9 cm × 3.4 cm in size, with clear borders, nodular calcifications in the interior, and obvious uneven enhancement on enhanced scan was seen. The imaging diagnosis was occupation of the gastric fundus and duodenum, GIST should be considered. (2) There were multiple round low-density lesions in the liver, the largest one was located in S2, and this was approximately 2.5 cm × 2.4 cm in size. There was no obvious abnormal enhancement on the enhanced scan, and the imaging diagnosis was multiple hepatic cysts. (3) The left kidney was not shown. (4) There were multiple subcutaneous soft tissue nodules in the chest and abdomen within the scan range, the largest one was located under the chest wall on the right dorsal side at the level of the flat 11 thoracic vertebrae, with clear boundaries, approximately 2.1 × 1.5 cm in size, with uniform internal density, and enhancements on the relevant (Fig. 12.7).

12.2.1.4 Preliminary Diagnosis

1. Stomach and duodenal masses, possible GIST
2. Gastrointestinal bleeding
3. NF1
4. Liver cyst
5. Mild anemia
6. Hypertension
7. Previous left nephrectomy

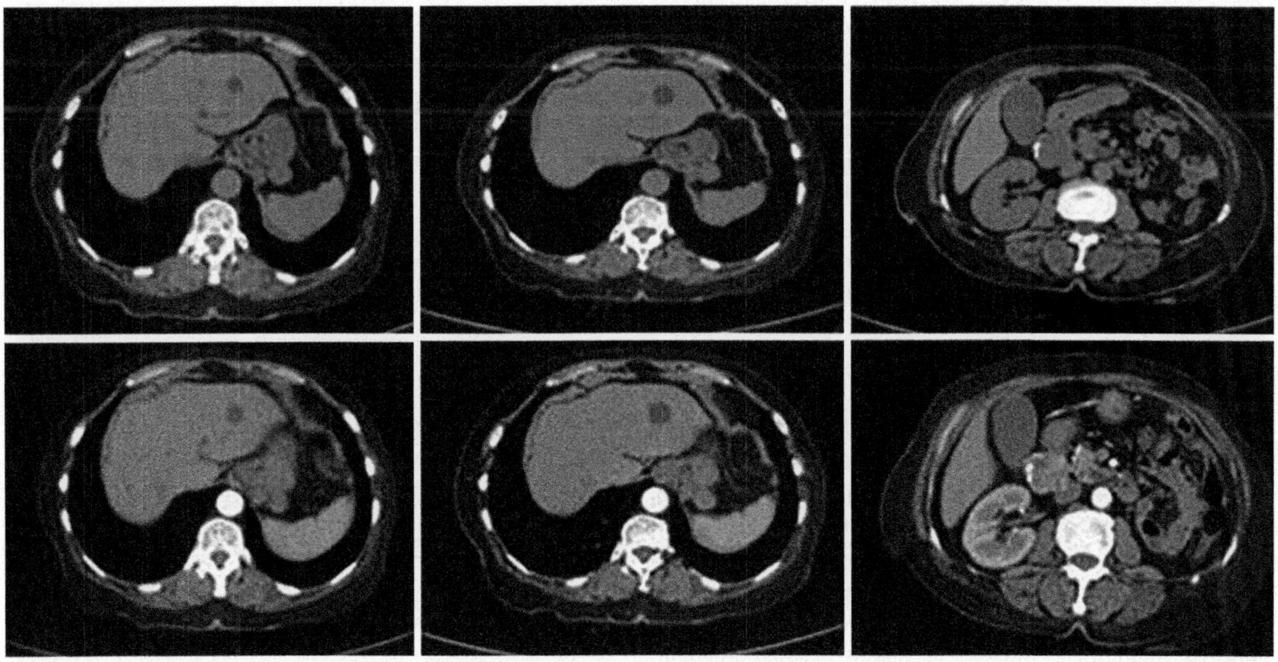

Fig. 12.7 CT of the abdomen revealed gastric and duodenal masses

12.2.2 Therapy

12.2.2.1 Case Analysis

The patient was an elderly woman who presented with gastrointestinal bleeding. After admission, combined with medical history, clinical manifestations, and auxiliary examination results, the clinical diagnosis was gastric and duodenal masses with high possibility of GIST. Abdominal enhanced CT showed no obvious peritoneal or liver metastases. There was no adhesion or infiltration of the surrounding important organs, nerves, or blood vessels. The preoperative evaluation was of a resectable mass. The patient was generally healthy, with good functions of important vital organs such as the heart, lung, liver, and kidney, and routine laboratory examinations demonstrated no obvious contraindications for surgery. It was determined that surgical treatment should be performed, and further postoperative treatment should be guided by postoperative pathological examination and molecular test results.

12.2.2.2 Treatment

An exploratory laparotomy was performed on November 30, 2016. The intraoperative findings were a small amount of light-yellow ascites in the abdominal cavity and mild adhesions, which were loosened. The liver size was normal, and multiple cyst-like changes were seen on the liver surface without metastatic nodules. The size of duct was not thick, the head of the pancreas was small and soft, and the spleen was normal in size. A subserosal mass was observed on the greater curvature of the gastric antrum, with a size of approximately 1.4 cm and a clear boundary. Additionally, a subserosal mass with a size of approximately 3 cm × 2.5 cm protruded from the posterior wall of the descending part of the duodenum, showing exogenous growth which was fragile with abundant blood supply, and the bile duct and pancreatic head were not involved. Twelve small nodules ranging in size from 0.2 to 1.4 cm were seen, positioned from 5 cm away from the hepatoduodenal ligament to about 80 cm of the small intestine. The boundary was still clear and the quality was tough. The largest nodule was located in the small intestine about 80 cm away from the ligament of flexion. There were no obviously swollen lymph nodes.

No mass or nodule was reached in the mesentery, omentum, colon, or pouch of Douglas. The intraoperative diagnosis was a gastric and duodenal mass, possible GIST, and multiple small bowel masses. A partial gastrectomy with partial duodenal resection and partial small bowel resection was performed. Considering that the duodenal mass was large and local suture after resection may have led to luminal stenosis, distal gastrectomy and gastrojejunostomy (Billroth II) were also performed. The operation process went smoothly, and the intraoperative bleeding was approximately 100 mL.

Surgical Specimens The gastric submucosal mass was located on the greater curvature of the gastric antrum, with a diameter of approximately 1.4 cm, clear borders and no mucosal involvement. The duodenal mass was located in the descending portion, with a diameter of approximately 3 cm, involving the mucosa, showing the "umbilical depression" sign and with surface bleeding. The small intestine masses were located 5–80 cm from the ligament of flexion. The mucosa was not involved. The largest nodule was approximately 1.4 cm in diameter and had a clear boundary.

12.2.2.3 Postoperative Pathology and Genetic Testing

Postoperative Pathology (1) Stomach, duodenum and jejunum GIST: stomach tumor, 1.8 cm × 1.8 cm × 1.4 cm, mitotic count 5/50 HPF; duodenal tumor, 3.5 cm × 3.3 cm × 2.9 cm in size, mitotic count 10/50 HPF; jejunal tumor, between 0.2 and 0.6 cm in size, mitotic count <5/50 HPF. (2) No tumor metastases were found in the mesenteric lymph nodes (0/1).

Immunohistochemistry Stomach: CD117 (+), DOG-1 (+), CD34 (+), desmin (−), S-100 (−), SOX10 (−), Ki-67 (Li: 5%+); Duodenum: CD117 (+), DOG-1 (focal +), CD34 (−), desmin (−), SMA (−), S-100 (−), SOX10 (−), p53 (−), Ki-67 (Li: 20%+); Jejunum: CD117 (+), DOG-1 (+), CD34 (−), desmin (−), S-100 (−), SOX10 (−), Ki-67 (Li: 2% +).

Genetic Testing Gastric tumors had detected *KIT* exon 11 mutations, the mutation type was c.1676 T > G The other tumors had no detected any *KIT* (including exons 9, 11, 13 and 17) or *PDGFRA* (Including exons 12 and 18) mutations.

12.2.3 Prognosis

The patient recovered and was discharged 12 days after surgery. Imatinib targeted therapy was not performed after the operation due to family financial conditions. As of October 2018, regular follow-up for 22 months, the patient's postoperative condition was stable, and no obvious signs of tumor recurrence or metastasis were found.

12.2.4 Experience of Diagnosis and Therapy

12.2.4.1 Incidence of NF1-Related GIST

Neurofibromatosis type 1, also known as von Recklinghausen disease, is a common autosomal dominant genetic disease, with an incidence of about 1/3000 in the general population [3]. Its main clinical manifestation are café-au-lait spots on the skin, multiple neurofibromas, and associated damage to the abdominal and pelvic viscera [3]. The incidence of sporadic GIST in the general population is 1–2/100,000, but in NF1 patients, the incidence of GIST increases significantly. According to the epidemiological survey of the Swedish National Cancer Registry, the probability of GIST in patients with NF1 can be as high as 7% [4]. Japanese scholars performed a CT scan of the whole abdomen of 95 NF1 patients with no clinical symptoms related to GIST and found six cases of GIST [2]. The incidence rate also supports the above data. Some researchers pointed out that NF1-related GIST often lack specific clinical manifestations due to their small size. This leads to the possibility of missed diagnoses, and nearly 50% of NF1-related GIST are discovered accidentally [5]. Therefore, in NF1 patients, the true incidence of GIST is may be higher than the above ratio, even up to 200 times that of sporadic GIST [2].

12.2.4.2 Pathogenesis of NF1-Related GIST

Most of GIST are caused by mutations in the exons of *KIT* or *PDGFRA*. However, most studies have pointed out that NF1-related GIST usually lacks mutations in *KIT* and *PDGFRA*, meaning these are wild-type GIST in the traditional sense, composing 1–2% of all GIST patients [6]. Neurofibromatosis type 1 is caused by a mutation in the *NF1* gene located on chromosome 17 (17q11.2), resulting in the loss of the expression of neurofibromin. Neurofibromin is a negative regulatory protein of Ras kinase. The loss of neurofibromin activates the activity of the proto-oncogene Ras, thereby promoting cell proliferation [7]. The potential molecular mechanism of GIST induced by *NF1* mutation has not yet been fully elucidated. Studies have pointed out that Ras activation caused by *NF1* gene mutation can further activate its downstream MEK-MAPK pathway, and then leads to the up-regulation in the expression of ETV1 [1]. ETV1 is an important regulatory factor in the GIST formation pathway, which can affect DNA transcription and *KIT* protein expression, and ultimately lead to the proliferation of Cajal cells.

12.2.4.3 Differential Diagnosis of NF1-Related GIST

Compared to sporadic GIST, multiple GIST is clinically rare, but it can still be roughly divided into three categories: sporadic multiple GIST, familial multiple GIST, and NF1-related GIST. Therefore, when multiple GIST are encountered in the clinic, differential diagnosis of these three conditions is required. Sporadic multiple GIST are caused by somatic mutations, which are mostly confined to one organ such as the stomach or small intestine. Familial multiple GIST are caused by genetic mutations in *KIT*. The tumors are often diffusely distributed throughout the digestive tract, and extensive proliferation of ICC cells can be seen. When NF1-related GIST is combined with skin café-au-lait spots and other manifestations outside of the digestive tract, tumors are often large and mostly confined to the jejunum. A large number of skeletal muscle fibers and amounts of ICC cell proliferation can be seen under the microscope [5].

12.2.4.4 Surgical Treatment Strategies for NF1-Related GIST

A major clinical feature of NF1-related GIST is that most cases show indolent growth, which is manifested by low mitotic count in GIST. A single-center retrospective study from Germany showed that the median survival time for patients with NF1-related GIST who undergo R0-R1 resection can reach 48 months [8]. Therefore, for NF1-related GIST, the best treatment plan is surgical resection. Another clinical feature of NF1-related GIST is that it may be accompanied by colon cancer, rectal cancer, and other gastrointestinal malignancies [2]. Therefore, gastroscopy, colonoscopy, and full-abdominal enhanced CT examination should be performed before surgery to fully evaluate the intra-abdominal lesions, so as not to miss any other malignant tumors in the gastrointestinal tract. It is necessary to fully explore the abdominal cavity intraoperatively, based on the preoperative imaging data, and ensure complete removal of the tumors. The prevalent sites such as duodenum and proximal jejunum need to be carefully explored to avoid missing small lesions that are not visible on imaging, which may lead to early tumor recurrence.

12.2.4.5 The Efficacy of Targeted Drugs for NF1-Related GIST

Different authors have different conclusions on whether targeted drug therapy for recurrent and metastatic NF1-related GIST is effective. Most scholars believe that since NF1-related GIST lacks *KIT* and *PDGFRA* mutations, this group of patients is not sensitive to the first-line targeted drug imatinib [9]. Of course, there are also some case reports that hold the opposite view. So far, a few studies have reported that point mutations in the *KIT* exon 11 have been detected in patients with NF1-related GIST [8]. For these patients, targeted therapy should be able to achieve clinical efficacy. Lee et al. reported that the case of a 65-year-old NF1 patient who suffered from small intestinal GIST with liver and peritoneal metastasis [10]. The postoperative treatment included 400 mg/d imatinib, which achieved a partial response and lasted for nearly 2 years. Therefore, there is no clear conclusion about targeted drug treatment for NF1-related GIST, and more basic research and clinical trials are still needed to explore this topic.

12.2.4.6 Wild-Type Duodenal GIST Can Also Be Aggressive

It has been reported that NF1-related GIST usually has an insidious onset, no obvious clinical symptoms, and the risk of recurrence is generally low [6]. In this case, the patient was treated for gastrointestinal bleeding. Although GIST was wild type, the pathology suggested high risk and invasive characteristics. This is similar to most of the previously reported wild-type GIST with hidden clinical manifestations. The manifestation of high-risk wild-type GIST in the duodenum suggests that in NF1-related GIST, even wild-type GIST can show aggressive clinical features. We suspect that the duodenal lesion in this case occurred earlier than the other lesions, and that the wild-type GIST in other areas may have been metastases of the duodenal GIST.

12.3 Expert Comments

Jian Li

NF1-related GIST is a rare subgroup of GIST. The two cases mentioned in this chapter are very valuable, demonstrating typical small bowel multiple GIST with neurofibromatosis. At the same time, genetic testing revealed no mutations in *KIT*, and also includes the rarer suspected NF1-related GIST combined mutation of *KIT*. Consequently, this chapter summarizes the clinicopathological characteristics of NF1, which will not be repeated here.

Since this subgroup of GIST is very rare, most clinicians do not encounter this type of disease, and it is easy to ignore its existence. Therefore, when clinically diagnosing and treating patients, the author has several suggestions: (1) Clinicians should consider the possibility of NF1 for patients with multiple stromal tumors of the small intestine; (2) Non-GIST patients who exhibit typical multiple subcutaneous nodules need to consider the possibility of neurofibromas. A routine CT scan of the abdominal and pelvic cavity, and regular physical examinations are recommended in such cases; (3) If possible, it is recommended to ask each patient about the family history of neurofibromas and the status of café-au-lait spots.

Most NF1-related GISTs are indolent. The several cases of NF1-related GIST have underwent radical surgery and no recurrence was seen. However, the absence of recurrence of GIST does not mean absolute safety, because most *NF1* gene mutations are germline mutations. Therefore, this group of patients may develop a second GIST or other gastrointestinal tumors a few years after surgery, and the lifetime follow-up of NF1-related GIST patients should be conducted.

In the absence of *KIT* or *PDGFRA* mutations, tyrosine kinase inhibitors (TKIs) might be not effective for NF1-related GIST. If it is confirmed that there are no *KIT/PDGFRA* mutations, postoperative imatinib is often not recommended. Once recurrence occurs and the opportunity for radical surgery is lost, anti-angiogenic drugs such as sunitinib or regorafenib can be administered to try to control tumor development [10]. For patients with slower development and lack of effective drug treatment, sometimes cytoreductive surgery has a certain effect in delaying the development of tumors. It is recommended that individualized choices should be made on the basis of multidisciplinary discussion for the treatment of this type of GIST.

References

1. Brems H, Beert E, de Ravel T, Legius E. Mechanisms in the pathogenesis of malignant tumours in neurofibromatosis type 1. Lancet Oncol. 2009;10(5):508–15. https://doi.org/10.1016/S1470-2045(09)70033-6.
2. Nishida T, Tsujimoto M, Takahashi T, Hirota S, Blay JY, Wataya-Kaneda M. Gastrointestinal stromal tumors in Japanese patients with neurofibromatosis type I. J Gastroenterol. 2016;51(6):571–8. https://doi.org/10.1007/s00535-015-1132-6.
3. Reynolds RM, Browning GG, Nawroz I, Campbell IW. Von Recklinghausen's neurofibromatosis: neurofibromatosis type 1. Lancet. 2003;361(9368):1552–4. https://doi.org/10.1016/s0140-6736(03)13166-2.
4. Zöller ME, Rembeck B, Odén A, Samuelsson M, Angervall L. Malignant and benign tumors in patients with neurofibromatosis type 1 in a defined Swedish population. Cancer. 1997;79(11):2125–31. https://pubmed.ncbi.nlm.nih.gov/9179058/
5. Andersson J, Sihto H, Meis-Kindblom JM, Joensuu H, Nupponen N, Kindblom LG. NF1-associated gastrointestinal stromal tumors have unique clinical, phenotypic, and genotypic characteristics. Am J Surg Pathol. 2005;29(9):1170–6. https://doi.org/10.1097/01.pas.0000159775.77912.15.
6. Miettinen M, Fetsch JF, Sobin LH, Lasota J. Gastrointestinal stromal tumors in patients with neurofibromatosis 1: a clinicopathologic and molecular genetic study of 45 cases. Am J Surg Pathol. 2006;30(1):90–6. https://doi.org/10.1097/01.pas.0000176433.81079.bd.
7. Basu TN, Gutmann DH, Fletcher JA, Glover TW, Collins FS, Downward J. Aberrant regulation of ras proteins in malignant tumour cells from type 1 neurofibromatosis patients. Nature. 1992;356(6371):713–5. https://doi.org/10.1038/356713a0.
8. Mussi C, Schildhaus HU, Gronchi A, Wardelmann E, Hohenberger P. Therapeutic consequences from molecular biology for gastrointestinal stromal tumor patients affected by neurofibromatosis type 1. Clin Cancer Res. 2008;14(14):4550–5. https://doi.org/10.1158/1078-0432.CCR-08-0086.
9. Huss S, Elges S, Trautmann M, Sperveslage J, Hartmann W, Wardelmann E. Classification of KIT/PDGFRA wild-type gastrointestinal stromal tumors: implications for therapy. Expert Rev Anticancer Ther. 2015;15(6):623–8. https://doi.org/10.1586/14737140.2015.1032941.
10. Lee JL, Kim JY, Ryu MH, Kang HJ, Chang HM, Kim TW, Lee H, Park JH, Kim HC, Kim JS, Kang YK. Response to imatinib in KIT- and PDGFRA-wild type gastrointestinal stromal associated with neurofibromatosis type 1. Dig Dis Sci. 2006;51(6):1043–6. https://doi.org/10.1007/s10620-006-8003-1.

Succinate Dehydrogenase Deficient GIST

13

Peng Zhang, Weizhen Liu, Yuqiang Du, and Bo Zhang

Keywords

Gastrointestinal stromal tumor · Succinate dehydrogenase · Wild type · Metastasis · Sunitinib · GIST · SDHB deficient · Surgery · Imatinib

13.1 Case 18 A 24-Year-Old Woman with SDHB Deficient GIST

Peng Zhang and Weizhen Liu

13.1.1 Introduction

Succinate dehydrogenase (SDH), also known as mitochondrial respiratory chain complex II, is located on the inner membrane of mitochondria and consists of four subunits A, B, C, and D [1]. It catalyzes the oxidation of succinate to fumarate in the tricarboxylic acid cycle and participates in electron transfer. The defect of any subunit in SDH complex will lead to the dysfunction of SDH, which results in the accumulation of succinate, abnormal activation of signal pathways related to tumorigenic response and angiogenesis, and promotes the occurrence of SDH defect related tumors, of which GIST are the most common. Compared to *KIT/PDGFRA* gene mutant GIST, SDH deficient GIST presents with particular clinicopathological manifestations, treatment, and prognosis [2].

P. Zhang · W. Liu (✉) · Y. Du
Department of Gastrointestinal Surgery, Union Hospital, Tongji Medical College, Huazhong University of Science and Technology, Wuhan, China
e-mail: zhangpengwh@hust.edu.cn; liuweizhen@hust.edu.cn

B. Zhang
Department of Gastrointestinal Surgery, Huaxi Hospital, Sichuan University, Chengdu, China

13.1.2 Case Background

The patient, a 24-year-old woman, presented to the local hospital in September 2015 for investigation of hematemesis for 3 h and bloody stool for 3 days. Abdominal CT showed (1) multiple high-density masses in the stomach, possible neoplastic lesions, gastric GIST and (2) multiple low-density shadows in the liver, probable intrahepatic hemangioma (Fig. 13.1). Gastroscopy revealed several spherical and hemispherical bulges of different sizes in the gastric body, gastric horn and gastric antrum, which were arranged like beads, and the largest one at the gastric antrum was approximately 7.0 cm × 7.0 cm with an erosive surface. A puncture biopsy exhibited several small clusters of spindle cells c; Immunohistochemistry indicated CD117 (+), CD34 (+), DOG-1 (+), SMA (−); Genetic testing was unavailable as only a small amount of tissue was retrieved. The immunohistochemistry results and clinical history were consistent with stomach GIST. She was scheduled treatment with imatinib 400 mg/d.

A repeat abdominal CT in December 2015 showed (1) multiple gastric masses, possibly gastric GIST, with no significant change in tumor size compared to that of 3 months earlier and (2) slightly low-density shadow in the liver, probable multiple intrahepatic hemangiomas (Fig. 13.2). The local doctor decided to continue the current treatment plan as the patient demonstrated stable disease with targeted treatment. A further abdominal CT on March 19, 2016, showed (1) multiple blood supply rich masses in gastric antrum, gastric lesser curvature, lateral wall, and hepatogastric space, which were considered to be gastrointestinal stromal tumors; (2) a left pelvic mass, considered to be a left ovarian tumor; and (3) slightly low density shadow in the liver, considered to be multiple hemangiomas. The tumors were significantly larger in size than they were 3 months earlier, and there was metastasis in hepatogastric space. In order to seek further treatment, the patient presented to the specialized disease outpatient department for GIST treatment at the Union Hospital,

K. Tao, H. Cao (eds.), *Clinical Management of Gastrointestinal Stromal Tumor*, https://doi.org/10.1007/978-981-99-9392-5_13

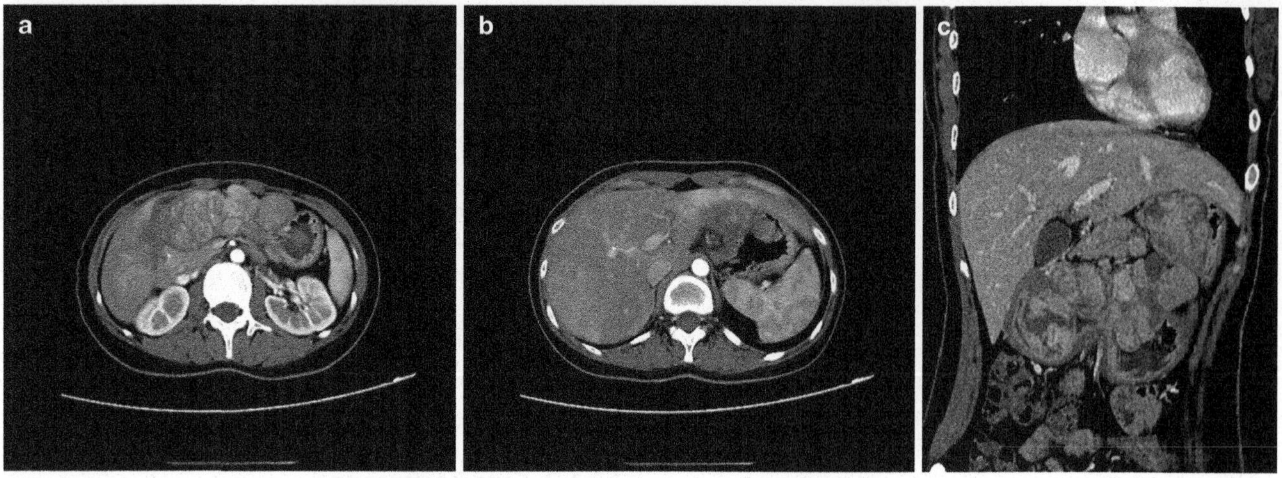

Fig. 13.1 Enhanced CT at the time of initial diagnosis. **a** and **b** Horizontal view; **c** Coronal view

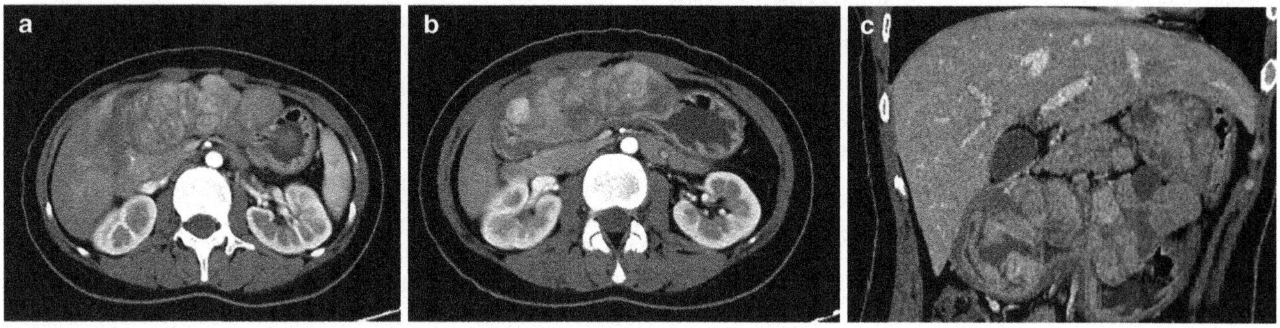

Fig. 13.2 Enhanced CT following treatment with imatinib for 3 months. **a** and **b** Horizontal view; **c** Coronal view

Tongji Medical College of Huazhong University of Science and Technology. The diagnosis at the time was stomach GIST after targeted treatment, with multiple space-occupying lesions in the liver and a space-occupying in the left ovary.

13.1.2.1 Past History and Family History

The patient had been previously healthy and reported no drug allergies. The patient's parents were alive and there was no similar medical history in the family.

13.1.2.2 Physical Examination

The patient's vital signs were stable, and the skin and sclera showed no yellow stain or pallor. The abdomen was flat, with no gastrointestinal shape or distinguishable peristaltic wave. There was slight tenderness in the upper abdomen and right lower abdominal quadrant. A mass about the size of a fist could be palpated under the xiphoid process; this mas had an unclear boundary, no rebound pain or muscle tension. The bowel sounds were normal.

13.1.2.3 Auxiliary Examination

Blood Routine LY 3.13×10^9/L ↓, RBC 3.02×10^{12}/L ↓, Hb 98 g/L ↓, PLT 282×10^9/L, NEUT% 38.88% ↓, LY% 42.4%.

Blood Biochemistry Creatinine 36.0 mmol/L ↓, urea nitrogen 2.88 mmol/L ↓, no other abnormalities were found.

Tumor Markers No abnormalities were found.

Whole Abdomen Enhanced CT (1) Multiple soft tissue density shadows could be seen in the gastric body, lateral wall of the gastric lesser curvature, gastric antrum and hepatogastric space, some of which were arranged in a beaded shape. The left and right diameter was approximately 12 cm; the anterior and posterior diameter was approximately 4.4 cm, and the largest mass in the gastric antrum was approximately 4.5 cm × 3.8 cm in size. The larger tumors in the gastric antrum appeared to be cystic, and the gastric cavity was blocked. The left hepatic artery, left gastric artery, and gastroduodenal artery were involved in the blood supply. Gastric GIST with hepatogastric space metastasis was considered. (2) Nodular, slightly low-density shadows were scattered in the liver, the larger nodules were located in the upper part of the right posterior lobe, with a length of 1.8 cm and gradual enhancement. It was difficult to distinguish whether these represented liver metastasis or hepatic hemangiomas. Further enhanced MR scanning was recommended. (3) A massive soft tissue density shadow was seen in the left accessory area, approximately

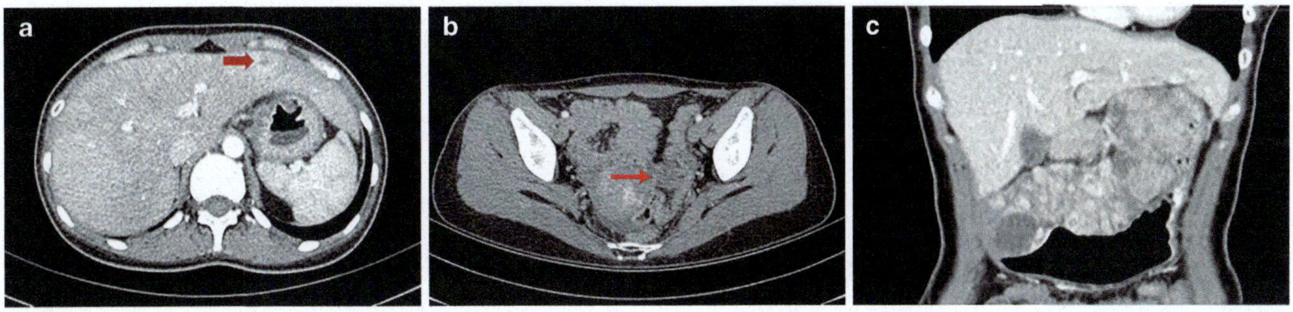

Fig. 13.3 Enhanced CT with imatinib for 6 months. **a** and **b** Horizontal view; **c** Coronal view

3.7 cm × 3.1 cm in size, it demonstrated mild uneven enhancement, and the possibility of left ovarian neoplastic lesions could not be excluded. Further MRI examination was recommended. (4) Small retroperitoneal lymph nodes were notably increased in size (Fig. 13.3).

Gynecological Ultrasound A mass of 2.4 cm × 1.9 cm could be seen in the left ovary with very low echo and reticular separation. This was considered to be a cystic lesion, the nature of which required investigation.

13.1.2.4 Preliminary Diagnosis

1. Gastric giant GIST with hepatogastric space metastasis, post imatinib targeted treatment
2. Liver space occupying lesions: possible GIST metastasis or hepatic hemangioma
3. Ovarian mass: possible metastasis or oophoritic cyst
4. Mild anemia

13.1.3 Therapy

13.1.3.1 Case Analysis

The patient was a young woman who presented with gastrointestinal bleeding. The local hospital diagnosed gastric GIST, and tumor progression occurred after 6 months of imatinib targeted treatment. Primary drug resistance of imatinib was considered. At present, the patient was diagnosed as gastric multiple GIST with progress after preoperative treatment, including possible metastasis in the liver and accessories. Although the operation could be risky, the patient was otherwise in good health. The ECOG score was 1 point, which was expected to be conducive for feasible and satisfactory tumor reduction surgery. Therefore, symptomatic treatment was given, and the surgery was performed after correcting anemia. The next treatment plan was to be decided postoperatively and would be determined based on the results of genetic testing.

13.1.3.2 Treatment

Laparoscopic abdominal exploration with distal gastrectomy (Roux-en-Y), liver tumor resection, and left oophorectomy were performed on April 1, 2016. During the operation, eight to ten nodules were observed in the gastric body and antrum, with a maximum size of 6 cm × 6 cm, and a nodule in the gastric antrum was significantly cystic. There were multiple enlarged lymph nodes surrounding the stomach, and multiple nodules of different sizes could be felt on the surface of the liver. The largest one of which was approximately 1.5 cm × 1.0 cm in size, located on the left outer lobe. The left ovary was large with necrotic tissue.

13.1.3.3 Postoperative Pathology and Genetic Testing

Pathological Diagnosis Gastric GIST post imatinib targeted treatment. (1) Distal stomach and liver GIST. Gastric tumor size: 14 cm × 4 cm; liver tumor size: 0.8 cm × 0.5 cm and 1.3 cm × 1.1 cm; mitotic count: 10/50 HPF (Fig. 13.4). No tumor involvement was found at the cut end of the gastric body and pylorus tissue or at the surgical margin of the liver. (2) Tumor metastasis was identified in the lymph nodes near the common hepatic artery (3/7), lesser curvature side (6/22), and greater curvature side (2/18) (Figs. 13.5 and 13.6). (3) Left ovarian follicular cyst.

Immunohistochemistry Stomach: CD117 (+), CD34 (+), DOG-1 (+), SMA (−), S-100 (−), Ki-67 (Li: 5%), SDHB (−). Liver: CD117 (+), CD34 (−), DOG-1 (+), SMA (−), S-100 (−), Ki-67 (Li: 5%), SDHB (−) (Fig. 13.7).

Genetic Testing Exon 9, 11, 13, and 17 of *KIT* and exon 12 and 18 of *PDGFRA* were wild type.

13.1.4 Prognosis

The patient recovered and was discharged 7 days after operation. The patient was diagnosed with wild type gastric GIST with multiple metastases of the liver and lymph nodes. During case screening in 2017, the MDT team determined that the patient's condition was consistent with SDH deficient GIST. Immunohistochemistry confirmed SDH deficiency. Considering the change of guidelines, sunitinib targeted therapy with 37.5 mg/d was initiated. In January 2022, the patients had been followed up for 69 months

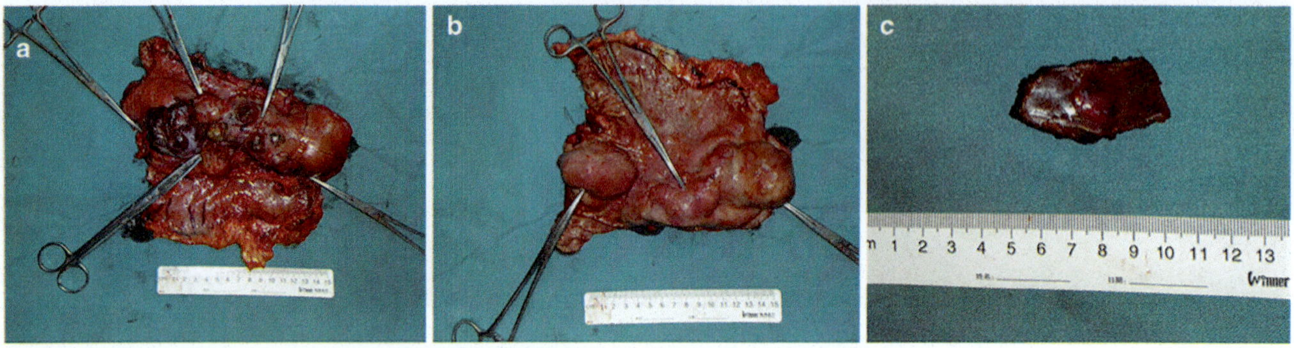

Fig. 13.4 The gross specimen. **a** View outside gastric wall; **b** View in gastric cavity; **c** Liver tumor

Fig. 13.5 H&E staining of the tumors

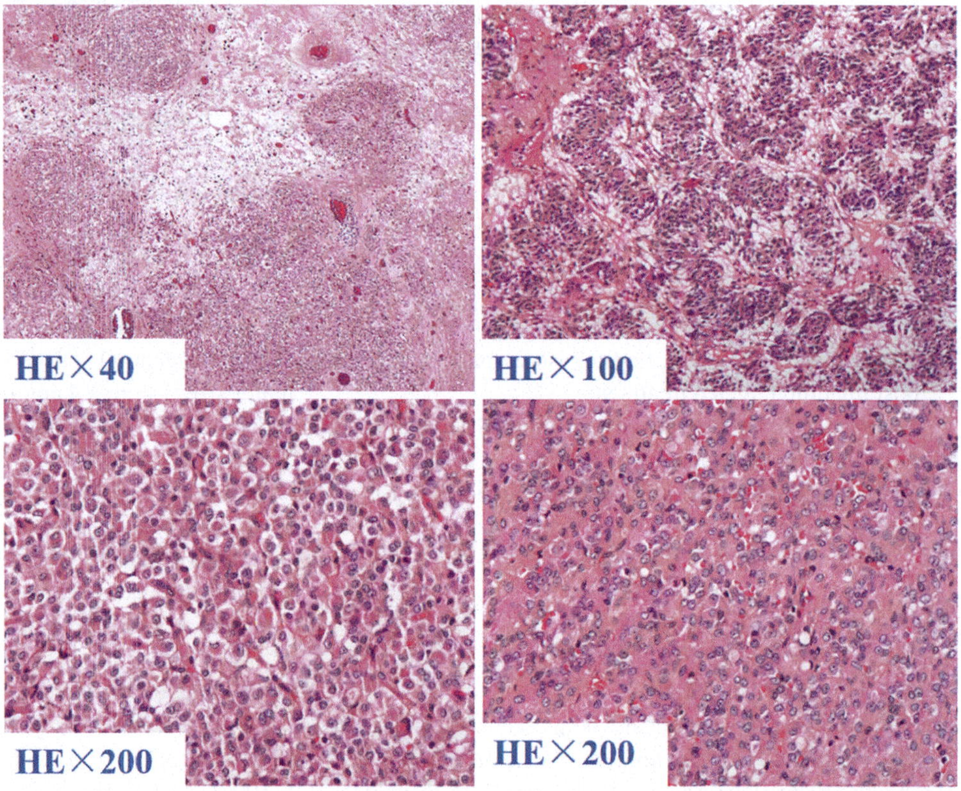

Fig. 13.6 H&E staining of the lymph nodes (**a**) and liver metastasis (**b**) tumor

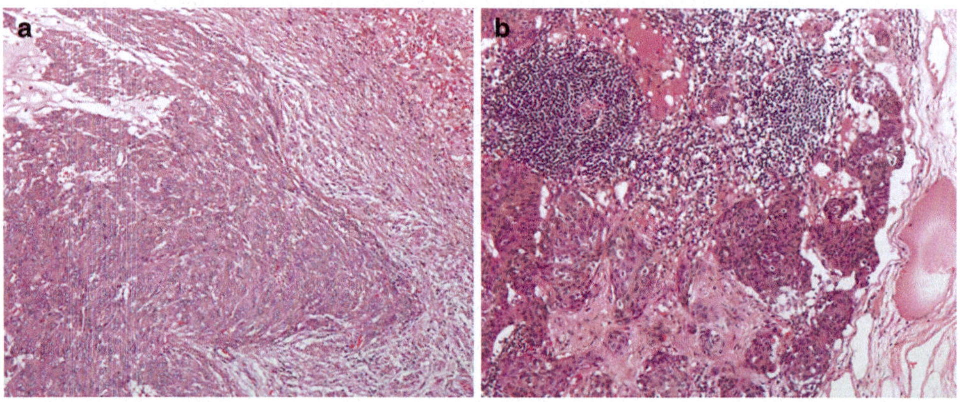

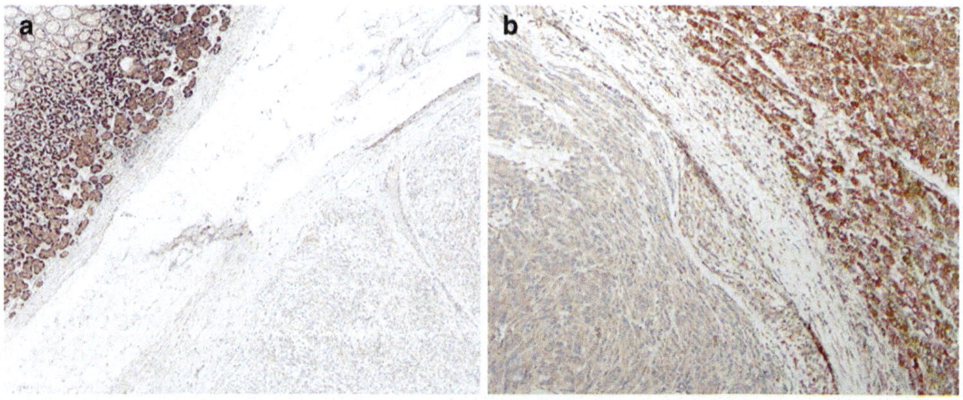

Fig. 13.7 IHC staining of SDHB. **a** CD117 staining; **b** CD34 staining

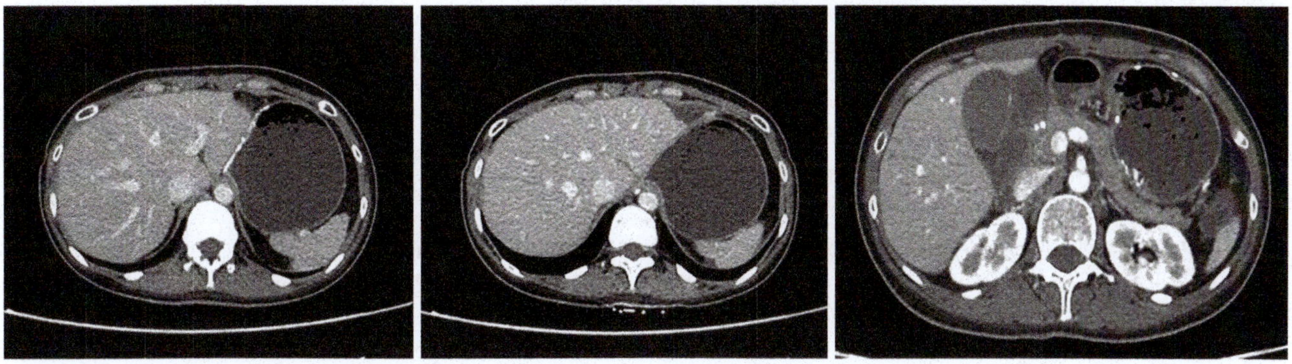

Fig. 13.8 Enhanced CT after surgical resection

(Fig. 13.8). The patients had no obvious adverse side reactions, the liver metastases were completely relieved, and no obvious signs of recurrence or metastasis were found elsewhere.

13.2 Case 19 A 20-Year-Old Man with SDHB Deficient GIST

Yuqiang Du and Peng Zhang

13.2.1 Case Background

The patient, a 20-year-old man, presented to the local hospital in July 2021 for investigation of abdominal pain with vomiting for 8 days. There was no obvious cause for epigastric pain or discomfort, the patient had vomited the stomach contents once, approximately 100 mL in volume and reported no diarrhea or constipation. Gastroscopy showed gastric space-occupying lesions. The patient attended Union Hospital, Tongji Medical College of Huazhong University of Science and Technology for further treatment.

13.2.1.1 Past History and Family History

The patient was previously healthy, and reported no drug allergies. The patient's parents were alive, and there was no similar medical history in the family.

13.2.1.2 Physical Examination

The vital signs were stable, and the skin and mucous membranes were not yellowish or pale. The abdomen was flat, and no gastrointestinal or peristaltic waves were seen. There was tenderness in the upper abdomen, with no rebound tenderness, guarding. The bowel sounds were normal.

13.2.1.3 Auxiliary Examination

Blood Routine and Blood Biochemistry No obvious abnormalities.

Tumor Markers No obvious abnormalities.

Full-Enhanced Three-Dimensional CT of the Entire Abdomen (1) There were multiple lump-like soft tissue density shadows on the lesser curvature of the gastric body, most of which showed a trend of fusion, some of which protruded into the gastric cavity, most of which protruded out of the gastric cavity. The enhanced scan showed mild to moderate enhancement, which was not uniform; these findings were suggestive of gastric GIST. Multiple lymph nodes, some of which appeared liquefied and necrotic, were observed in the perigastric space. The relationship to the lesions was unclear; (2) The spleen was slightly enlarged; (3) An accessory spleen was identified; (4) Scattered small lymph nodes were identified in the ileocolon.

PET/CT Imaging of Glucose Metabolism of the Entire Body The stomach wall was thickened and metabolism was abnormally increased. There were multiple enlarged lymph nodes in the hepatogastric and pancreatic gastric spaces, and the metabolism was also abnormally increased. These findings were considered to indicate malignant tumors, and malignant lymphoma infiltration.

Ultrasound Gastroscopy The gastric corpus-antrum lesions originated from the muscularis propria, showed uniform hypoechoic changes, and clear boundaries, and the lesions grew in and out of the gastric cavity. The largest cross-section size was approximately 42.8 mm × 32.9 mm. Doppler showed no obvious blood flow inside the lesion. Multiple swollen hypoechoic nodules were seen outside the stomach wall (Fig. 13.9). Biopsy samples were collected from the perigastric lymph nodes and gastric wall lesions for pathological examination.

Gastric Body Mucosal Biopsy The perigastric puncture biopsy and gastric puncture biopsy findings were consistent with GIST (mainly epithelioid morphology).

Immunohistochemistry CD117 (+), CD34 (+), DOG-1 (+), SMA (−), Desmin (−), S-100 (−), PCK (−), Ki-67 (Li: 5%).

13.2.2 Primary Diagnosis

1. Space-occupying lesions of lesser curvature of the gastric body, GIST
2. Gastrointestinal bleeding

13.2.3 Therapy

13.2.3.1 Case Analysis

The patient was a young man who presented with abdominal pain with vomiting, and was diagnosed with a space-occupying lesion in the lesser curvature of the gastric corpus, considered to be a possible GIST. The patient was otherwise generally healthy, had an ECOG score 0, and should be treated with surgery. Then patient was given symptomatic treatment, prepared for elective surgery, and guided postoperative treatment was subsequently based on the results of pathology and genetic testing.

13.2.3.2 Treatment

On August 17, 2021, the patient underwent laparoscopic abdominal cavity exploration and distal gastrectomy (Roux-en-Y). The intraoperative findings were several tumors of different sizes positioned from the body of the stomach to the posterior wall of the gastric antrum, approximately 2–3 cm in diameter, and multiple tumors on the gastric wall.

13.2.3.3 Postoperative Pathology and Genetic Testing

Pathological Diagnosis (1) Small curvature of the gastric body GIST with SDH deficiency. The tumor was a multinodular growth with an infiltrating border, was mainly located in the serosal layer, with local involvement of the mucosa with ulcer formation. Intravascular tumor thrombus and nerve

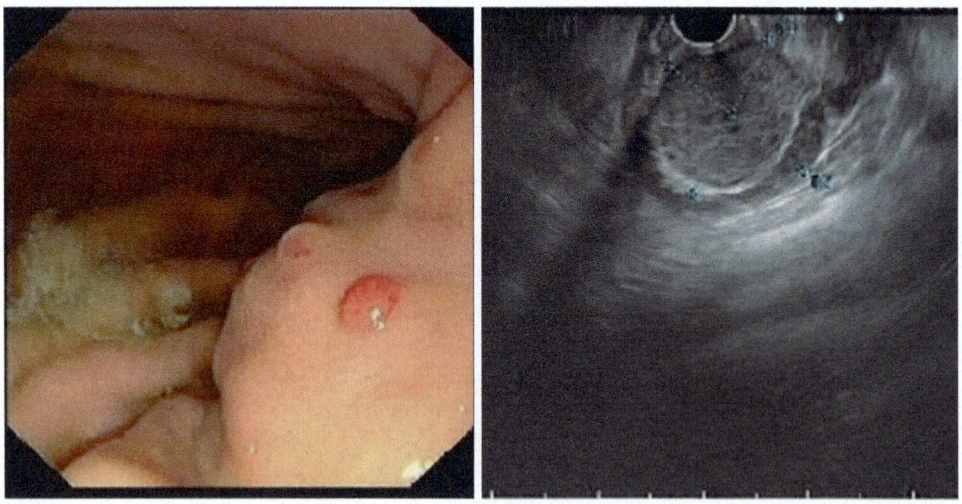

Fig. 13.9 Ultrasound gastroscopy pictures from August

invasion were seen around the tumor. There was no evidence of tumor involvement on the lateral resection margin of the gastric body or the lateral resection margin of the pylorus. The tumor demonstrated a multinodular growth pattern, and nodules varied in size from 0.6 cm × 0.5 cm × 0.5 cm to 7.6 cm × 4.7 cm × 2.9 cm. The histological morphology was of epithelial-spindle cell mixed type (mainly epithelioid morphology). The presence of mitotic count was 15/5 mm^2. There was no tumor metastasis on the sections of lesser curvature lymph nodes, greater omental lymph nodes, the greater curvature lymph nodes, or the mesenteric lymph nodes (2) (Figs. 13.10 and 13.11).

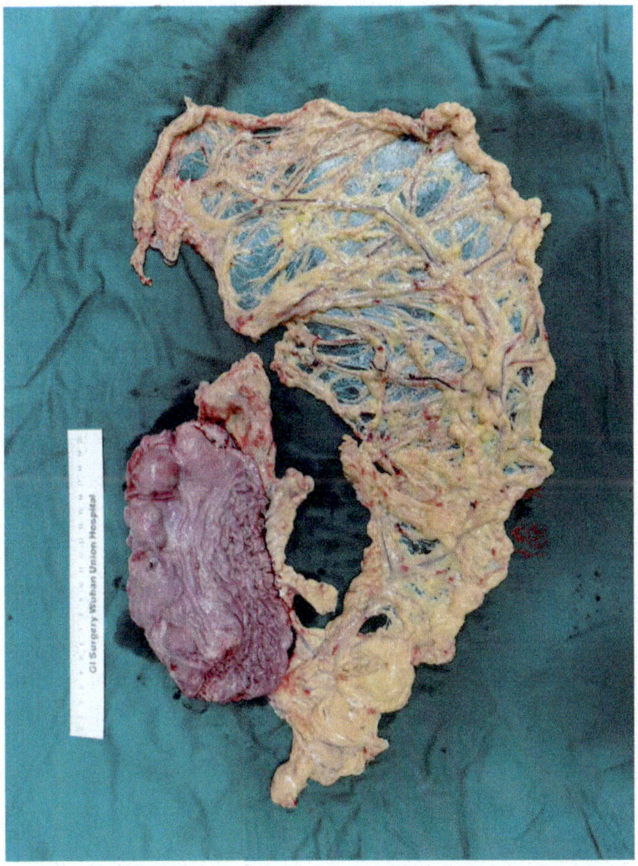

Fig. 13.10 The gross specimen

Immunohistochemistry CD117 (+), CD34 (+), DOG-1 (+), SDHB (−), SMA (−), S-100 (−), ALK (−), Ki-67 (Li: 20%).

Genetic Testing A mutation in exon 7 of *SDHB* was identified, and the mutation type was c.G725A_p.Arg242His.

13.2.4 Prognosis

The postoperative recovery was smooth. Considering that SDH-deficient GIST is usually resistant to imatinib, postoperative imatinib treatment was not administered, and regular follow-up observations were scheduled. At the last follow-up in January 2022, no tumor recurrence or metastasis were observed.

13.2.5 Experience of Diagnosis and Therapy

13.2.5.1 What Are Wild-Type GIST? What Are the Characteristics of SDH Deficient GIST?

Wild-type GIST lacks *KIT* and *PDGFRA* mutations but is often accompanied by an abnormal structure or expression of other genes, such as *SDH*, *BRAF*, or NF1 mutations and multiple gene fusion. Different mutant types of wild-type GIST have different clinical manifestations, epidemiological characteristics, and pathological characteristics.

About 20–40% of wild-type GIST are characterized by SDH deficiency. These patients often have the following characteristics: most are found in young people, most tumors occur in the stomach, tumor progress is relatively slow, the incidence of lymph node metastasis is high, and the prognosis is quite different. In addition, SDH deficient GIST is often accompanied by insulin-like growth factor 1 receptor upregulation, so these tumors are more sensitive to sunitinib, which may become the therapeutic target for this type of GIST [3, 4]. Dr. Kaixiong Tao's team from Union Hospital, Tongji Medical College of Huazhong University of Science and Technology summarized cases of SDH deficient GIST

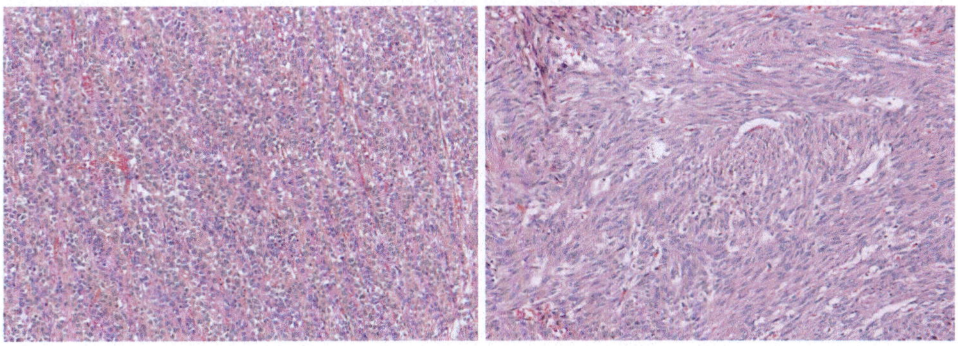

Fig. 13.11 H&E staining of primary tumor

and found that SDH deficient GIST is a special subtype of GIST, and its biological behavior and treatment scheme differ from ordinary GIST [5]. For GIST without *KIT* or *PDGFRA* mutation, especially for young patients with primary gastric cancer, SDHB immunohistochemical examination is recommended. Additionally, visibly enlarged lymph nodes should be resected during operation for this type of GIST. Patients with this type of GIST are usually resistant to imatinib, but may have a higher response rate to sunitinib.

Therefore, at the time of initial GIST diagnosis, preoperative biopsy and genetic testing are of great value for the diagnosis, treatment, and risk evaluation of the disease. We suggest that for patients with preoperative biopsy, clinicians should fully communicate with endoscopists and pathologists, take more tissues, and conduct genetic testing under the condition of ensuring safety.

13.2.5.2 How to Choose Postoperative Targeted Therapy for Wild-Type GIST?

This patient was diagnosed with SDH deficient GIST, which is a wild-type GIST. Whether wild-type GIST will benefit from adjuvant therapy with imatinib is controversial, but some small sample studies have found that SDH deficient GIST patients are usually resistant to imatinib and have a higher response rate to sunitinib [5, 6]. For this patient, imatinib was ineffective and led to tumor progression before surgery. Sunitinib therapy was commenced postoperatively, and good curative effect was achieved. Therefore, we suggest that for wild-type GIST, especially patients with abnormal structure or expression of other genes, such as NF1 and BRAF, second-generation sequencing could be considered if economic conditions permit, and appropriate targeted drugs should be selected according to the sequencing results.

13.3 Expert Comments

Bo Zhang

Commonly, SDH deficient GIST only occurs in the stomach and is multifocal and is prone to liver and lymph node metastasis. Additionally, with SDH deficient GIST, there are no mutations in *KIT* or *PDGFRA*. Most patients have systemic mutations involving different SDH subunit genes, which are characterized by a loss of SDH expression in immunophenotype. Therefore, detecting SDH deletion by immunohistochemistry is the most effective method to identify SDH deficient GIST. In addition, histologically, SDH deficient GIST is mostly strip-shaped or features solid, sheet nested epithelioid tumor cells, which grow in clusters or multiple nodules between smooth muscle or are mixed with spindle tumor cells [2]. The cells display mild to moderate heterogeneity, mitotic count is common, and the tumors are often accompanied by lymphatic invasion or regional lymph node metastasis.

In terms of treatment approach, complete surgical resection and regional lymph node dissection are the most important treatment methods for SDH deficient GIST. Because most of these GIST are resistant to imatinib, and some small sample studies have shown that they have better response to sunitinib, sunitinib could be selected for targeted treatment after surgery. Even if there is metastasis, the clinical process of such GIST tends to be stable. The number of mitotic bodies has no clear relationship with the risk of tumor metastasis. Even in cases with liver metastasis, there is good long-term survival for patients with SDH deficient GIST. Therefore, it is not recommended to use conventional risk assessment criteria (mitotic number and tumor size) to evaluate the malignant potential of this subtype GIST.

In addition, through the diagnosis and treatment of this case, the following points are worth learning:

1. Before preoperative treatment, GIST patients should undergo biopsy and genetic testing to ensure a definitive diagnosis is made and determine the initial dose of imatinib according to the genetic testing results.
2. During preoperative treatment, the treatment effect should be evaluated regularly (every 2–3 months). The Choi standard or RECIST1.1 standard is recommended for assessment of GIST [7]. The condition of patients with tumor progression after imatinib treatment should be comprehensively evaluated. If it is possible to remove the progressive lesions, stopping targeted drug therapy and conducting early surgical intervention could be considered.
3. Lymph node metastasis rarely occurs in GIST. Generally, routine dissection is not necessary. However, in cases with pathologically enlarged lymph nodes, the possibility of SDH deficient GIST should be considered and pathological lymph nodes should be removed [5].

References

1. Huang S, Millar AH. Succinate dehydrogenase: the complex roles of a simple enzyme. Curr Opin Plant Biol. 2013;16(3):344–9. https://doi.org/10.1016/j.pbi.2013.02.007.
2. Ibrahim A, Chopra S. Succinate dehydrogenase-deficient gastrointestinal stromal tumors. Arch Pathol Lab Med. 2020;144(5):655–60. https://doi.org/10.5858/arpa.2018-0370-RS.
3. Chou A, Chen J, Clarkson A, Samra JS, Clifton-Bligh RJ, Hugh TJ, Gill AJ. Succinate dehydrogenase-deficient GISTs are characterized by IGF1R overexpression. Mod Pathol. 2012;25(9):1307–13. https://doi.org/10.1038/modpathol.2012.77.
4. Tarn C, Rink L, Merkel E, Flieder D, Pathak H, Koumbi D, Testa JR, Eisenberg B, von Mehren M, Godwin AK. Insulin-like growth factor 1 receptor is a potential therapeutic target for gastrointestinal stromal tumors. Proc Natl Acad Sci USA. 2008;105(24):8387–92. https://doi.org/10.1073/pnas.0803383105.

5. Liu WZ, Zeng XY, Wu XL, He J, Gao JB, Shuai XM, Wang GB, Zhang P, Tao KX. Clinicopathologic study of succinate-dehydrogenase-deficient gastrointestinal stromal tumors: a single-institutional experience in China. Medicine (Baltimore). 2017;96(32):e7668. https://doi.org/10.1097/MD.0000000000007668.
6. Boikos SA, Pappo AS, Killian JK, LaQuaglia MP, Weldon CB, George S, Trent JC, von Mehren M, Wright JA, Schiffman JD, Raygada M, Pacak K, Meltzer PS, Miettinen MM, Stratakis C, Janeway KA, Helman LJ. Molecular subtypes of KIT/PDGFRA wild-type gastrointestinal stromal tumors: a report from the National Institutes of Health Gastrointestinal Stromal Tumor Clinic. JAMA Oncol. 2016;2(7):922–8. https://doi.org/10.1001/jamaoncol.2016.0256.
7. Shinagare AB, Jagannathan JP, Kurra V, Urban T, Manola J, Choy E, Demetri GD, George S, Ramaiya NH. Comparison of performance of various tumour response criteria in assessment of regorafenib activity in advanced gastrointestinal stromal tumours after failure of imatinib and sunitinib. Eur J Cancer. 2014;50(5):981–6. https://doi.org/10.1016/j.ejca.2013.11.037.

KIT Mutant Gastrointestinal Stromal Tumors with Lymphatic Metastasis

14

Yongzhou Huang, Xiangyu Zeng, and Ye Zhou

Keywords

Lymph node metastasis · *KIT* · Gene mutation · Imatinib Blood concentration · Preoperative biopsy

14.1 Case 20 A 59-Year-Old Woman Diagnosed with GIST Accompanied by Lymphatic Metastasis

Yongzhou Huang and Xiangyu Zeng

14.1.1 Introduction

Lymph node metastasis of GIST is very rare, especially in adult GIST patients. However, there is a higher incidence of lymph node metastasis in pediatric patients with SDH-deficiency. The Chinese GIST diagnosis and treatment expert consensus and NCCN guidelines both recommend that routine lymph node dissection is not necessary for GIST surgery. At present, the relationship between GIST lymph node metastasis and prognosis remains less clear. This case reports a gastric GIST with *KIT* mutation and lymph node metastasis for reference.

14.1.2 Case Background

The patient, a 59-year-old woman, presented to the local hospital on January 8, 2017, for investigation of intermittent abdominal distension and pain for more than 1 week. A CT scan of the abdomen showed that the stomach was not well filled, and the stomach wall was thickened. Gastroscopy showed that there was a large mass on the lesser curvature of the stomach, identified as a possible gastric tumor. The patient's care was transferred to the Department of Gastrointestinal Surgery, Union Hospital Affiliated to Tongji Medical College, Huazhong University of Science and Technology on April 10, 2017. During the course of the disease, the patient experienced no discomfort such as nausea and vomiting, constipation, diarrhea, hematemesis, or melena. The patient was admitted to hospital for further treatment.

14.1.2.1 Past History and Family History

The patient had a >10-year history of type 2 diabetes, which was well controlled with medication. The patient reported no history of surgery or trauma. There was no similar medical history in the family.

14.1.2.2 Physical Examination

The patient's skin was pale, with no jaundice, and no palpable superficial lymphadenopathy. The abdomen was flat, and there were no abdominal wall varicose veins, gastrointestinal patterns, or peristaltic waves. The abdomen, with no resistance, the liver and spleen are not palpable below the costal margin, and no obvious abdominal mass. Murphy sign was negative, there was no shifting dullness, and bowel sounds were normal. There was slight edema in both lower limbs.

14.1.2.3 Auxiliary Examination

Blood Routine WBC 5.93 × 10^9/L, RBC 3.70 × 10^9/L ↓, Hb 97 g/L ↓, PLT 341 × 10^9/L, NEUT % 49.0%, LY% 37.6%.

Blood Biochemistry TP 61.3 g/L ↓, ALB 34.8 g/L ↓, ALT 10 U/L, AST 14 U/L. Other indicators were within the normal range.

Y. Huang · X. Zeng (✉)
Department of Gastrointestinal Surgery, Union Hospital, Tongji Medical College, Huazhong University of Science and Technology, Wuhan, China
e-mail: xiangyuzeng@hust.edu.cn

Y. Zhou
Department of Gastric Surgery, Fudan University Cancer Hospital, Shanghai, China

K. Tao, H. Cao (eds.), *Clinical Management of Gastrointestinal Stromal Tumor*, https://doi.org/10.1007/978-981-99-9392-5_14

Tumor Markers No obvious abnormalities.

Full-Enhanced Three-Dimensional CT of the Entire Abdomen (1) Uneven thickening of the stomach wall on the fundus-lesser curvature, multiple ulcer formations, a slightly fuzzy and rough serosal surface. There were a few lymph nodes in the liver and stomach ligament; one of the enlarged lymph nodes had a fuzzy appearance and the long edge was approximately 1.1 cm. Gastric cancer was considered the most likely diagnosis, and the imaging stage was T3-4aN1Mx. (2) There was a slightly rounded, slightly low-density shadow with unclear margins in the right posterior lobe of the liver, with a diameter of approximately 1.1 cm, and the enhancement was not obvious. The possibility of metastases was not excluded, and MR examination was recommended. (3) No obvious abnormal density in the uterus and bilateral appendages. (4) No enlarged lymph nodes were observed in the abdominal pelvic cavity and retroperitoneum.

Liver and Spleen Enhanced MRI (1) A round-shaped long T1 long T2 signal shadow with a diameter of approximately 1.2 cm was identified in the junction of liver S6–7. The central T2 signal was higher, and the DWI was circular with limited diffusion. Enhanced scanning provided edge enhancement, which was suggestive of liver metastasis. (2) In the enhanced scanning arterial phase, scattered small nodules and small patches in the liver were obviously enhanced, and the other phases demonstrated iso-signals, and transient perfusion abnormalities should be considered. (3) Uneven thickening of the stomach wall on the gastric fundus-small curvature of the gastric body was observed, wide ulcers were seen, the serosal surface was not smooth, and a few lymph nodes were seen on the gastric curvature. These findings were consistent with gastric cancer, and it was recommended that these be assessed in conjunction with the endoscopy findings (4) No obvious enlarged lymph nodes were observed in the hilar or retroperitoneal regions. (Fig. 14.1).

Electronic Gastroscopy Huge new masses were observed on the lesser curvature of the stomach and on the front and rear walls. The surface of the mass was ulcerated, uneven, and coated in dirty moss. Five biopsy tissue samples were collected, and the tissue was soft in consistency. No other abnormalities were observed (Fig. 14.2).

Gastric Body Mucosal Biopsy Immunohistochemistry staining showed DOG-1 (+), CD117 (+), CD34 (+), S-100 (−), PCK (−), CK8/18 (−), LCA (−), Syn (−), SDHB (+), Ki-67 (Li: 30%). Further pathological examination was recommended after complete removal of the tumor.

14.1.3 Primary Diagnosis

1. Gastric GIST with liver metastasis
2. Mild anemia
3. Type 2 diabetes

14.1.4 Therapy

14.1.4.1 Case Analysis

The patient was a middle-aged woman who was admitted to the hospital for investigation of intermittent abdominal pain and abdominal distension for more than 1 week. Abdominal CT showed a high possibility of gastric cancer (imaging stage T3-4aN1Mx), possibly accompanied by lymph node metastasis, but liver metastasis was not excluded. Liver and spleen MRI examination was then performed, and the results were also suggestive of gastric cancer accompanied by liver metastasis. Tissue biopsies revealed that the primary gastric tumor was GIST. Based on this investigation, the patient was diagnosed with: gastric body GIST with liver metastasis. After evaluation, it was determined that the primary tumor and metastatic tumor could be completely resected. In addi-

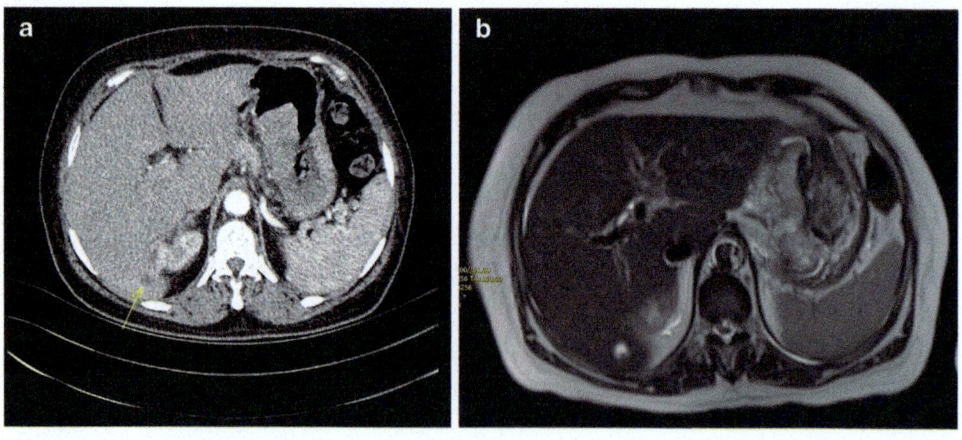

Fig. 14.1 Abdominal imaging showed liver metastases. **a** CT image; **b** MRI image

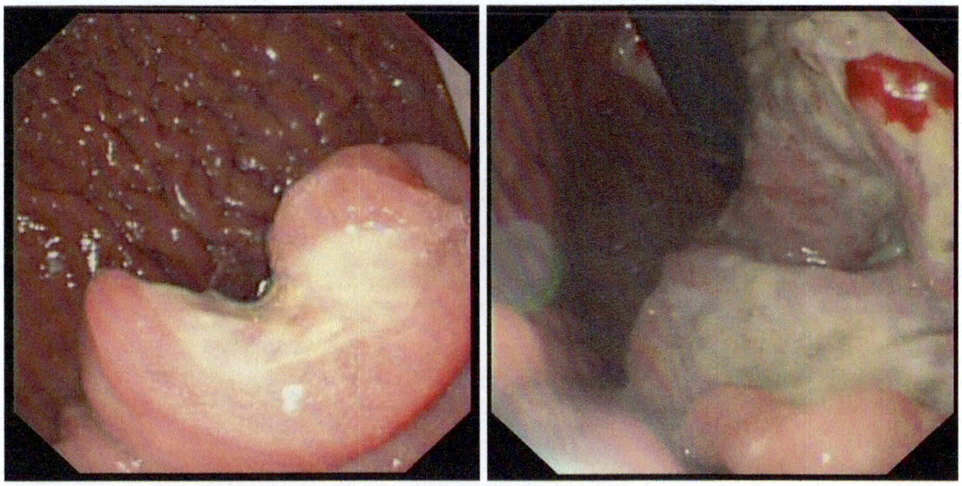

Fig. 14.2 Electronic gastroscope showed that huge new masses were visible on the lesser curvature of the stomach and on the anterior and posterior walls, with an ulcerated surface

tion, the patient was currently in a stable condition and would be able to tolerate the procedure. Therefore, surgery was considered for this patient, with the primary gastric tumor and liver metastases to be removed together, and with possible postoperative targeted drug therapy based on the results of further pathological examination and genetic testing.

14.1.4.2 Treatment

An exploratory laparotomy was performed on January 21, 2017. During the operation, a raised mass, approximately 5 cm × 6 cm in size, was found in the lesser curvature of the stomach, and there was a clear boundary with the surrounding tissues. A partial gastrectomy was performed to remove the gastric tumor. For the liver mass, displacing the falciform ligament fully exposed the lesion. The lesion was located above the upper pole of the kidney in the right posterior lobe of the liver, with a diameter of about 2 cm and a slightly hardened texture. A pre-cut line was drawn with an electric knife along the outer edge of the lesion with a margin of 1.5 cm. Subsequently, an incision was made to the liver parenchyma, and the tumor was resected. Intraoperative bleeding was approximately 200 mL, both tumors were completely removed, and the surgery process went smoothly.

14.1.4.3 Postoperative Pathology and Genetic Testing

Pathological Diagnosis (1) Gastric body GIST with interstitial mucus change, tumor metastasis on the peri gastric lymph nodes (1/9), and no tumor involvement on the surgical margins on both sides. The tumor was 8.5 cm × 8 cm × 5 cm, mitotic count >10/50HPF. (2) Liver metastatic GIST with reactive hyperplasia of lymphoid tissue. Combined with medical history, morphology and immunohistochemistry, the findings were consistent with gastric origin. There was no tumor involvement at the surgical margin (Fig. 14.3).

Immunohistochemistry Gastric body GIST: CD117 (+), DOG-1 (+), S-100 (−), Ki-67 (Li: 30%), SDHB (+). Liver metastasis: CD117 (+), DOG-1 (+), SDHB (+), Ki-67 (Li: 30%), CD3 (+), and CD20 (+) (indicating the mixed presence of T cells and B cells), and CD21 (+) and CD23 (+) (indicating the presence of the FDC network of proliferative B cells).

Genetic Testing The primary gastric lesions and liver metastases exhibited *KIT* exon 11 mutations; the mutation type was c.1673_1674insTCC. *PDGFRA* exons 12 and 18 were wild type.

14.1.5 Prognosis

The patient recovered and was discharged on the 12th day postoperative. The patient started adjuvant treatment with imatinib at 400 mg/d one month after surgery. During this period, severe edema around the orbit, scattered rashes on both upper limbs, diarrhea and other adverse reactions to imatinib therapy occurred. After corresponding symptomatic and supportive treatments such as diuresis, acid suppression and stomach protection, the adverse reactions were not alleviated. In May 2017, the blood concentration of imatinib was 2423.2 ng/mL, and the dose was reduced to 300 mg/d. The adverse reactions were reduced, and the patient could tolerate ongoing therapy. Two weeks later, the blood concentration of imatinib was 1548.3 ng/mL, and the patient continued imatinib 300 mg/d until March 2020. As of January 2022, after 60 months of follow-up, the patient showed no signs of tumor recurrence or metastasis.

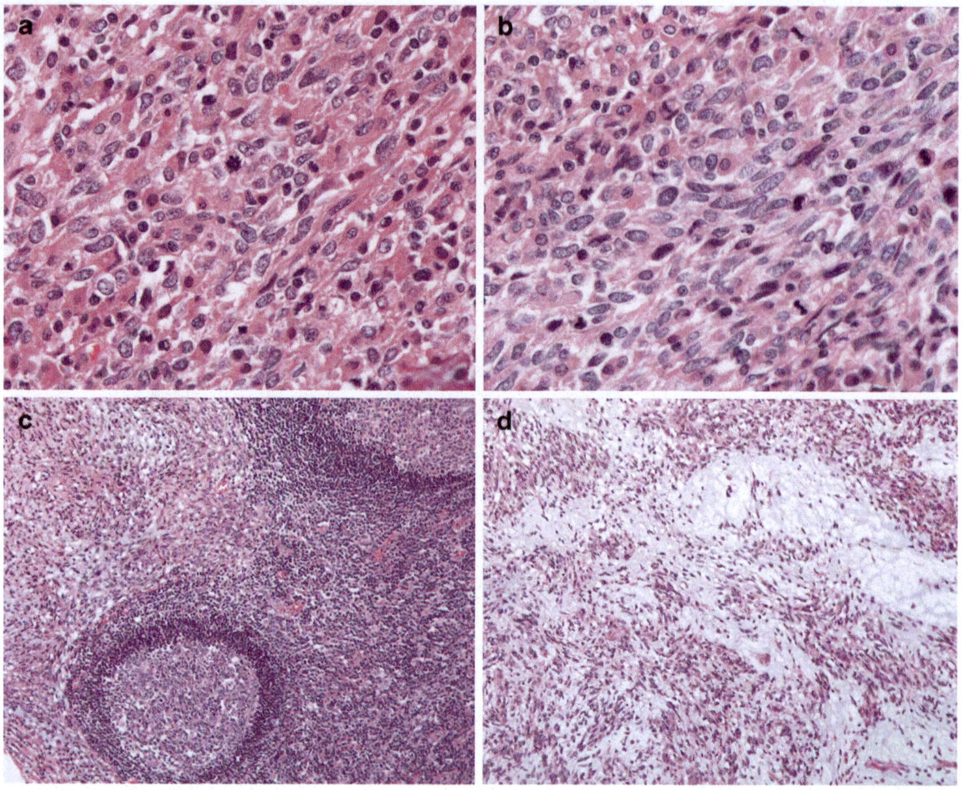

Fig. 14.3 Pathological diagnosis. **a** Primary tumor; **b** Liver metastasis; **c** Lymph node metastasis; **d** Mucus

14.1.6 Experience of Diagnosis and Therapy

14.1.6.1 Is Lymph Node Metastasis a Late Event in the Development of GIST Disease?

The main routes of GIST metastasis occurs are through blood transport to the liver or direct dissemination through the peritoneum. Lymph node metastasis of GIST is relatively rare [1]. There are many classification and staging standards for the risk assessment of primary GIST, such as NIH classification, AFIP classification, and the most widely used modified NIH classification. These standards do not include lymph node metastasis as an evaluation parameter. In the American Joint Committee on Cancer (AJCC) TNM staging system published in 2009, for the first time, lymph node metastasis was used as a factor for assessing the biological behavior and prognosis of GIST. Subsequently, this staging considered the presence of lymph node metastasis to indicate stage IV disease, which conflicts with traditional understanding, and has been disputed. Some scholars believe that lymph node metastasis is a relatively late event in the pathogenesis of GIST which occurs after blood metastasis. Once lymph node metastasis occurs, the disease often progresses or exhibits local invasion or distant metastasis. This may be one of the reasons why AJCC classified lymph node metastasis as an indicator of stage IV disease. Some scholars also believe that, unlike gastrointestinal epithelial tumors, the status of lymph node metastasis in the course of GIST is not very clear. Some patients with lymph node metastasis do not exhibit liver metastasis or develop liver metastasis later. Therefore, lymph node metastasis may not be a late event in the course of GIST.

A study analyzed the prognosis of GIST patients with lymph node metastasis from 2004 to 2014 in the National Cancer Institute database (The Surveillance, Epidemiology, and End Results database), and found that patients with distant metastases were more likely to develop lymph node metastasis. Moreover, the study also found that lymph node metastasis had no effect on the overall survival of patients with primary GIST. For patients with distant metastasis, lymph node metastasis was an independent prognostic factor, and the overall survival for these patients was significantly shorter than that of patients with lymph node metastasis alone [2]. This case was diagnosed with simultaneous liver and lymph node metastasis. After the operation, targeted drug therapy was performed in accordance with the doctor's instructions and follow-up revealed no signs of tumor recurrence or metastasis.

14.1.6.2 The Dose of Imatinib Should Be Adjusted According to the Blood Concentration

The pharmacokinetic study of the B2222 trial found that for patients with advanced GIST, the therapeutic effect of imatinib was significantly reduced when plasma trough concentration of imatinib was lower than 1100 ng/mL [3]. Therefore, maintaining a certain plasma drug concentration is essential for the efficacy of imatinib.

Imatinib is well tolerated in most patients. The common adverse reactions include edema, gastrointestinal reactions, leukopenia, anemia, and skin rash. Most side effects are mild to moderate in severity and can be improved or relieved with symptomatic treatment. However, for some patients, serious adverse reactions may occur during treatment with a standard dose of imatinib [4]. During the period of taking imatinib 400 mg/d, this patient experienced a series of local and systemic adverse reactions which seriously affected the quality of life, and did not resolve after symptomatic and supportive treatment. The NCCN guidelines point out that for patients with serious adverse reactions, the drug may be temporarily ceased or the dose may be reduced to 300 mg/d. Therefore, after measuring the blood concentration of imatinib, we recommend that the patient reduce the dose to 300 mg/d. Subsequently, the plasma concentration of imatinib dropped to 1548.3 ng/mL, and the adverse reactions improved. After 60 months of follow-up, no signs of tumor recurrence or metastasis were found.

Therefore, it may be a more reasonable choice for adjuvant treatment of GIST to monitor the plasma drug concentration of imatinib and customize a personalized drug dosage regimen according to the individual situation of the patient [5–7].

14.2 Expert Comments

Ye Zhou

GIST, as a kind of soft tissue sarcoma, has a low lymph node metastasis rate, and it does not require routine lymph node dissection. However, young women with multinodular gastric GIST, SDHB (−) accompanied by adrenal tumors or pulmonary chondroma, which might be Carney triad or Carney Stratakis syndrome, lymph node dissection should be considered, because lymph node metastasis is more common in this situation. Lymph node dissection is also recommended for patients with lymph node swelling found during preoperative CT or during surgery. Because of the differences in biological behavior of such patients, the prognosis cannot be evaluated using common risk assessment criteria. Some patients, despite the presence of lymph node or liver metastasis, have a better prognosis than those with other types of GIST. However, in non-SDHB-deficient GIST, lymph node metastasis is an independent factor predicting prognosis. This patient had *KIT* exon 11 mutant GIST, which is not SDHB-deficient GIST, and not only has lymph node metastasis, but also liver metastasis. These factors indicated that targeted therapy should be actively conducted.

References

1. von Mehren M, Randall RL, Benjamin RS, Boles S, Bui MM, Ganjoo KN, George S, Gonzalez RJ, Heslin MJ, Kane JM, Keedy V, Kim E, Koon H, Mayerson J, McCarter M, McGarry SV, Meyer C, Morris ZS, O'Donnell RJ, Pappo AS, Paz IB, Petersen IA, Pfeifer JD, Riedel RF, Ruo B, Schuetze S, Tap WD, Wayne JD, Bergman MA, Scavone JL. Soft tissue sarcoma, version 2.2018, NCCN clinical practice guidelines in oncology. J Natl Compr Cancer Netw. 2018;16(5):536–63. https://doi.org/10.6004/jnccn.2018.0025.
2. Gaitanidis A, El Lakis M, Alevizakos M, Tsaroucha A, Pitiakoudis M. Predictors of lymph node metastasis in patients with gastrointestinal stromal tumors (GISTs). Langenbeck's Arch Surg. 2018;403(5):599–606. https://doi.org/10.1007/s00423-018-1683-0.
3. Demetri GD, Wang Y, Wehrle E, Racine A, Nikolova Z, Blanke CD, Joensuu H, von Mehren M. Imatinib plasma levels are correlated with clinical benefit in patients with unresectable/metastatic gastrointestinal stromal tumors. J Clin Oncol. 2009;27(19):3141–7. https://doi.org/10.1200/JCO.2008.20.4818.
4. Li J, Wang M, Zhang B, Wu X, Lin TL, Liu XF, Zhou Y, Zhang XH, Xu H, Shen LJ, Zou J, Lu P, Zhang D, Gu WJ, Zhang MX, Pan J, Cao H, Chinese Society of Surgeons for Gastrointestinal Stromal Tumor of the Chinese Medical Doctor Association. Chinese consensus on management of tyrosine kinase inhibitor-associated side effects in gastrointestinal stromal tumors. World J Gastroenterol. 2018;24(46):5189–202. https://doi.org/10.3748/wjg.v24.i46.5189.
5. Yu H, Steeghs N, Nijenhuis CM, Schellens JH, Beijnen JH, Huitema AD. Practical guidelines for therapeutic drug monitoring of anticancer tyrosine kinase inhibitors: focus on the pharmacokinetic targets. Clin Pharmacokinet. 2014;53(4):305–25. https://doi.org/10.1007/s40262-014-0137-2.
6. Verheijen RB, Yu H, Schellens JHM, Beijnen JH, Steeghs N, Huitema ADR. Practical recommendations for therapeutic drug monitoring of kinase inhibitors in oncology. Clin Pharmacol Ther. 2017;102(5):765–76. https://doi.org/10.1002/cpt.787.
7. Gao B, Yeap S, Clements A, Balakrishnar B, Wong M, Gurney H. Evidence for therapeutic drug monitoring of targeted anticancer therapies. J Clin Oncol. 2012;30(32):4017–25. https://doi.org/10.1200/JCO.2012.43.5362.

Gastrointestinal Stromal Tumors with *PDGFRA* Exon 18 D842V Mutation

15

Liwu Zeng, Peng Zhang, and Kailin Cai

Keywords

GIST · *PDGFRA* D842V mutation · Dasatinib Avapritinib

15.1 Case 21 GIST with *PDGFRA* Exon 18 D842V Mutation

Liwu Zeng and Peng Zhang

15.1.1 Introduction

The *PDGFRA* gene is located on human chromosome 4 and belongs to the type III tyrosine kinase receptor family. The D842V mutation is a point mutation in exon 18 of the activation loop domain encoded by *PDGFRA*, which will lead to abnormal *PDGFRA* structure, abnormal transmission of its downstream signal pathway, and finally lead to GIST [1]. The D842V mutation is the most common mutation of the *PDGFRA* gene [2]. Compared to other mutation types, GIST with a *PDGFRA* D842V mutation demonstrate a unique pattern of occurrence, development, and required treatment, which needs more attention from clinicians.

15.1.2 Case Background

The patient, a 55-year-old man, presented to local hospital with severe knife cutting pain in the middle abdomen and heavy feeling, with no obvious inducement on July 11, 2018. Abdominal ultrasonography performed at the local hospital showed was a huge mass shadow in the middle and upper abdominal cavity. In order to seek further treatment, the patient was admitted to the Department of gastrointestinal surgery of Union Hospital, Tongji Medical College Huazhong University of Science and Technology on July 12 for investigation of the diagnosed abdominal mass.

15.1.2.1 Past History and Family History

The patient had a 10-year history of hypertension, the highest blood pressure was about 170/90 mmHg, but this was well controlled with medicine. Tonsillectomy was performed to treat tonsillitis 30 years previously. There was no history of blood transfusion, and the patient reported no food or drug allergies. The patient's parents were deceased and there was no similar medical history in the family.

15.1.2.2 Physical Examination

The patient has an acute ill-looking, pale skin and sclera, no jaundice, no swelling of superficial lymph nodes, and no swelling of the lower limbs. The abdomen was full, with visible surgical scars, no varicose veins, no gastrointestinal shape, or peristaltic wave. The abdomen was slightly hard, with tenderness but no rebound pain. A large mass with irregular shape was palpated in the middle and upper abdomen. The texture was slightly hard, the size was difficult to estimate, and the mobility is poor. The liver and spleen could not be touched beneath the ribs. The patient exhibited no Murphy sign or mobile dullness. Bowel sounds were heard about six times/min.

15.1.2.3 Auxiliary Examination

Blood Routine WBC 11.87 × 10^9/L ↑, RBC 4.42 × 10^9/L, Hb 151 g/L, PLT 220 × 10^9/L, NEUT% 71.6%, LY% 19.4%.

Blood Biochemistry Fasting blood glucose was 6.91 mmol/L ↑, TP and ALB levels were normal, and liver and kidney function and electrolytes were normal.

L. Zeng · P. Zhang (✉) · K. Cai
Department of Gastrointestinal Surgery, Union Hospital, Tongji Medical College, Huazhong University of Science and Technology, Wuhan, China
e-mail: zhangpengwh@hust.edu.cn; caikailin@hust.edu.cn

K. Tao, H. Cao (eds.), *Clinical Management of Gastrointestinal Stromal Tumor*, https://doi.org/10.1007/978-981-99-9392-5_15

High Sensitivity C-Reactive Protein 29.54 mg/L ↑.

Tumor Markers Carbohydrate antigen 72–4 9.93 U/mL ↑, no other abnormalities were detected.

Coagulation Function No abnormality.

CTA of Abdominal Aorta (1) Mild atherosclerosis of abdominal aorta. Calcified and non-calcified plaques were detected in the main abdominal aorta, and the lumen was slightly narrowed. The main branches (celiac trunk, superior mesenteric artery and renal artery) were not significantly narrowed or locally dilated. (2) A heterogeneous mass was seen on the greater curvature of the gastric body, approximately 12.4 cm × 5.9 cm × 16.4 cm in size, with an unclear boundary with gastric body. The left, right gastric and right gastroepiploic arteries seem to send out branches to supply blood to the above mass. In the arterial phase, tortuous and thickened blood vessels could be seen in the mass, which was connected to the right gastric vein. The right gastric vein was thickened, and the portal vein was early, suggesting an arteriovenous fistula.

Total Abdominal and Pelvic Contrast-Enhanced CT (1) An irregular soft tissue mass was identified in the middle and upper abdominal cavity, approximately 12.4 cm × 5.9 cm × 16.4 cm in size. The enhancement scan showed obvious uneven enhancement. The left gastric artery, right gastric artery, and right gastroepiploic artery seemed to send out branches to supply blood to the above mass. In the arterial phase, tortuous and thickened blood vessels were seen within the mass and these were connected to the right gastric artery. The right gastric vein was thickened, and the portal vein appeared early, suggesting an arteriovenous fistula. The boundary between the local part of the mass and the gastric wall on the greater curvature of the stomach and the adjacent intestinal canal was unclear, the surrounding fat space was clear, and no obvious enlarged lymph nodes were observed. The above image characteristics are mostly considered as neoplastic lesions, possible GIST. (2) No obvious abnormal density shadows were found in the liver, gallbladder, spleen, pancreas, or kidneys. (3) The sigmoid colon was excessively long. (4) The bladder was well filled and the wall was smooth; (5) No obvious enlarged lymph nodes were found in the abdominal cavity or retroperitoneum (Fig. 15.1).

Electronic Gastroscope Scattered erosion was apparent at the bottom of the stomach, multiple erosion was seen in the gastric antrum, and no other obvious abnormalities were detected (Fig. 15.2).

Electronic Colonoscopy No obvious abnormalities were found.

15.1.2.4 Preliminary Diagnosis

1. Abdominal mass: possible stomach GIST
2. Hypertension, grade II, very high risk
3. Mild atherosclerosis of abdominal aorta
4. Superficial erosive gastritis

15.1.3 Therapy

15.1.3.1 Case Analysis

The patient was a middle-aged man who was experiencing acute knife-like abdominal pain. He had a history of hypertension for more than 10 years and needed to be vigilant regarding possible abdominal aortic aneurysm. After admission, he underwent emergency abdominal CTA, which ruled out the possibility of a ruptured abdominal aortic aneurysm. Abdominal contrast-enhanced CT showed that there was a mass of approximately 12.4 cm × 5.9 cm × 16.4 cm in the upper abdominal cavity, closely related to the stomach, considered to be GIST. Electronic gastroscopy identified only partial erosion in the gastric cavity. It was recommended that a biopsy be taken to clarify the nature of the lesion, but this was rejected by the patient.

The mass was located on the greater curvature of the stomach. Although it was large, it did not invade the surrounding organs. After evaluation, it was expected that the mass could be completely removed, and the risk of serious complications after resection was low. Therefore, the patient agreed to surgical resection. Since the patient had Rh-negative blood, known as "panda blood" in China, and the blood type is relatively rare, it was decided that surgery should be performed as soon as possible after full preparation to avoid bleeding and dissemination caused by tumor rupture. After surgical resection of the tumor, adjuvant targeted therapy was guided by the results of pathological examination and gene detection.

15.1.3.2 Treatment

After adequate preoperative preparation, laparotomy was performed on July 20, 2018. During the operation, severe intra-abdominal adhesion was found, and a cystic solid mass size of approximately 16 cm × 18 cm was visible in the upper abdomen. The mass was irregularly shaped, and closely related to the greater curvature of the gastric antrum and the greater omentum but did not invade other organs. After loosening the intra-abdominal adhesions and fully exposing the mass, partial gastrectomy was performed to completely

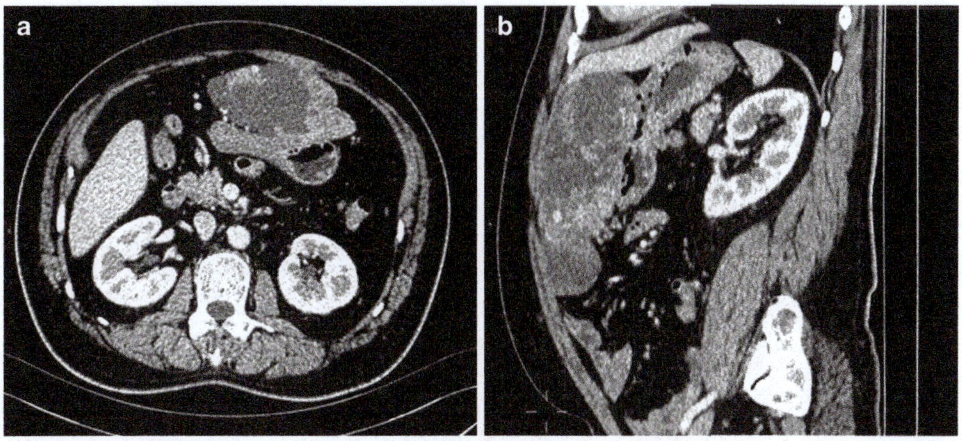

Fig. 15.1 Enhanced CT at the time of initial diagnosis. **a** Horizontal view; **b** Sagittal view

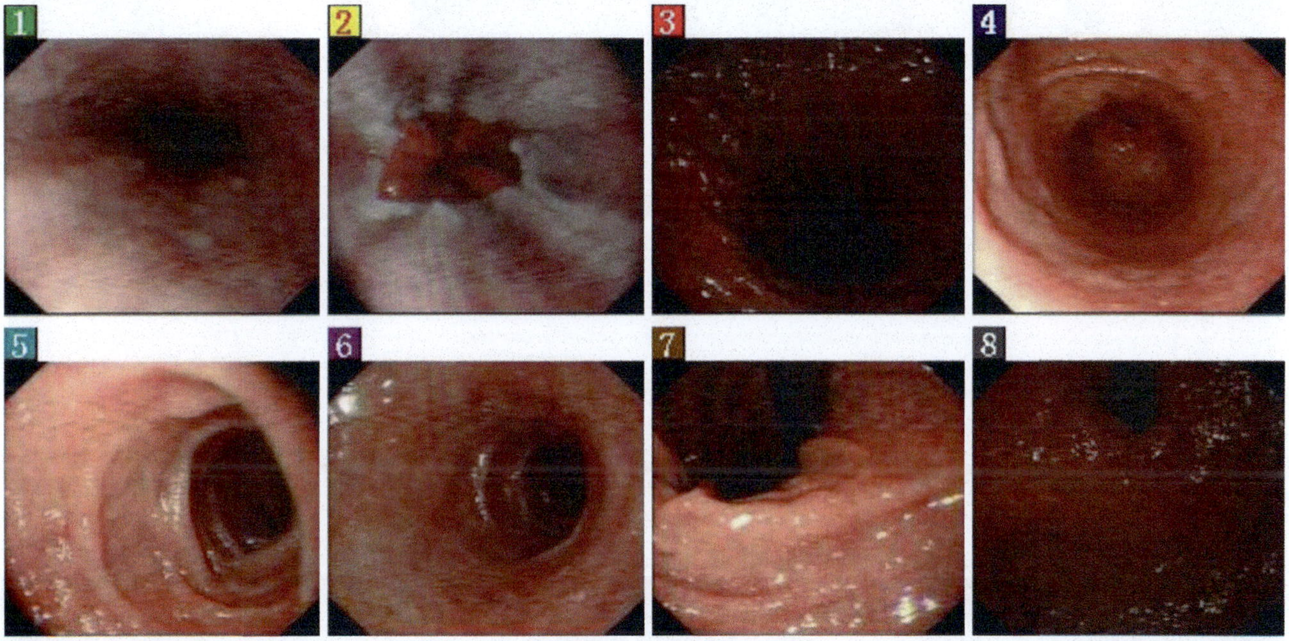

Fig. 15.2 Represented photograph of the electronic gastroscope

remove the mass. The intraoperative bleeding was approximately 50 mL, and the operation process was smooth. (Fig. 15.3).

15.1.3.3 Postoperative Pathology and Genetic Testing

Pathological Diagnosis Stomach GIST with cystic changes. The cell morphology was epithelioid cell spindle cell mixed type. The maximum diameter of the tumor was 19 cm, mitotic count 0–1/50HPF, and the modified NIH risk grade was high risk. No tumor cells were present at the surgical margin.

Immunohistochemistry CD117 (−), CD34 (+), DOG-1 (+), SMA (−), S-100 (−), SDHB (+), Ki-67 (Li < 2%).

Genetic Testing Exon 18 of *PDGFRA* was mutated, and the mutation type was c.2525a > t (p.D842V). (Fig. 15.4).

15.1.4 Prognosis

The patient recovered smoothly and was discharged on the 10th postoperative day. Dasatinib 50 mg/d was prescribed at the time of discharge. Mild periorbital edema occurred during the administration of dasatinib, which was tolerated by the patient. To January 2022, the patient had been followed up for 42 months, and there were no signs of tumor recurrence or metastasis (Fig. 15.5).

15.1.5 Experience of Diagnosis and Therapy

About 5–10% of GIST exhibit mutations in *PDGFRA*, and the D842V mutation is the most common [2]. Most patients with *PDGFRA* D842V mutation also present with a CD117 positive molecular phenotype, but a few show a weak positive, partial positive or negative result in CD117 testing. The

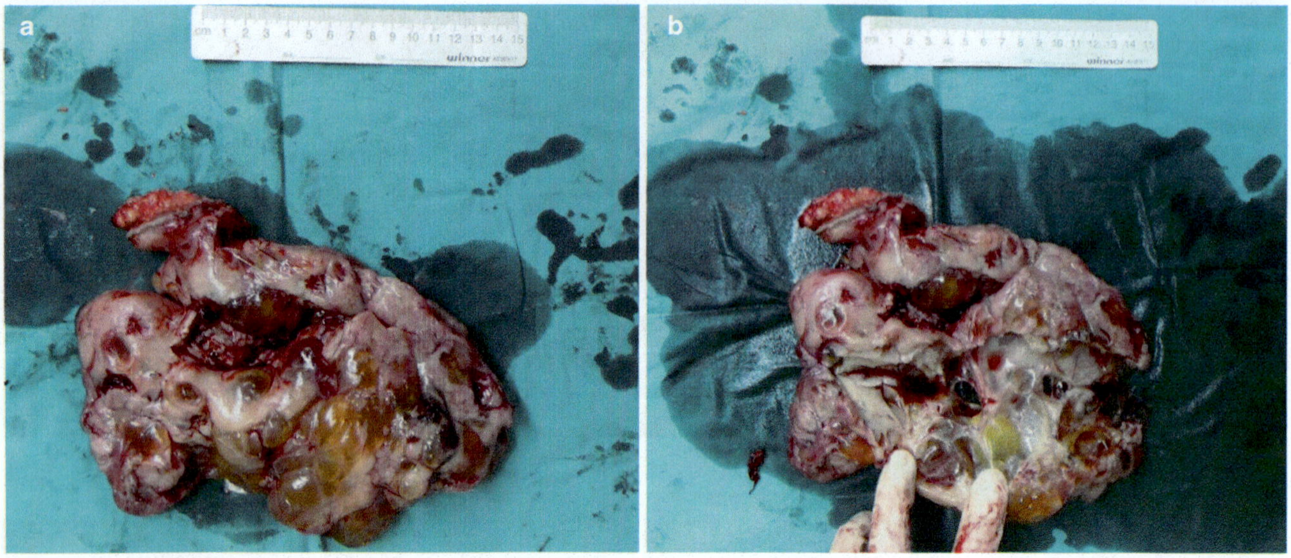

Fig. 15.3 The gross specimen. **a** Before incision; **b** After incision

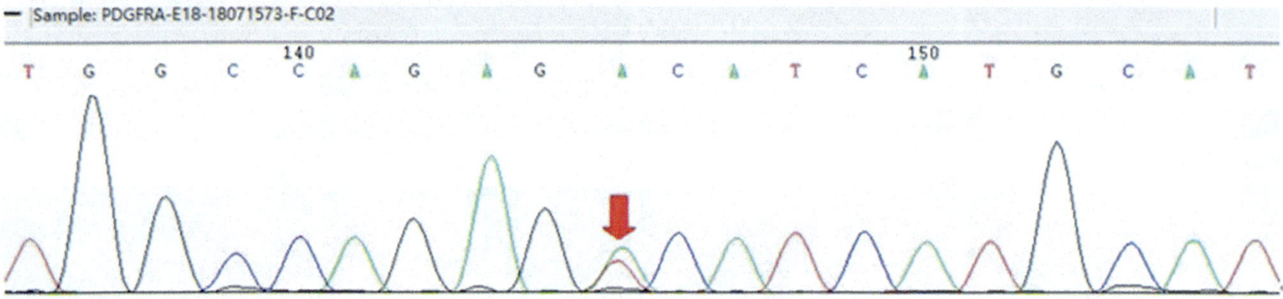

Fig. 15.4 Results of Sanger sequencing

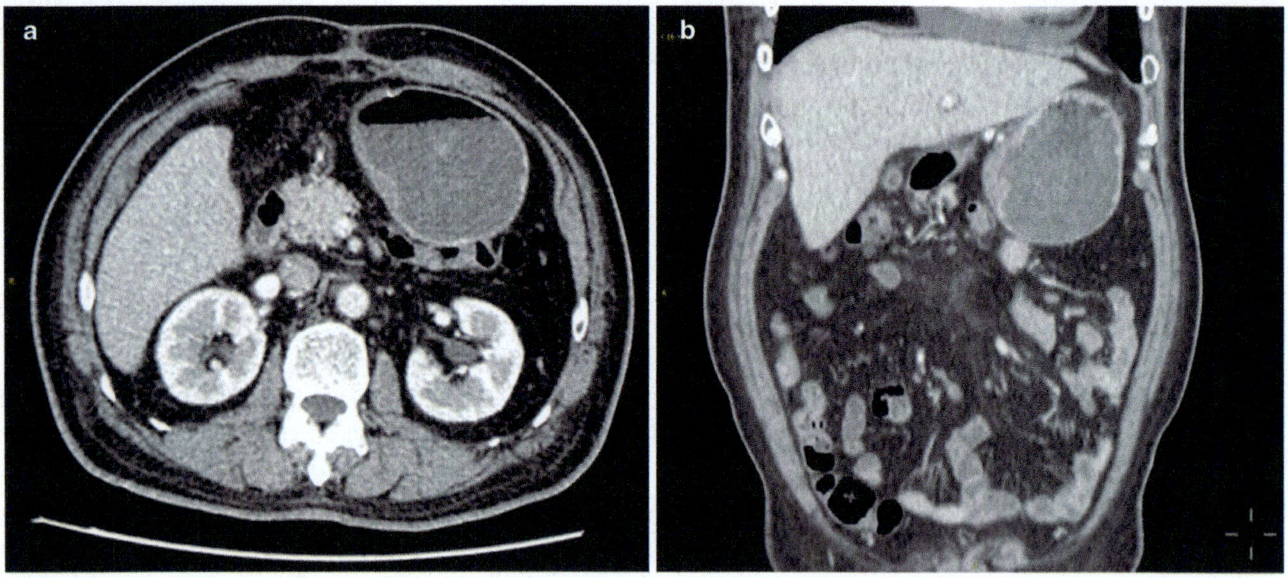

Fig. 15.5 Enhance CT at the follow-up. **a** Horizontal view; **b** Sagittal view

latest released ESMO/EURACAN Clinical Practice Guidelines and Consensus on the Diagnosis and Treatment of GIST in China indicate that *KIT/PDGFRA* mutation detection is recommended for patients with CD117 (−) and DOG-1 (+) to achieve a clear diagnosis. The patient's post-operative pathological immunohistochemistry showed CD117 (−) and DOG-1 (+). In order to further clarify the diagnosis and guide postoperative targeted therapy, genetic testing was recommended. Finally, a D842V mutation in exon 18 of *PDGFRA* was confirmed.

The *PDGFRA* D842V mutation cause a conformational change in the activation ring of the tyrosine kinase receptor, so that imatinib cannot bind and thereby inhibiting its activity [2]. Therefore, patients with this type of mutation are resistant to imatinib therapy. Guidelines in China and Western countries indicate that imatinib is not recommended for postoperative adjuvant treatment of patients with *PDGFRA* D842V mutation. Dasatinib is a second-generation oral Bcr-Abl tyrosine kinase inhibitor that can effectively inhibit BCR-ABL and SRC gene families encoding tyrosine kinase and can also inhibit *KIT* and *PDGFRA* [3]. It was approved by China National Medical Products Administration (NMPA) in 2012. Dasatinib has been applied for patients with chronic myeloid leukemia who were resistant or intolerable to imatinib in all stages (chronic stage, accelerated stage, lymphoid cell blast stage or myeloid cell blast stage) [4]. In this case, high-risk recurrence was determined by pathological diagnosis. Given the fact that there is no recommended targeted therapy for GIST with *PDGFRA* D842V mutation at that time and the patient had a strong desire for dasatinib treatment. The patient was scheduled with dasatinib treatment and was relapse-free at the 9-month follow-up.

In recent years, great progress has been achieved in research of targeted drugs for *PDGFRA* D842V mutation. Avapritinib is a high-specific *KIT* and *PDGFRA* tyrosine kinase inhibitor that can bind to active conformation loop of downstream signaling of *KIT* and *PDGFRA* [5]. The US FDA approved avapritinib for treating *PDGFRA* exon 18 mutation, including adult patients with unresectable or metastatic *PDGFRA* exon 18 mutations GIST in 2020 [6]. Subsequently, avapritinib was recommended as first-line therapy for unresectable/metastatic GIST with *PDGFRA* exon 18 mutations according to the NCCN Guidelines (v2021). Furthermore, avapritinib was recommended as neoadjuvant therapy for resectable GIST with *PDGFRA* exon 18 mutations, including the D842V mutation. Avapritinib was approved by China NMPA in March 2021, and was recommended in CSCO Guidelines.

15.2 Expert Comments

Kailin Cai

D842V mutation is the most common form of *PDGFRA* mutation, accounting for approximately 60% of all *PDGFRA* mutations [2]. Different from GIST with *KIT* mutation, D842V mutant GIST almost exclusively occurs in the stomach. Tumor cells usually show epithelioid morphology and a low mitotic count. Moreover, patients with primary D842V mutation are resistant to TKI drugs; therefore, these patients do not benefit from targeted therapy with drugs such as imatinib. The molecular mechanism of drug resistance in patients with D842V mutation is not very clear. At present, the preferred treatment strategy for GIST patients with D842V mutation is surgical complete resection, and postoperative imatinib adjuvant treatment is not recommended. Avapritinib, a new *KIT/PDGFRA* inhibitor, has achieved excellent efficacy in the treatment of unresectable GIST with *PDGFRA* D842V mutation, and is recommended as a first-line therapy for the treatment of unresectable D842V mutation GIST by NCCN and CSCO Guidelines. Avapritinib provides an effective and safe treatment and opens a new era of precision medicine for GIST based on genetic testing [5]. Therefore, physician should attach great importance to genetic testing of GIST to schedule precise therapy for patients. Further research is needed to explore whether avapritinb should be provided as adjuvant therapy for complete surgical resection GIST with *PDGFRA* exon 18 mutations.

References

1. Rizzo A, Pantaleo MA, Astolfi A, Indio V, Nannini M. The identity of PDGFRA D842V-mutant gastrointestinal stromal tumors (GIST). Cancers (Basel). 2021;13(4):705–12. https://doi.org/10.3390/cancers13040705.
2. Corless CL, Schroeder A, Griffith D, Town A, McGreevey L, Harrell P, Shiraga S, Bainbridge T, Morich J, Heinrich MC. PDGFRA mutations in gastrointestinal stromal tumors: frequency, spectrum and in vitro sensitivity to imatinib. J Clin Oncol. 2005;23(23):5357–64. https://doi.org/10.1200/JCO.2005.14.068.
3. Zhou Y, Zhang X, Wu X, Zhou Y, Zhang B, Liu X, Wu X, Li Y, Shen L, Li J. A prospective multicenter phase II study on the efficacy and safety of dasatinib in the treatment of metastatic gastrointestinal stromal tumors failed by imatinib and sunitinib and analysis of NGS in peripheral blood. Cancer Med. 2020;9(17):6225–33. https://doi.org/10.1002/cam4.3319.
4. Abbott BL. Dasatinib: from treatment of imatinib-resistant or -intolerant patients with chronic myeloid leukemia to treatment of patients with newly diagnosed chronic phase chronic myeloid leukemia. Clin Ther. 2012;34(2):272–81. https://doi.org/10.1016/j.clinthera.2012.01.009.

5. Heinrich MC, Jones RL, von Mehren M, Schöffski P, Serrano C, Kang YK, Cassier PA, Mir O, Eskens F, Tap WD, Rutkowski P, Chawla SP, Trent J, Tugnait M, Evans EK, Lauz T, Zhou T, Roche M, Wolf BB, Bauer S, George S. Avapritinib in advanced PDGFRA D842V-mutant gastrointestinal stromal tumour (NAVIGATOR): a multicentre, open-label, phase 1 trial. Lancet Oncol. 2020;21(7):935–46. https://doi.org/10.1016/S1470-2045(20)30269-2.
6. Dhillon S. Avapritinib: first approval. Drugs. 2020;80(4):433–9. https://doi.org/10.1007/s40265-020-01275-2.

16 Multiple Gastrointestinal Stromal Tumors

Peng Zhang, Yuan Yin, Xinyu Zeng, Qun Zhao, and Jun Zhang

Keywords

Gastrointestinal stromal tumors · Multiple · Surgery

16.1 Case 22 An 80-Year-Old Man with Multiple Primary Sporadic GISTs

Peng Zhang and Yuan Yin

16.1.1 Introduction

GIST is generally found as a single tumor, and multiple GISTs are usually seen in familial GISTs or in some syndromes, such as NF1 and Carney syndrome. Multiple primary sporadic GISTs are relatively rare, sometimes difficult to detect with preoperative imaging examination or endoscopy, and there may be missed diagnosis or misdiagnosis. Therefore, attention should be paid to the possibility of multiple GIST in clinic. In addition, the pathogenesis and pathological risk classification schemes for multiple GIST are still inconclusive, and treatment is controversial. Here, we will share our experience in the diagnosis and treatment of two patients with primary multiple sporadic GIST from the perspectives of clinical manifestations, relevant examinations, surgical treatment, and pathological diagnosis.

16.1.2 Case Background

The patient, an 80-year-old man, had suffered from repeated melena over the past 1 month without obvious inducement, accompanied by mild abdominal pain, bloating, but no hematemesis. The patient's symptoms were slightly relieved after taking stomach medicine. Yesterday, the patient experienced melena again. The patient visited the Department of Gastrointestinal Surgery of West China Hospital for investigation and treatment of upper gastrointestinal bleeding.

16.1.2.1 Past History and Family History

No special medical history, and no family history of tumor.

16.1.2.2 Physical Examination

The patient's vital signs were stable, and the abdomen was full, soft, without rebound tenderness. There was no palpable mass in the abdomen, and no edema in the lower limbs.

16.1.2.3 Auxiliary Examination

Abdominal Enhanced CT Two mass shadows with mixed density, approximately 5 and 3 cm in size, were observed in the gastric cardia and body, respectively. The enhanced scan of the two masses showed uneven enhancement, and the masses were considered to be GISTs (Fig. 16.1).

Laboratory Examination Hb 85 g/L↓, Na^+ 126.3 mmol/L↓, K^+ 2.93 mmol/L↓, Cl^- 95.6 mmol/L↓, C-reactive protein 75.30 mg/L↑, total prostate specific antigen 39.150 ng/mL↑, others were within the normal range.

P. Zhang · X. Zeng
Department of Gastrointestinal Surgery, Union Hospital, Tongji Medical College, Huazhong University of Science and Technology, Wuhan, China
e-mail: zhangpengwh@hust.edu.cn; zengxy@hust.edu.cn

Y. Yin (✉)
Department of Gastrointestinal Surgery, West China Hospital, Sichuan University, Chengdu, China
e-mail: yinyuan10@wchscu.cn

Q. Zhao (✉)
Department of General Surgery, The Fourth Hospital of Hebei Medical University, Shijiazhuang, China
e-mail: zhaoqun@hebmu.edu.cn

J. Zhang
Department of Gastrointestinal Surgery, The First Affiliated Hospital of Chongqing Medical University, Chongqing, China

K. Tao, H. Cao (eds.), *Clinical Management of Gastrointestinal Stromal Tumor*, https://doi.org/10.1007/978-981-99-9392-5_16

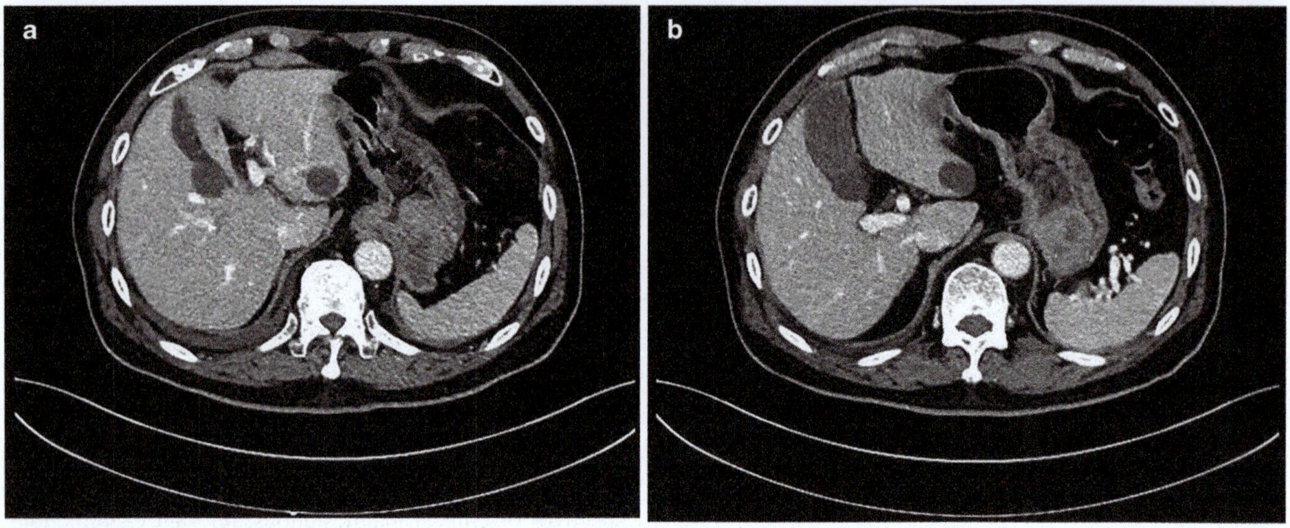

Fig. 16.1 Preoperative abdominal CT images of gastric tumors. **a** Fundus and Cardia of stomach, **b** Body of stomach

16.1.2.4 Preliminary Diagnosis

1. Multiple stomach masses: possible GIST
2. Moderate anemia
3. Hypokalemia

16.1.3 Therapy

16.1.3.1 Case Analysis

The patient was an elderly man with repeated melena in the past month. Abdominal CT examination revealed tumors in the cardia and gastric body. From the CT examination, the possibility of GIST was considered surgical removal was needed. It was recommended that the patient undergo surgical resection of the gastric mass to clarify the nature of the tumor and guide postoperative treatment. The patient was in poor condition, and it was determined that anemia and the water-electrolyte imbalance should be corrected, relevant preoperative examination should be performed.

16.1.3.2 Treatment

After completing preoperative preparation, the patient underwent open radical gastrectomy under general anesthesia. Intraoperative findings were the following: no ascites in the abdominal cavity, smooth pelvic peritoneum, cysts in the liver, no solid nodules, no abnormalities in the pancreas or spleen, and no abnormalities in the small intestine or mesangium. Two large masses, from the gastric cardia near great curvature and anterior wall of body, were observed, with diameters of 5 cm × 4 cm × 4 cm and 3 cm × 3 cm × 3 cm. The masses originated from the submucosa of the gastric wall and grew into and out of the gastric cavity in the shape of dumbbell. There were normal gastric wall tissue intervals between the two tumors (Fig. 16.2). The tumor was completely resected with a 2 cm margin. Intraoperative fast frozen pathology revealed a gastric spindle cell tumor. In addition, an exogenous nodule with a diameter of 1 cm was also observed on the serosal surface of the gastric wall, which was removed (Fig. 16.3). The operation went well. Parenteral nutrition, fasting, fluid replacement, and other symptomatic supportive treatment were given after the operation. The patient recovered well and was discharged smoothly.

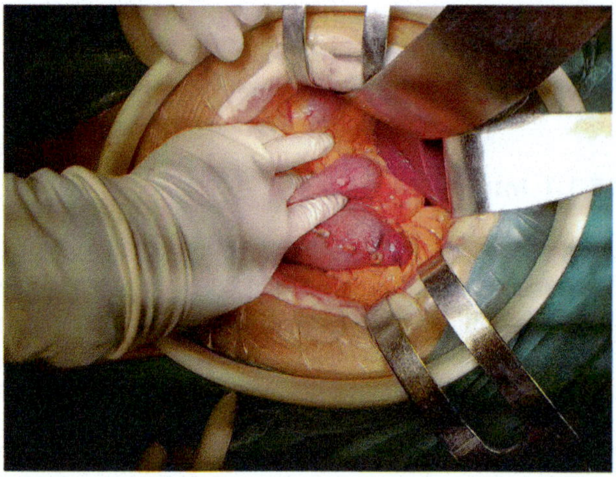

Fig. 16.2 Intraoperative findings

16.1.3.3 Postoperative Pathology and Genetic Testing

Pathological Diagnosis All three tumors were GIST. Tumor 1 was 5.2 cm × 4.5 cm × 3.0 cm in size, mitotic count 3/50HPF, spindle cell type, and large necrosis was seen in the tumor. Tumor 2 was 3.5 cm × 2.5 cm × 2.0 cm in size, mitotic count 6/50HPF, epithelial cell type. Tumor 3 was approximately 0.6 cm × 0.5 cm × 0.4 cm in size, mitotic count 1/50 HPF, epithelial cell type. Modified NIH recur-

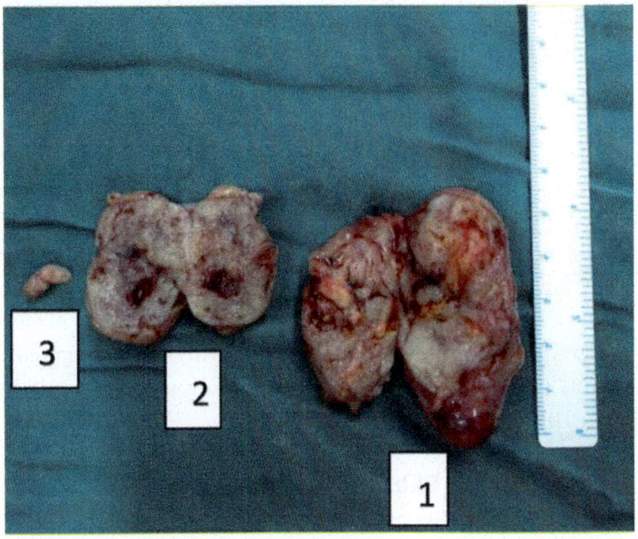

Fig. 16.3 The gross specimens

rence risk classification for tumors 1 and 2 was intermediate risk, and tumor 3 was very low risk.

Immunohistochemistry CD117 (+), DOG-1 (+), VIM (+), SMA (−), SDHB (+), Caldesmon (+), DES (−), S-100 (−), Ki-67 (Li: about 10%).

Genetic Testing Heterozygous mutation in exon 11 of *KIT*, mutation type c.1734_1735insCAATAT. Exons 9, 13, and 17 of *KIT* and exons 12 and 18 of *PDGFRA* were wild type.

16.1.4 Prognosis

The patient received adjuvant treatment with imatinib after surgery, and no signs of recurrence or metastasis were found up to the last follow-up (10 months after surgery).

16.1.5 Experience of Diagnosis and Therapy

The onset of GIST has no specific symptoms. Most patients seek medical treatment for common gastrointestinal symptoms such as abdominal distension, abdominal pain, and gastrointestinal bleeding. Complete tumor resection is the main treatment and diagnosis method for GIST and imatinib treatment has greatly improved the prognosis of GIST. Generally, GIST are found as single tumors, and sporadic multifocal GIST is rare [1]. The clinical symptoms and treatment of multiple GIST are the same as those for general single GIST. At present, the pathogenesis of primary multiple GIST is still unclear. According to the different disease manifestations, primary multiple GIST can be divided into three categories: (1) Familial multiple GIST, such GIST with a clear family history. These are mostly caused by embryonal mutations, and are characterized by young onset, mostly small intestinal GIST, and are accompanied by intestinal Cajal cell proliferation [2]. (2) NF1 and Carney triad related GIST. These GISTs usually have no mutation in *KIT* or *PDGFRA*, and the expression of CD34, CD117 and DOG-1 was negative by immunohistochemistry [3]. (3) Primary multiple sporadic GIST, generally caused by somatic mutations. The clinical manifestations are generally the same as solitary GIST, and these are mostly found in elderly patients. Based on the medical history, physical examination, and pathological results, the patient was given a preliminary diagnosis of multiple sporadic GIST, which is common in the stomach and small intestine, or both locations. The pathology of this patient was particularly special. The cell morphology of tumor 1 was different from that of tumor 2 and 3. The former was spindle cell type, while the latter two were epithelial cell type. Different cell morphology suggests different cytological origins of tumor. Unfortunately, we have not yet obtained the results of multiple tumor gene tests of this patient. Currently, there is no unified pathological risk classification for primary multiple GIST in clinic. The modified NIH and AFIP classification do not specify a pathological risk classification standard for multiple GIST, and final risk is generally taken as that of the tumor with highest risk classification in clinical practice [4, 5].

In practice, multiple GISTs are usually diagnosed by exclusion. The first step is to determine if the patient has primary metastasis, and then make a final diagnosis based on the clinical characteristics of the GIST and the pathological results. At present, complete surgical resection of the tumor is still the main treatment method for multiple GIST. At the same time, the postoperative risk grade is used to determine whether patients should receive adjuvant treatment with imatinib.

16.2 Case 23 Primary Multiple Sporadic GIST

Xinyu Zeng and Qun Zhao

16.2.1 Case Background

The patient, a 49-year-old man, was admitted to the Fourth Affiliated Hospital of Hebei Medical University on May 15, 2017, for investigation of a stomach mass found in physical examination 14 days previously. The patient reported no acid reflux, heartburn, nausea, vomiting, abdominal pain, or diarrhea. Gastroscopy diagnosis: An eminence lesion was found at the fundus of stomach, possibly as GIST. Endoscopic ultrasound showed that there was an obvious bulge of about

1.5 cm in diameter at the gastric fundus, the mucosa was intact, and the upper margin was about 4–5 cm away from the dentate line. In the fourth layer, there is a well-defined circular hypoechoic circle, approximately 15.6 mm × 9.9 mm in size. A hyperechoic spot could be seen in the center, blood flow signals could be seen, and elastic imaging showed that the mass was hard. Full-abdominal enhanced CT revealed soft tissue nodules in the fundus of the stomach, which were possible gastric GIST and multiple small cysts on the top of the liver. For further diagnosis and treatment, the patient was admitted to the hospital with the diagnosis of a gastric fundus mass.

16.2.1.1 Past History and Family History

Previously healthy, the patient reported no history of surgery, trauma, or food and drug allergies. The patient's father died due to cerebral infarction, and the patient's mother was alive.

16.2.1.2 Physical Examination

The patient's vital signs were stable, cardiopulmonary examination showed no obvious abnormalities. The abdomen was flat, with no observable gastrointestinal or peristaltic waves. The abdomen was soft, with no rebound tenderness, and there were no palpable masses in the abdomen. There was no shifting dullness and bowel sounds were normal.

16.2.1.3 Auxiliary Examination

Endoscopic Ultrasound The gastric cavity was empty, the fundus of the stomach was visibly uplifted by approximately 1.5 cm, the mucosa was intact, and the upper distance from the dentate line was about 4–5 cm. Ultrasound: 7.5–12 MHZ explores the first 1–3 layers of the lesion to be continuous and complete. In the fourth layer, there was a circular hypoechoic circle with a clear boundary, approximately 15.6 mm × 9.9 mm in size. A hyperechoic spot could be seen in the center, blood flow signals could be seen, and elastic imaging showed that it was hard. Gastroscopy diagnosis: fundus mass in muscle layer (considering as gastric GIST) (Fig. 16.4).

Full-Abdominal Enhanced CT Soft tissue nodules were visible in the fundus of the stomach, considered to be possible gastric GIST. Multiple small cysts were observed on the top of the liver (Fig. 16.5).

Blood Routine WBC 3.85 × 10^9/L, NEUT 2.35 × 10^9/L, RBC 4.46 × 10^{12}, Hb 144.2 g/L, PLT 165 × 10^9/L.

Blood Biochemistry ALP 38.8 U/L, but no other abnormalities were detected.

Urine and Stool Routine There were no abnormalities detected.

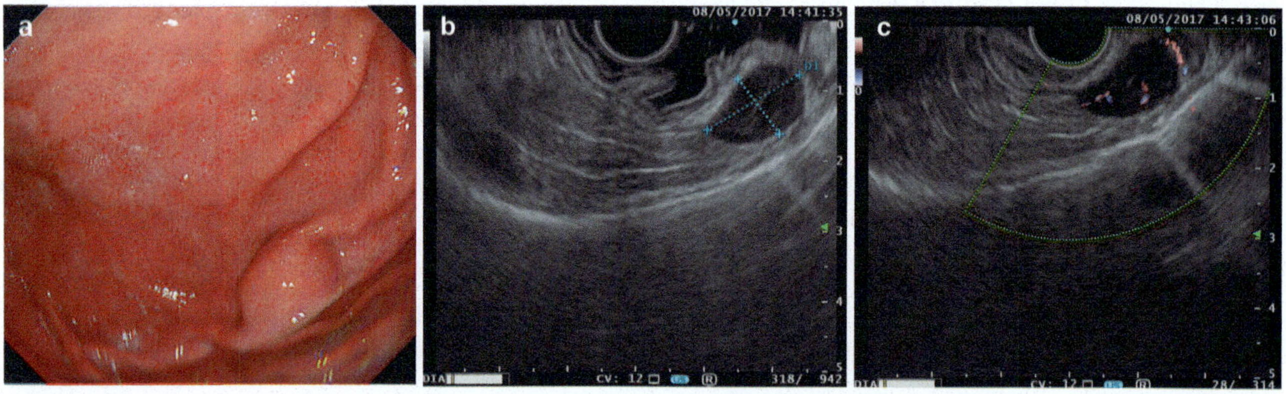

Fig. 16.4 Ultrasound gastroscopy. **a** Tumor under gastroscopy. **b, c** Tumor under ultrasound gastroscopy

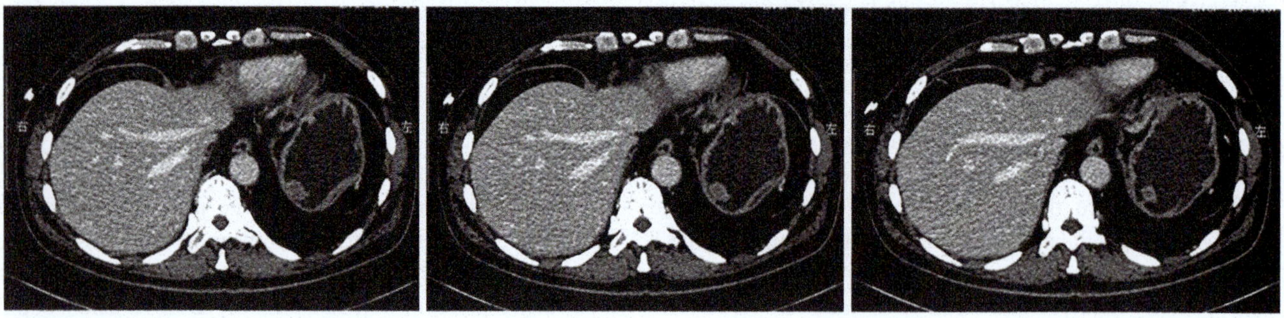

Fig. 16.5 Abdominal enhanced CT

Heart Color Doppler Ultrasound No obvious abnormalities were observed in the shape, structure, or function of the heart.

Lung Function No abnormalities were detected.

16.2.1.4 Preliminary Diagnosis

1. Gastric fundus mass: possible GIST
2. Multiple cysts in the liver

16.2.2 Therapy

16.2.2.1 Case Analysis

The patient was a middle-aged man who was admitted to the hospital with a "stomach mass found in physical examination for 14 days." On admission, it was diagnosed as gastric fundus mass, approximately 15.6 mm × 9.9 mm in size. Considering the possibility of small gastric GIST, and the presence of uneven mass echoes on ultrasound gastroscopy, and adverse factors, surgical resection should be considered. The patient was generally in good health and no obvious abnormalities were found in cardiopulmonary function assessments. The ECOG score was 1 point. Laparoscopic resection of gastric fundus mass was considered feasible. Considering the small size of the tumor, intraoperative gastroscopy was prepared, so that this technique could be used to locate the tumor under intraoperative endoscopy if necessary. Further therapeutic schedule would be determined by pathological diagnosis.

16.2.2.2 Treatment

A 3D laparoscopic wedge-resection of gastric fundus mass and part of gastric wall was performed on May 19, 2017. The intraoperative findings were as follows: No obvious metastatic nodules were found in the exploration of the abdomen and pelvis, the mass was located in the greater curvature of the anterior wall of the fundus of the stomach, and was approximately 1.5 cm × 1 cm in size. The fundus of the stomach was freed, and another mass was found in the great curvature of the posterior wall of the fundus of the stomach, this was approximately 0.5 cm in size (Fig. 16.6). The remaining gastric wall was fully explored laparoscopically, and no other masses were found. The two masses were completely removed with a straight intraluminal cutting and closing device (Fig. 16.7). The gastric cavity was carefully examined under gastroscopy during the operation, and no other masses were seen.

16.2.2.3 Postoperative Pathology and Genetic Testing

Postoperative Pathology Mass on the anterior wall of the stomach: the stomach tissue and mass tissue was 4 cm × 3 cm × 1.5 cm in total, and a 1.5 cm × 1 cm × 1 cm mass was observed after incision, with brittle gray matter on the cut surface. Immunohistochemistry: CD34 (+), CD117 (+), DOG-1 (+), desmin (−), Act (−), Ki-67 (Li: 2%), S100 (−), Vim (+), mitotic count <5/50 HPF.

Mass on the posterior wall of the stomach: The stomach tissue and the tumor tissue section was 3.5 cm × 2.5 cm × 1 cm in total, and a nodule with a diameter of approximately 0.6 cm was observed after incision, with brittle gray matter on the cut surface. Immunohistochemistry: CD34 (+), CD117 (+), DOG-1 (+), desmin (−), Act (−), Ki-67 (Li: 2%), S100 (−), Vim (+), mitotic count 3/50 HPF.

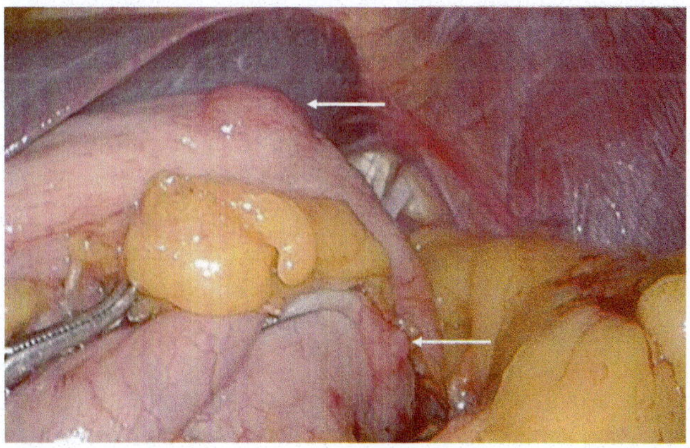

Fig. 16.6 Intraoperative tumor location

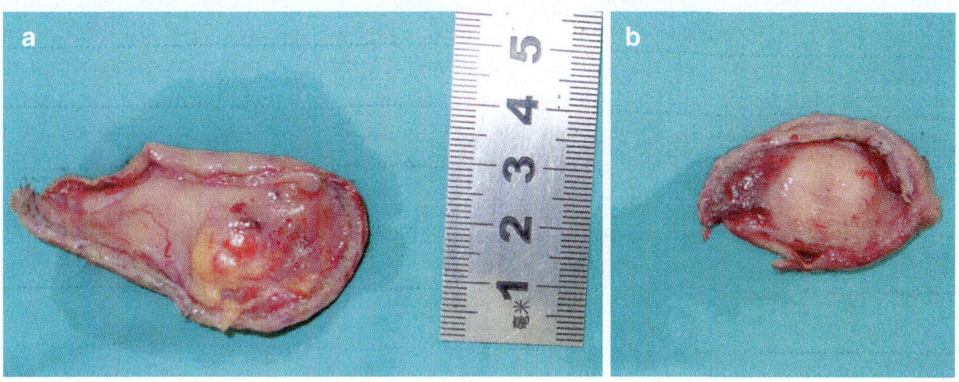

Fig. 16.7 The gross specimen of the resected tumor. **a** Posterior stomach wall mass, **b** Anterior stomach wall mass

Genetic Testing Heterozygous mutation in exon 11 of *KIT*, mutation type is c.1742_1743insCCCAACACAACTTCCTT ATGATCACAA (p.H580_K581insNPTQLPYDH). Exons 9, 13, and 17 of *KIT* and exons 12 and 18 of *PDGFRA* were wild type.

16.2.3 Prognosis

The patient recovered well and was discharged on the 4th postoperative day. The patient's condition was diagnosed as double-focal gastric GIST, very low risk. According to the Chinese Consensus on Diagnosis and Treatment of Gastrointestinal Stromal Tumors (2013 edition), the tumors were classified as very low risk, and no adjuvant imatinib treatment was required after surgery. As of September 2019, 28-month follow-up, no signs of recurrence or metastasis were found.

16.2.4 Experience of Diagnosis and Therapy

16.2.4.1 Does Small Gastric GIST Need Surgery? If Surgery Is Required, How to Choose the Surgical Method?

Currently, surgery is the main treatment for GIST [6]. Surgical treatment is still the first choice for localized stromal tumors with a diameter of >2 cm originating from the stomach. For small gastric GIST with diameter ≤2 cm, the indications for different surgical methods are still controversial. Some scholars believe that most small gastric GISTs have a benign clinical process, which can be observed regularly and do not require radical surgery. Other scholars believe that small gastric GIST may be malignant. Once discovered, early surgical treatment is recommended [7]. The NCCN guidelines point out that gastric GIST with a diameter of <2 cm, but in the presence of unregular borders, ulceration, strong echoes, heterogeneity, and other adverse factors, resection should be considered; if there are no adverse factors, the patient can be regularly reviewed with ultrasound endoscopy [8]. However, ESMO recommends surgical resection even for gastric GIST with a maximum diameter of <2 cm. Based on a retrospective study of 90 cases of gastric GIST, one author believed that early detection and timely intervention for gastric GIST not only has the advantages of minimal trauma and swift recovery, but can also effectively reduce the recurrence of GIST after surgery and improve patient prognosis [9]. Early radical surgical intervention is an ideal and reasonable treatment for small gastric GIST. Through a retrospective study of 63 cases of gastric GIST, Zhang Hongwei et al. from Xijing Digestive Disease Hospital suggested that small gastric GIST have malignant potential and recommended surgical resection following GIST diagnosis [10].

The dispute between serosal surgery and mucosal surgery in small GIST has been ongoing for a long time. The detection rate of small gastric GIST under endoscopy is gradually increasing, and with the rapid development of endoscopic treatment technology, endoscopists have been able to achieve full-thickness resection of gastric wall masses, and some gastric GIST can be directly removed endoscopically to avoid surgery. However, the characteristics of GIST determine that it originates in the muscularis propria of the stomach, which makes GIST far more difficult to treat than mucosal lesions. Insufficient resection may lead to tumor damage and a high incidence of perforation. Severe bleeding perforation may endanger the lives of patients. Therefore, the Chinese Consensus on Diagnosis and Treatment of Gastrointestinal Stromal Tumors (2017 Edition) did not recommend routine endoscopic treatment of GIST [11]. The author believes that in practical clinical work, each unit should appropriately match the endoscopy and endoscopy forces according to the technical strength of specific departments and carry out dual-lens combined technology with the goal of maximizing the clinical benefit for patients. This author believes that for the rational treatment of small gastric GIST, the patient's condition (including tumor size, site, general growth pattern, and patient's treatment willingness) and the physician's technology (including the hardware and software capabilities of endoscopic and laparoscopic treatment) should be taken into consideration to make individual decisions with the goal of maximizing the clinical benefit of patients.

16.2.4.2 How to Avoid Missed Diagnosis and Misdiagnosis in Clinical Practice?

GIST is usually single, and multiple GIST is relatively rare. There is no typical clinical manifestation of GIST in the early stage, and GISTs are mostly found accidentally while investigating symptoms such as upper abdomen and upper gastrointestinal bleeding or on gastroscopy or abdominal CT examination during physical examination. It is easier to diagnose large GIST using abdominal CT or gastroscopy, but tumors less than 1 cm, and sometimes in the presence of poor gastric filling, are difficult to identify using abdominal CT, similarly, it is difficult to find tumors growing out of the cavity by gastroscopy. Based on this, we should not trust the imaging examination completely, but should be alert to the possibility of multiple gastric GIST, and fully explore the gastric wall during surgery to avoid missing small tumors, resulting in poor prognosis for patients.

16.3 Expert Comments

Jun Zhang

Multiple primary sporadic GISTs are rare, the locations and clinical manifestations are not significantly different to those of single GIST, and tumors often appear in the stomach and small intestine [12]. Often, additional lesions are found when a patient presents with symptoms caused by a larger GIST or during intraoperative exploration. GIST has strong heterogeneity. There are different reports and opinions about the differences in clinicopathological features between primary multiple GIST at home and abroad. However, existing results tend to suggest that primary multiple GIST originates from different Cajal cell subsets in the gastrointestinal stroma, leading to the diversity of clinicopathological features. The treatment of primary multiple GIST is also based on complete surgical resection. The current risk assessment methods for postoperative GIST are mainly modified NIH classification and AFIP standards, but these methods are all aimed at single GIST. Although retrospective studies have shown that the efficacy of adjuvant therapy for patients with multiple GIST is similar to that of single GIST after using the above-mentioned evaluation methods, there may be some limitations in the evaluation of patients with complex multiple primary GIST by applying the current criteria. How to accurately judge the risk of postoperative recurrence in such patients and formulate a reasonable adjuvant treatment plan needs to attract the attention of clinicians and be investigated in corresponding research.

References

1. Gasparotto D, Rossi S, Bearzi I, Doglioni C, Marzotto A, Hornick JL, Grizzo A, Sartor C, Mandolesi A, Sciot R, Debiec-Rychter M, Dei Tos AP, Maestro R. Multiple primary sporadic gastrointestinal stromal tumors in the adult: an underestimated entity. Clin Cancer Res. 2008;14(18):5715–21. https://doi.org/10.1158/1078-0432.CCR-08-0622.
2. Li FP, Fletcher JA, Heinrich MC, Garber JE, Sallan SE, Curiel-Lewandrowski C, Duensing A, van de Rijn M, Schnipper LE, Demetri GD. Familial gastrointestinal stromal tumor syndrome: phenotypic and molecular features in a kindred. J Clin Oncol. 2005;23(12):2735–43. https://doi.org/10.1200/JCO.2005.06.009.
3. Andersson J, Sihto H, Meis-Kindblom JM, Joensuu H, Nupponen N, Kindblom LG. NF1-associated gastrointestinal stromal tumors have unique clinical, phenotypic, and genotypic characteristics. Am J Surg Pathol. 2005;29(9):1170–6. https://doi.org/10.1097/01.pas.0000159775.77912.15.
4. Joensuu H. Risk stratification of patients diagnosed with gastrointestinal stromal tumor. Hum Pathol. 2008;39(10):1411–9. https://doi.org/10.1016/j.humpath.2008.06.025.
5. Miettinen M, Lasota J. Gastrointestinal stromal tumors: pathology and prognosis at different sites. Semin Diagn Pathol. 2006;23(2):70–83. https://doi.org/10.1053/j.semdp.2006.09.001.
6. Nishida T, Yoshinaga S, Takahashi T, Naito Y. Recent progress and challenges in the diagnosis and treatment of gastrointestinal stromal tumors. Cancers (Basel). 2021;13(13):3158. https://doi.org/10.3390/cancers13133158.
7. Wang M, Xue A, Yuan W, Gao X, Fu M, Fang Y, Wang L, Shu P, Li H, Hou Y, Shen K, Sun Y, Qin X. Clinicopathological features and prognosis of small gastric gastrointestinal stromal tumors (GISTs). J Gastrointest Surg. 2019;23(11):2136–43. https://doi.org/10.1007/s11605-018-04070-3.
8. von Mehren M, Randall RL, Benjamin RS, Boles S, Bui MM, Ganjoo KN, George S, Gonzalez RJ, Heslin MJ, Kane JM, Keedy V, Kim E, Koon H, Mayerson J, McCarter M, McGarry SV, Meyer C, Morris ZS, O'Donnell RJ, Pappo AS, Paz IB, Petersen IA, Pfeifer JD, Riedel RF, Ruo B, Schuetze S, Tap WD, Wayne JD, Bergman MA, Scavone JL. Soft tissue sarcoma, version 2.2018, NCCN clinical practice guidelines in oncology. J Natl Compr Cancer Netw. 2018;16(5):536–63. https://doi.org/10.6004/jnccn.2018.0025.
9. Zhao Q, Li Y, Yang P, Zang Y, Fan L, Tan B, Tian Y. Evaluation for therapeutic measures to small gastric stromal tumor: a retrospective study of 90 cases. Curr Probl Cancer. 2018;42(1):107–14. https://doi.org/10.1016/j.currproblcancer.2018.01.012.
10. Yang J, Feng F, Li M, Sun L, Hong L, Cai L, Wang W, Xu G, Zhang H. Surgical resection should be taken into consideration for the treatment of small gastric gastrointestinal stromal tumors. World J Surg Oncol. 2013;11(1):273. https://doi.org/10.1186/1477-7819-11-273.
11. Li J, Ye Y, Wang J, Zhang B, Qin S, Shi Y, He Y, Liang X, Liu X, Zhou Y, Wu X, Zhang X, Wang M, Gao Z, Lin T, Cao H, Shen L, Chinese Society of Clinical Oncology Csco Expert Committee on Gastrointestinal Stromal Tumor. Chinese consensus guidelines for diagnosis and management of gastrointestinal stromal tumor. Chin J Cancer Res. 2017;29(4):281–93. https://doi.org/10.21147/j.issn.1000-9604.2017.04.01.
12. Li K, Tjhoi W, Shou C, Yang W, Zhang Q, Liu X, Yu J. Multiple gastrointestinal stromal tumors: analysis of clinicopathologic characteristics and prognosis of 20 patients. Cancer Manag Res. 2019;11:7031–8. https://doi.org/10.2147/CMAR.S197560.

Hereditary Gastrointestinal Stromal Tumors

17

Xiaoqi Li, Linxi Yang, and Gang Zhao

Keywords

Gastrointestinal stromal tumors · Germline mutation Targeted therapy

17.1 Case 24 A 49-Year-Old Woman with Familial Hereditary GIST

Xiaoqi Li and Linxi Yang

17.1.1 Introduction

GIST is predominantly driven by gain-of-function mutations of either *KIT* or *PDGFRA* genes, with the majority of these mutations being somatic. However, a minority of GIST cases exhibit germline mutations of these genes. This kind of GIST often presents with some characteristic clinical manifestations and needs clinicians' attention.

17.1.2 Case Background

A 49-year-old woman presented to the doctor with abdominal pain. Gastroscopy and CT scan showed a 2.7 cm × 3.4 cm mass occupied the descending part of the duodenum. Neuroendocrine tumors could not be excluded. She underwent duodenal tumor resection on May 26, 2016. Postoperative pathology showed GIST, with a tumor size of 3.5 cm × 3 cm × 3 cm, without mitoses. Genetic testing revealed a mutation in exon 13 of *KIT*, 654 AAA > GAA (heterozygosity). The patient did not receive adjuvant therapy and was followed up with regular CT scans. 1 year after surgery, follow-up CT scans showed multiple enhancement lesions in the horizontal and initial segments of the jejunum with a maximum diameter of 1.8 cm, considered to be possible GIST. Repeat CT scans during the follow-up period showed that the lesions were all similar in size. A CT scan in April 2019 showed that the multiple masses in the duodenum and jejunum had increased in size, with a maximum diameter of 2.5 cm. The patient was referred to our hospital for further treatment. After inquiring about the relevant medical history, we learned that the patient's mother had undergone surgery at a local hospital for GIST in June 2018. A GIST was found on the greater curvature of the stomach with multiple disseminated nodules in the bowel wall. Genetic testing also revealed a mutation in exon 13 of *KIT*, 654 AAA > GAA (heterozygosity). Her mother received imatinib targeted therapy after surgery and had stable disease.

X. Li · L. Yang (✉) · G. Zhao
Department of Gastrointestinal Surgery, Renji Hospital, Shanghai Jiaotong University School of Medicine, Shanghai, China

17.1.2.1 Past History and Family History

The patient was previously healthy and reported no drug allergies. The patient's parents were alive and the patient's mother also suffered from GIST.

17.1.2.2 Physical Examination

The patient's vital signs were stable, and the skin and mucous membranes were not yellowish or pale. The abdomen was flat, and no gastrointestinal pattern or peristaltic wave was observed. The abdomen was soft, with no palpable masses. The bowel sounds were normal.

17.1.2.3 Auxiliary Examination

Abdominal CT The small intestinal wall in the abdominal cavity was thickened, and the multiple masses in the duodenum and jejunum were larger than before, with a maximum diameter of 2.5 cm. The findings were consistent with multiple GIST (Fig. 17.1).

17.1.2.4 Preliminary Diagnosis

Postoperative recurrence and metastasis of duodenal GIST, possible hereditary GIST.

K. Tao, H. Cao (eds.), *Clinical Management of Gastrointestinal Stromal Tumor*, https://doi.org/10.1007/978-981-99-9392-5_17

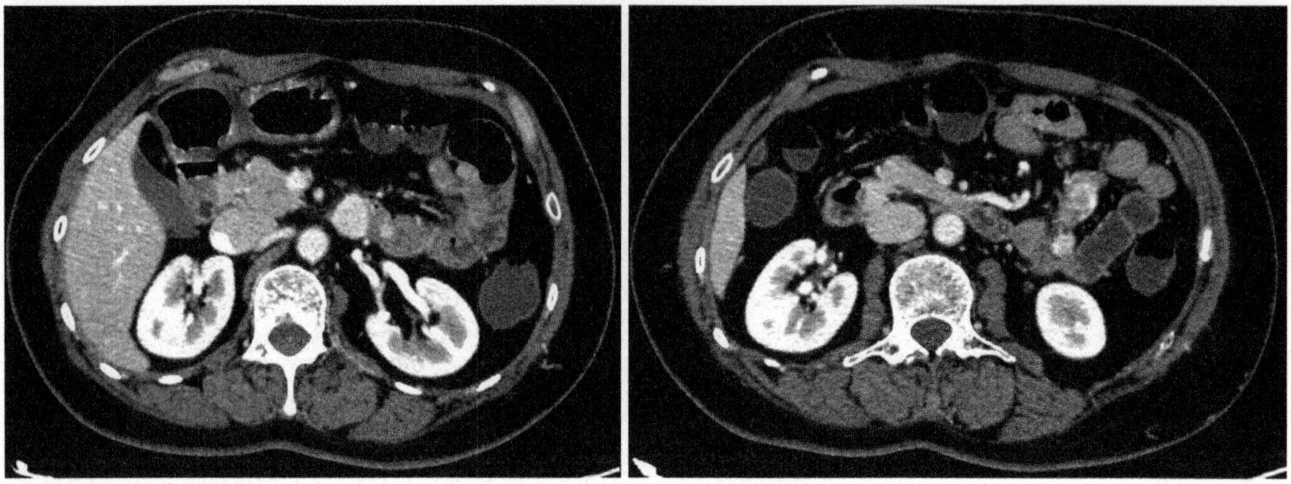

Fig. 17.1 CT from April 2019 demonstrated multiple masses in the duodenum and jejunum

17.1.3 Therapy

17.1.3.1 Case Analysis

The patient had low-risk duodenal GIST and received radical surgery 3 years ago and with multiple mass-occupying lesions on the small intestinal wall in the abdominal cavity. The possibility of recurrence and metastasis of the original tumor was considered. Given that her mother also suffered from GIST and the mother and daughter had the same genetic mutation, the possibility of familial hereditary multiple GIST could not be ruled out. Surgical exploration to clarify the pathology, and peripheral blood genetic testing on the immediate family members were recommended.

17.1.3.2 Treatment

The patient underwent laparotomy, duodenal tumor resection and small bowel tumors resection on April 14, 2019. We found that the omentum below the original incision in her abdominal cavity was widely adhered to the abdominal wall, and there were dozens of tumors of various sizes in the duodenum and jejunum. The largest tumor was approximately 3 cm in diameter and the smallest one was approximately 2 mm in diameter. The two largest tumors were located at Treitz's ligament and the jejunum, 50 cm from the Treitz's ligament, respectively (Fig. 17.2). We removed all tumors larger than 2 mm which were visible and tried not to damage the intestinal mucosa. Liquid biopsy of peripheral blood by next-generation sequencing was performed on the patient, her mother and their immediate family.

17.1.3.3 Postoperative Pathology and Genetic Testing

Pathological Diagnosis Duodenal GIST (2 cm × 1.5 cm × 1.5 cm), mitotic count <5/50 HPF. Four small intestinal GIST (2 cm × 1.5 cm × 1 cm; 0.3 cm; 0.5 cm; 0.5 cm), mitotic count <5/50 HPF.

Immunohistochemistry CD117 (+), DOG-1 (+), CD34 (+), S-100 (−), Ki-67 (LI: 5%), SDHB (+).

Genetic Testing Heterozygous mutations in exon 13 of *KIT*, 654 AAA > GAA, the encoded amino acid was converted from lysine to glutamic acid. Exons 9, 11, and 17 of *KIT* and exons 12 and 18 of *PDGFRA* were all wild type.

Liquid biopsy Heterozygous mutation in exon 13 of *KIT*, 654 AAA > GAA, was found in the patient and her mother. No other family members had this mutation (Fig. 17.3).

17.1.4 Prognosis

The patient recovered well after the operation, and imatinib 400 mg/d treatment was started 2 weeks after discharge. As of follow-up in December 2021, all lesions in the abdominal cavity of the patient and her mother were stable (Fig. 17.4).

17.1.5 Experience of Diagnosis and Therapy

Multiple GIST caused by germline *KIT* mutation is an extremely rare autosomal dominant disorder. So far, more than 30 families involving mutations at 8, 11, 13 and other *KIT* sites have been reported [1–5]. In addition to intra-abdominal multiple GIST, families with germline *KIT* mutations may present with a variety of clinical symptoms, including hyperpigmentation, urticaria pigmentosa, and dysphagia [6]. In this case, the patient and her mother did not have any skin symptoms or swallowing problems. Like other sporadic mutant GIST, imatinib is also effective for heredi-

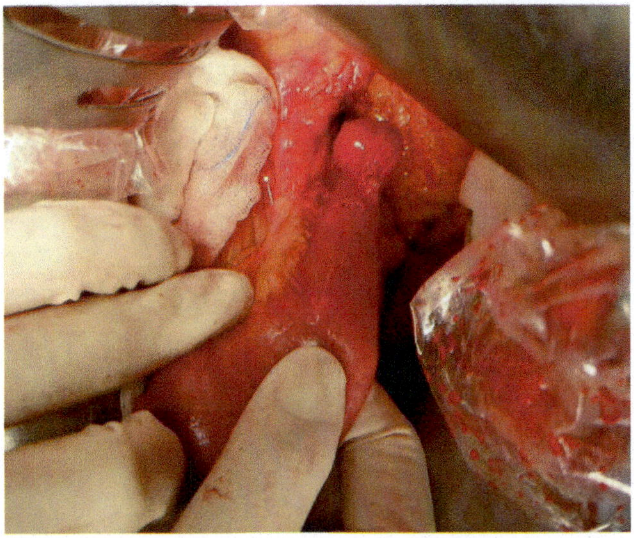

Fig. 17.2 Intraoperative findings

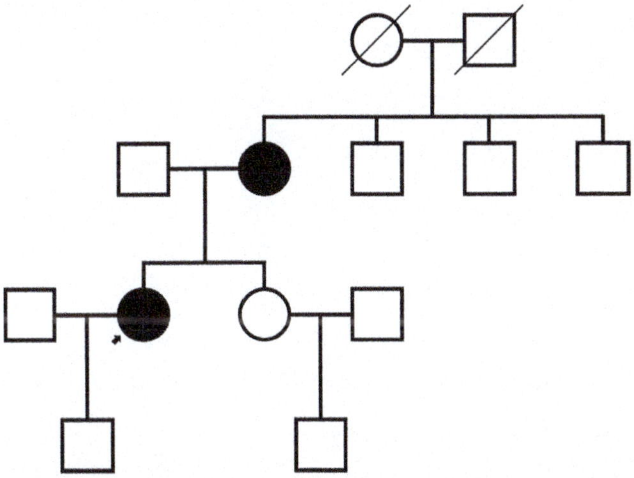

Fig. 17.3 Family tree

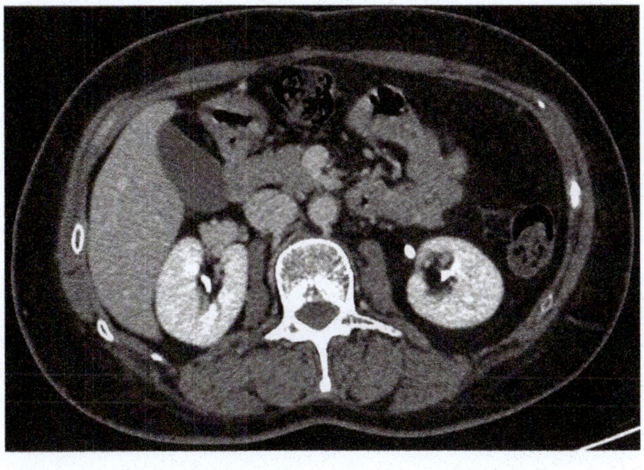

Fig. 17.4 CT 3 years after surgery

tary GIST. In the reported cases, the tumors progressed relatively slowly, and imatinib was effective for a long time. Some patients have disease control for nearly 10 years with imatinib therapy [4, 5].

In this case, both the patient and her mother had multiple intra-abdominal GIST, and the disease control time was more than 3 years. For follow-up treatment of hereditary advanced GIST, it is still recommended to formulate the treatment plan according to the specific gene mutation site.

17.2 Expert Comments

Gang Zhao

GIST with germline *KIT* mutation only accounts for a very small number of GIST, but it often has characteristics different from sporadic GIST, such as multiple primary lesions, primary mutation in exon 13 of *KIT,* and inert biological behavior. This also suggests that we need to consider the possibility of hereditary GIST when we encounter patients with atypical features. Genetic counseling and screening are very important for GIST with germline mutations [7]. The popularization of next-generation sequencing technology greatly improves the accuracy and accessibility of genetic screening [8], which will contribute to accurate treatment for patients with relevant pathogenic gene mutations.

References

1. Halpern AL, Torphy RJ, McCarter MD, Sciotto CG, Glode LM, Robinson WA. A familial germline mutation in KIT associated with achalasia, mastocytosis and gastrointestinal stromal tumors shows response to kinase inhibitors. Cancer Genet. 2019;233–234:1–6. https://doi.org/10.1016/j.cancergen.2019.02.001.
2. Ke H, Kazi JU, Zhao H, Sun J. Germline mutations of KIT in gastrointestinal stromal tumor (GIST) and mastocytosis. Cell Biosci. 2016;6:55. https://doi.org/10.1186/s13578-016-0120-8.
3. Meir M, Maurus K, Kuper J, Hankir M, Wardelmann E, Rosenwald A, Germer CT, Wiegering A. The novel KIT exon 11 germline mutation K558N is associated with gastrointestinal stromal tumor, mastocytosis, and seminoma development. Genes Chromosomes Cancer. 2021;60(12):827–32. https://doi.org/10.1002/gcc.22988.
4. Bachet JB, Landi B, Laurent-Puig P, Italiano A, Le Cesne A, Lévy P, Safar V, Duffaud F, Blay JY, Emile JF. Diagnosis, prognosis and treatment of patients with gastrointestinal stromal tumor (GIST) and germline mutation of KIT exon 13. Eur J Cancer. 2013;49(11):2531–41. https://doi.org/10.1016/j.ejca.2013.04.005.
5. Engin G, Eraslan S, Kayserili H, Kapran Y, Akman H, Akyuz A, Aykan NF. Imatinib response of gastrointestinal stromal tumor patients with germline mutation on KIT exon 13: a family report. World J Radiol. 2017;9(9):365–70. https://doi.org/10.4329/wjr.v9.i9.365.
6. Li FP, Fletcher JA, Heinrich MC, Garber JE, Sallan SE, Curiel-Lewandrowski C, Duensing A, van de Rijn M, Schnipper LE,

Demetri GD. Familial gastrointestinal stromal tumor syndrome: phenotypic and molecular features in a kindred. J Clin Oncol. 2005;23(12):2735–43. https://doi.org/10.1200/JCO.2005.06.009.

7. Kuroda N, Tanida N, Hirota S, Daum O, Hes O, Michal M, Lee GH. Familial gastrointestinal stromal tumor with germ line mutation of the juxtamembrane domain of the KIT gene observed in relatively young women. Ann Diagn Pathol. 2011;15(5):358–61. https://doi.org/10.1016/j.anndiagpath.2010.05.003.
8. Vanden Bempt I, Vander Borght S, Sciot R, Spans L, Claerhout S, Brems H, Lehnert S, Dehaspe L, Fransis S, Neuville B, Topal B, Schöffski P, Legius E, Debiec-Rychter M. Comprehensive targeted next-generation sequencing approach in the molecular diagnosis of gastrointestinal stromal tumor. Genes Chromosomes Cancer. 2021;60(4):239–49. https://doi.org/10.1002/gcc.22923.

Part IV

Gastrointestinal Stromal Tumors with Other Malignant Tumors

18 Intermediate-Risk Gastrointestinal Stromal Tumor with Advanced Gastric Cancer

Tianlong Ling, Haibo Qiu, and Leping Li

Keywords

Gastrointestinal stromal tumors · Gastric cancer
Intestinal cancer · Adjuvant therapy · Imatinib

18.1 Case 25 An 80-Year-Old Man with Synchronous GIST and Gastric Cancer

Tianlong Ling and Haibo Qiu

18.1.1 Introduction

GIST is a kind of unique mesenchymal tumor which displays positive CD117. It is rare for a GIST to occur concurrently with another type of gastrointestinal (GI) tumor. There is minimal knowledge on the causes. Some scholars believe the etiology for GIST with another GI tumor is long-term exposure to unknown pathogens. In these conditions, both mesenchymal and epithelial cells of patients with GIST are subject to carcinogenic transformation, leading to the development of synchronous tumors. Some other scholars propose that the two malignant tumors have the same mutated tumor suppressor genes. For patients with dual tumors, it is necessary to comply to the principle of individualized treatment, carry out multidisciplinary team (MDT) discussion, and develop suitable treatment regimens. On the other hand, the presence of synchronous tumors may increase the risk of metastasis. Thus, it is necessary to arrange close follow-up for patient with dual tumors.

T. Ling
Department of Gastrointestinal Surgery, Renji Hospital, Shanghai Jiaotong University School of Medicine, Shanghai, China

H. Qiu (✉)
Department of Gastric Surgery, Sun Yat-sen University Cancer Center, Guangzhou, China
e-mail: qiuhb@sysucc.org.cn

L. Li
Department of Gastrointestinal Surgery, Shandong Provincial Hospital, Jinan, China
e-mail: Lileping@medmail.com.cn

18.1.2 Case Background

An 80-year-old man was admitted to our hospital in July 2014. He had been diagnosed with an abdominal mass following a routine screening test at a local hospital. He received a series of examinations in our hospital. The abdominal CT scan showed a mass at the gastric cardia close to the lesser curvature. The mass appeared to be a GIST originating from the gastric wall (Fig. 18.1). A low-density lesion in liver segment II, likely to be a liver cyst was also observed. Gastroscopy revealed an ulcerated mass between the cardia and the fundus of the stomach (Fig. 18.2). The pathology findings identified a gastric adenocarcinoma with moderate differentiation.

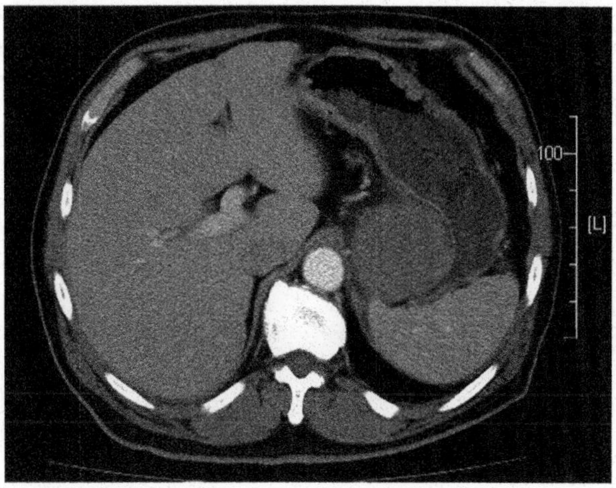

Fig. 18.1 Abdominal CT

K. Tao, H. Cao (eds.), *Clinical Management of Gastrointestinal Stromal Tumor*, https://doi.org/10.1007/978-981-99-9392-5_18

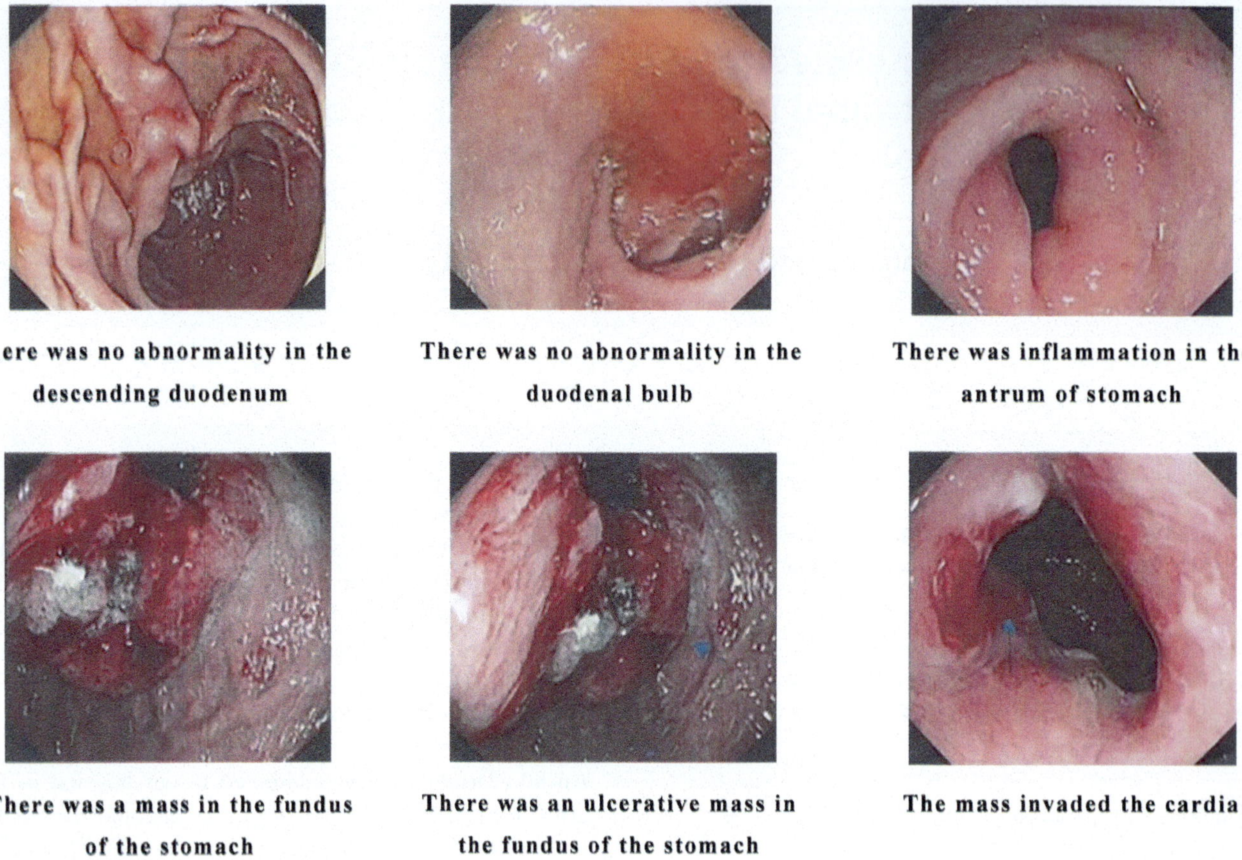

Fig. 18.2 Gastroscopic findings

18.1.2.1 Past History and Family History

The patient was previously healthy and reported no history of drug allergies. There was no similar medical history in the family.

18.1.2.2 Physical Examination

The patient's vital signs were stable, and the skin and sclera were not yellowish or pale. The abdomen was flat, and no gastrointestinal or peristaltic waves were seen. The abdomen was soft, with no tenderness, rebound pain, or palpable abdominal masses and the bowel sounds were normal.

18.1.2.3 Auxiliary Examination

Gastroscopy An ulcerated mass between the cardia and the fundus of the stomach.

Abdominal CT There was a mass in the gastric cardia, close to the lesser curvature, which appeared to be a GIST originating from the gastric wall. Additionally, there was a low-density lesion in liver segment II, likely to be a liver cyst.

Blood (Routine) White blood cells 24.5 × 10^9/L; hemoglobin 92 g/L; platelets 90.9 × 10^9/L.

Liver and Renal Function Normal.

Coagulation Test Normal.

Cardiac Ultrasound Unremarkable.

18.1.2.4 Preliminary Diagnosis

1. Type III adenocarcinoma of the esophagogastric junction (AEG)
2. Leukocytosis with unknown cause

18.1.3 Therapy

18.1.3.1 Case Analysis

The patient was an elderly man. The diagnosis of type III AEG was confirmed by gastroscopy, pathology findings, and CT scans. However, the cause of leukocytosis was unknown. Thus, a bone marrow biopsy was performed, and a hematology consultation was requested. The biopsy revealed active bone marrow hyperplasia, in which the granulosa system had slightly maturation and left shift. No malignant tumor cells were found in the smear. As a result, the hematologist ruled out chronic myeloid leukemia and believed the AEG was the main cause of leukocytosis. The subsequent MDT meeting, considering that both tumors had no distant metastasis and were expected to be completely resected, concluded that surgical intervention should be performed.

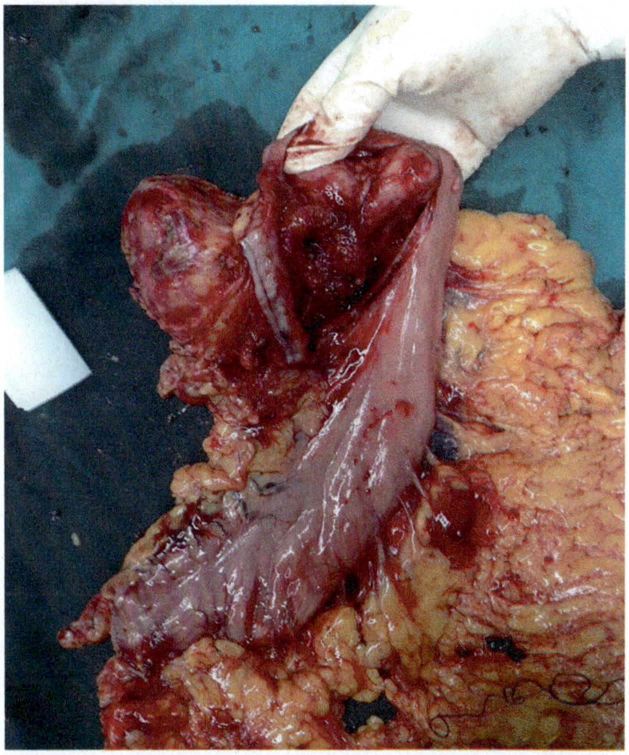

Fig. 18.3 An ulcerative mass between the fundus and the cardia of the stomach

18.1.3.2 Treatment

The patient underwent total gastrectomy with D2 lymph node dissection, esophagojejunal Roux-en-Y anastomosis, and splenectomy on July 12, 2014. During the surgery, the primary tumor was assessed and was found to be 7 cm × 6 cm in size and located between the fundus and the cardia of the stomach. The tumor had invaded the retroperitoneum and splenic hilus but not the pancreas, the colon or the liver. Gross observation of the postoperative specimen revealed an ulcerative mass, 4 cm × 3 cm in size, between the fundus and the cardia of the stomach (Fig. 18.3). Another mass, 6 cm × 7 cm in size, was also identified at right side of the cardia, not attached to the primary tumor (Fig. 18.4).

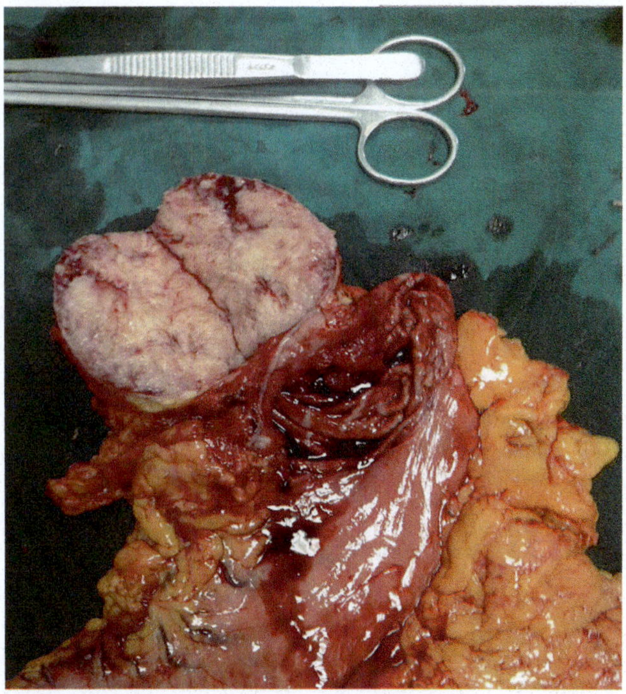

Fig. 18.4 A mass at right side of the cardia not attached to the primary tumor

18.1.3.3 Postoperative Pathology

Pathological Diagnosis (Tumor 1) AEG, 3.5 cm × 3 cm × 1 cm, intestinal type, with poor to moderate differentiation. The tumor infiltrated the superficial muscularis. There was no evidence of vascular or neural invasion and there were no tumor cells in the omentum majus or spleen. Lymph node invasion: 1/45. The tumor was located at the cardia of the stomach. The mass resembled a cauliflower in appearance, was greyish white in color and was firm.

Immunohistochemistry (Tumor 1) VEGF (+), Her-2 (3+), CEA (+), CD56 (+), Syn (−), CgA (−), NSE (−), Ki-67 (Li: 15%).

Pathological Diagnosis (Tumor 2) Gastric GIST, 7 cm × 4 cm × 6 cm in size, mitotic count <5/50 HPF. The tumor located at the right of the gastric cardia, and was firm. The cross-section appeared greyish white and the mass had a partial capsule. The tumor consisted of spindle cells in bundle and spiral patterns. Slight hyperplasia was observed.

Immunohistochemistry (Tumor 2) CD117 (+), CD34 (+), DOG-1 (+), S-100 (−), desmin (−), HHF35 (−), Ki-67 (Li >5%).

18.1.4 Prognosis

The patient recovered well. The WBC reduced from 42×10^9/L on surgery day to 36×10^9/L. The neutrophil level was 61.89% on postoperative day 9. After the consultation with the hematologist, the hematology consultant recommended expectant management regarding the WBC. The sutures were removed, and the patient was discharged on postoperative day 9. The patient did not experience symptoms of fever, cough, or abdominal pain in the postoperative recovery period.

18.1.5 Experience of Diagnosis and Therapy

18.1.5.1 Synchronous GI Carcinoma and GIST

According to reports, approximately 20–30% of the population have a small GIST, <2 cm in size. Most of these GIST are discovered during autopsy. In fact, it is common to see synchronous GI carcinoma with GIST. These small GIST are often present on the gastrectomy specimen for gastric cancer [1, 2]. Usually, these GIST are low risk and do not require further treatment. However, it is unusual to see synchronous GI carcinoma with high or intermediate risk GIST, as in this case [3].

18.1.5.2 Choices of Surgical Procedure for Synchronous GI Carcinoma with GIST

Having diagnosed synchronous GI carcinoma with GIST, it is mandatory to confirm the location and the size of the tumors. In addition, preoperative assessment is required to determine the appropriate resection margin. In general, a sufficient resection margin and lymph node dissection is mandatory during gastrectomy for gastric cancer [4]. However, there are no such requirements for GIST surgery, provided R0 resection is achieved [5]. Therefore, having obtained a proper resection margin and lymph node dissection for gastric cancer, it is only necessary to achieve R0 resection for the GIST.

18.1.5.3 Adjuvant Therapy

This patient had gastric cancer at stage pT2N1M0, IIA. He also had GIST with intermediate risk by modified NIH classification. The AFIP was 3.6%. Based on the grading, adjuvant therapy was indicated for both tumors in this case. It was possible for the patient to receive tegafur and 400 mg/d imatinib at the same time [6]. However, the patient was 80 years old and the two tumors were at relatively early stage, so the prognosis was expected to be good with low risk for GIST recurrence. After consulting with the patient and their family regarding the pros and cons of treatment, the patient postponed adjuvant therapy. He was advised to comply with close follow up.

18.2 Expert Comments

Leping Li

About 20% of patients with GIST have synchronous tumors, of which 25% are GI tumors. Colorectal cancer and AEG are the most common. Most synchronous GIST are small with low risk. The patient in this case was diagnosed with cardia cancer and intermediate risk GIST. The WBC showed leukocytosis both pre- and postoperatively, which was probably caused by the cancer in the cardia. The patient should be subject to further examination and monitoring to rule out hematological diseases. It is especially worth noting that the WBC remained high after surgery. Only a small proportion of patients with synchronous tumors receive adjuvant therapy because most patients have small, low-risk GIST. Furthermore, these patients usually exhibit low compliance. According to the NCCN guidelines, oral imatinib therapy is recommended for 1 year following resection [7]. It is common to administer platinum- or fluorouracil-based adjuvant treatment for advanced gastric cancer [8]. The overlap for the systematic treatment of the two diseases is low. When prescribing an adjuvant regimen for such patients, it is necessary to consider the drug interactions of the treatments for both tumors. It is also important to evaluate the efficacy and side effects of the joint regimen on patients. Extending patient's life expectancy is also as important as ensuring quality of life.

References

1. Liu Z, Liu SS, Zheng GZ, Yang JJ, Hong L, Sun L, Fan DM, Zhang HW, Feng F. Clinicopathological features and prognosis of coexistence of gastric gastrointestinal stromal tumor and gastric cancer.

Medicine (Baltimore). 2016;95(45):e5373. https://doi.org/10.1097/MD.0000000000005373.
2. Liu S, Liu HY, Dong YL, Wang FB, Wang HJ, Chen J. Gastric carcinoma with a gastrointestinal stromal tumor – a case report and literature review. Med Sci (Paris). 2018;34:15–9. https://doi.org/10.1051/medsci/201834f103.
3. Giuliani J, Bonetti A. The occurrence of gastrointestinal stromal tumors and second malignancies. J Gastrointest Cancer. 2015;46(4):408–12. https://doi.org/10.1007/s12029-015-9759-3.
4. Smyth EC, Nilsson M, Grabsch I, Van Grieken NCT, Lordick F. Gastric cancer. Lancet. 2020;396(10251):635–48. https://doi.org/10.1016/S0140-6736(20)31288-5.
5. Akahoshi K, Oya M, Koga T, Shiratsuchi Y. Current clinical management of gastrointestinal stromal tumor. World J Gastroenterol. 2018;24(26):2806–17. https://doi.org/10.3748/wjg.v24.i26.2806.
6. Lin M, Lin JX, Huang CM, Zheng CH, Li P, Xie JW, Wang JB, Lu J. Prognostic analysis of gastric gastrointestinal stromal tumor with synchronous gastric cancer. World J Surg Oncol. 2014;12:25. https://doi.org/10.1186/1477-7819-12-25.
7. von Mehren M, Randall RL, Benjamin RS, Boles S, Bui MM, Ganjoo KN, George S, Gonzalez RJ, Heslin MJ, Kane JM, Keedy V, Kim E, Koon H, Mayerson J, McCarter M, McGarry SV, Meyer C, Morris ZS, O'Donnell RJ, Pappo AS, Paz IB, Petersen IA, Pfeifer JD, Riedel RF, Ruo B, Schuetze S, Tap WD, Wayne JD, Bergman MA, Scavone JL. Soft tissue sarcoma, version 2.2018, NCCN clinical practice guidelines in oncology. J Natl Compr Cancer Netw. 2018;16(5):536–63. https://doi.org/10.6004/jnccn.2018.0025.
8. Wagner AD, Syn NL, Moehler M, Grothe W, Yong WP, Tai BC, Ho J, Unverzagt S. Chemotherapy for advanced gastric cancer. Cochrane Database Syst Rev. 2017;8(8):CD004064. https://doi.org/10.1002/14651858.CD004064.pub4.

Gastrointestinal Stromal Tumors with Kidney Cancer

19

Chen Huang, Ruizhi Zhang, and Yong Li

Keywords

Gastrointestinal stromal tumors · Renal cancer Synchronous tumor · Targeted Therapy · Preoperative treatment · Imatinib · Sunitinib

19.1 Case 26 A 55-Year-Old Woman with Synchronous GIST and Kidney Cancer

Chen Huang and Ruizhi Zhang

19.1.1 Introduction

GIST is a common GI tumor originating from mesenchymal tissue. The incidence of synchronous tumors involving GIST is not as low as it appears to be. According to long term follow-up data from the MD Anderson cancer center, approximately 20% of patients with GIST also have another synchronous tumor. It remains rare that non-familial or general GIST are accompanied by another malignant tumor synchronously. Synchronous renal cancer with GIST is also uncommon. Recent studies have shown a connection between the pathogenesis and treatment for these two malignancies as described in this chapter.

C. Huang
Department of Gastrointestinal Surgery, Renji Hospital, Shanghai Jiaotong University School of Medicine, Shanghai, China

R. Zhang (✉)
Department of Gastrointestinal Surgery, Union Hospital, Tongji Medical College, Huazhong University of Science and Technology, Wuhan, China
e-mail: ruizhizhang@hust.edu.cn

Y. Li
Department of General Surgery, The Fourth Hospital of Hebei Medical University, Shijiazhuang, China

19.1.2 Case Background

A 55-year-old woman received an abdominal MRI scan which showed an unusual signal posterior to the gastric lesser curvature, considered to be a possible GIST. There was also another unusual signal in the right renal parenchyma. She was admitted to Union Hospital, Tongji Medical College, Huazhong University of Science and Technology for further treatment in July 2017.

19.1.2.1 Past History and Family History

The patient had type II diabetes mellitus which, to her best knowledge, was well controlled with medication. The patient reported no history of drug allergies and there was no similar medical history in the family.

19.1.2.2 Physical Examination

The patient's vital signs were stable. The abdominal physical examinations were normal.

Abdominal CT A round mass was observed 5.7 cm × 4.0 cm × 4.6 cm in size, positioned superiorly and posteriorly to the wall of gastric antrum. The mass was progressively enhanced under contrast. The mass was low-density, without internal enhancement. A GIST was suspected (Fig. 19.1). A further mass, 3.4 cm × 3.7 cm in size, was located in the middle of the right kidney with uneven enhancement under contrast and attenuated enhancement during the delayed phase. A renal cancer was suspected (Figs. 19.2 and 19.3).

Kidney Emission Computed Tomography (ECT) Perfusion of both kidneys was normal. Glomerular filtration was slightly decreased with rates of 32.6 mL/min and 32.9 mL/min in the left and right kidney, respectively.

Ultrasound Gastroscopy A hypoechoic semi-spherical bulge was observed at the lesser curvature near the gastric antrum. The bulge originated from the muscularis propria

K. Tao, H. Cao (eds.), *Clinical Management of Gastrointestinal Stromal Tumor*, https://doi.org/10.1007/978-981-99-9392-5_19

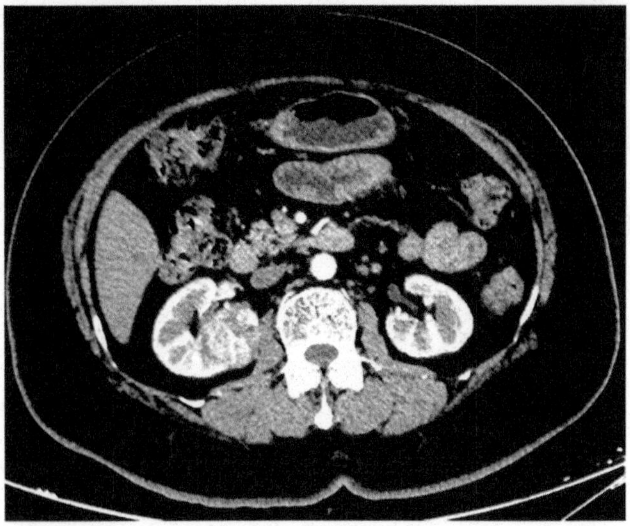

Fig. 19.1 Cross section of the round mass positioned superiorly and posteriorly to the wall of gastric antrum which was visible on enhanced CT

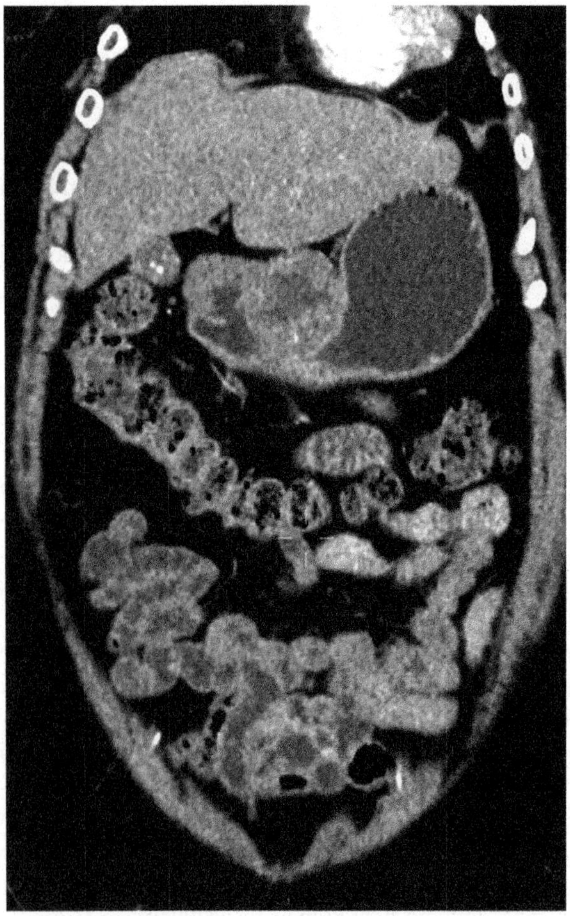

Fig. 19.2 A cross-section of the mass at middle right kidney, which was visible on enhanced CT

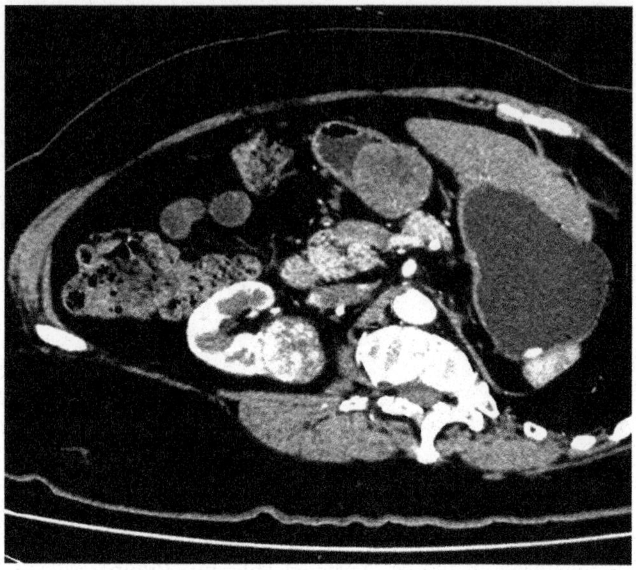

Fig. 19.3 Enhanced CT showed synchronous tumors at the two different sites

and contained an anechoic area. The mass had a distinct border and protruded toward and away from the gastric lumen. The cross-sectional diameter was 4.9 cm × 3.8 cm. Elastography showed that the mass was hard (Fig. 19.4). An abdominal ultrasound showed a patchy, hypoechoic shadow, 2.2 cm in size, in the right kidney with a slightly indistinct border (Fig. 19.4).

19.1.2.3 Preliminary Diagnosis

1. Gastric mass
2. Right kidney mass
3. Type II diabetes mellitus

19.1.3 Therapy

19.1.3.1 Case Analysis

A routine MRI scan showed synchronous tumors in the stomach and the right kidney. The patient received an enhanced abdominal CT scan after being admitted to hospital, which showed a possible GIST and a right kidney mass of unknown origin. Ultrasound gastroscopy showed a possible GIST in the stomach. The cause of the right kidney mass was highly unlikely to be either a distant metastasis or infiltration of the GIST by the primary evaluation based on the usual biological behaviors and common metastatic sites of GIST. The kidney mass was then determined to be a primary renal cancer. The consultation with

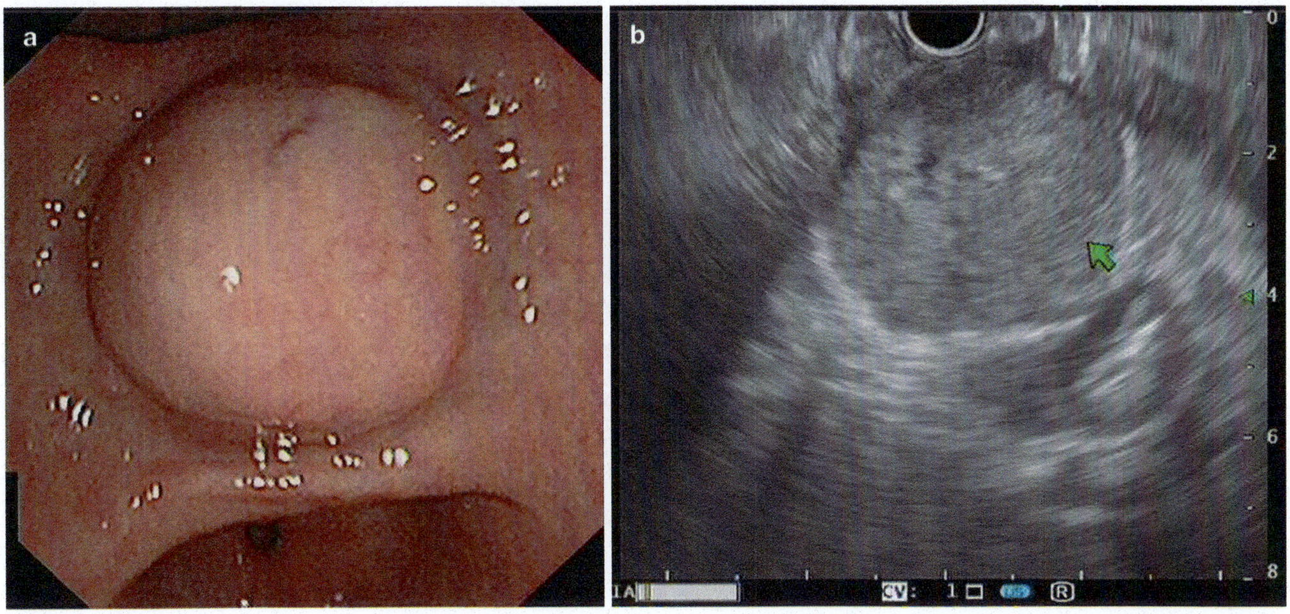

Fig. 19.4 Gastroscope: **a** Gastric mass. The location of the mass. **b** The layer of the gastric wall from which the mass originated

a urologist showed that the renal mass was located near the renal hilum. Total renal resection was indicated. The patient suffered diabetes Mellitus with ECOG 0 and ASA II. Multi-staged surgery would likely hamper the postoperative recovery. Overall, synchronous resection of both tumors was advised.

19.1.3.2 Treatment

The patient underwent laparoscopic gastric tumor resection and total right renal resection in July 2017. Laparoscopically, one of the tumors, 5 cm in size, was located at the posterior wall of the gastric antrum. The second tumor, 3 cm in size, was located close to the right renal hilum.

19.1.3.3 Postoperative Pathology and Genetic Testing

Pathological Diagnosis (Tumor 1) Submucosal gastric GIST, 7.0 cm × 6.0 cm × 4.0 cm in size, with focal necrosis, and cystic degeneration. The resection margin showed no tumor involvement. Mitotic count <5/50 HPF. The tumor was intermediate risk by the modified NIH classification.

Immunohistochemistry (Tumor 1) CD117 (+), CD34 (+), DOG-1 (+), SMA (−), S-100 (−), Ki-67 (LI: 3%) (Fig. 19.5).

Pathological Diagnosis (Tumor 2) Clear cell carcinoma of right kidney, nucleolus classification 2/4. There was no evidence of tumor cells in the right ureter resection margin, the renal hilum lumen, the renal pelvis, or the peri-renal fat (Fig. 19.6).

19.1.4 Prognosis

The patient received enteral nutrition on postoperative day 3. The nasogastric tube was removed on postoperative day 7. The patient also received routine anticoagulation treatment postoperatively. She recovered well and was discharged on postoperative day 12. The patient was advised to undergo genetic testing in accordance with the Chinese Expert Consensus on Diagnosis and Treatment of GIST, 2017 edition. Due to financial issues, the patient did not receive targeted therapy after discharge. The follow-up imaging examinations were taken regularly, and demonstrated 17 months of disease-free survival.

19.1.5 Experience of Diagnosis and Therapy

The overall incidence of synchronous tumors involving GIST and other tumors is 5–30%, according to different studies [1–3]. It can be assured that the incidence is not as low as reported. Due to the limited numbers of patients, studies on the prognosis of such patients are rare. Union Hospital Affiliated to Tongji Medical College of Huazhong University of Science and Technology conducted a survival analysis comparing more than 70 patients with GIST who underwent sole tumor resection to synchronous resection involving another malignant tumor during the same period. The results showed the prognosis of the synchronous patients was inferior to that of patients with GIST only, which is similar to the findings of other studies [4]. With the mechanisms of *KIT*

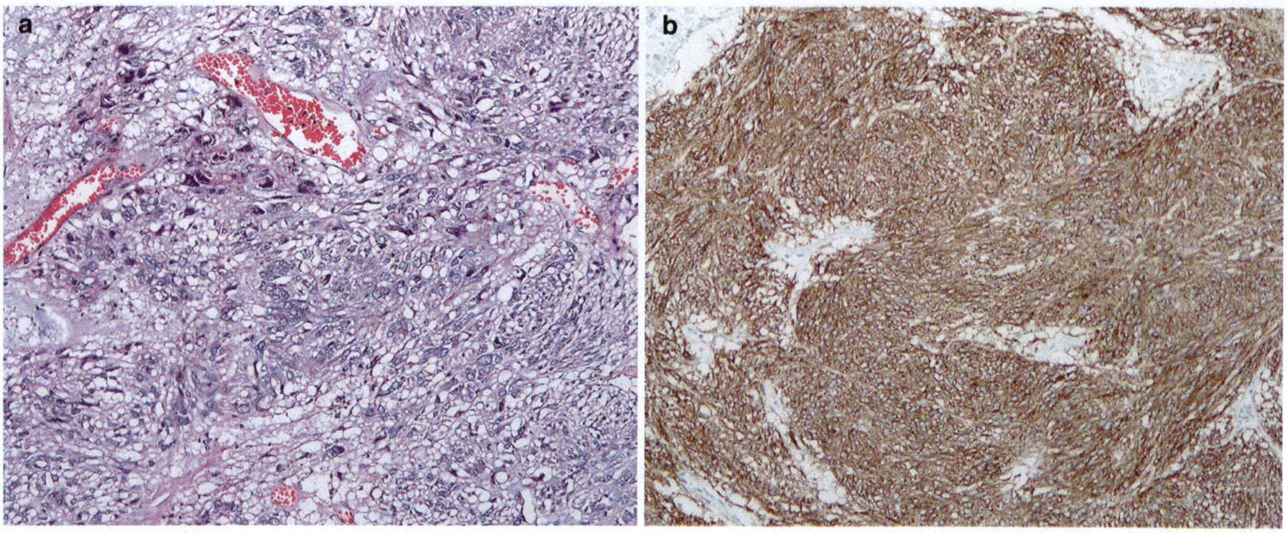

Fig. 19.5 GIST immunohistochemistry. **a** H&E staining; **b** CD117 staining

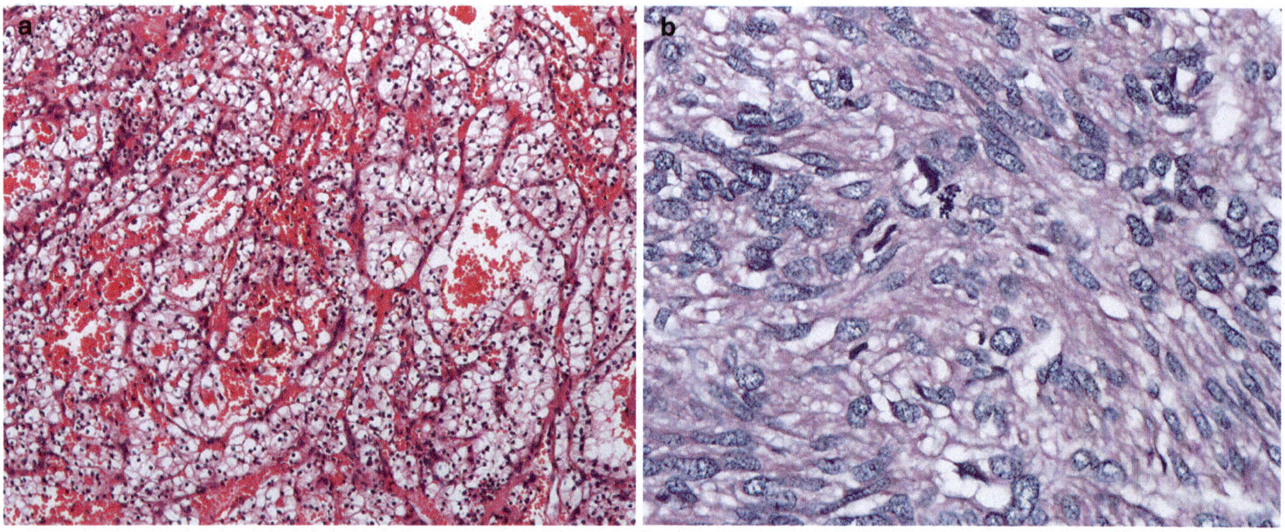

Fig. 19.6 Immunohistochemistry of clear cell carcinoma of right kidney. **a** H&E staining; **b** Mitosis

and *PDGFRA* in the pathogenesis of GIST being learned, most of the biological behaviors of these tumors have been determined. In fact, GIST still has high heterogeneity. A study conducted in 2018, which included 405 patients, raised the possibility of a potential connection between GIST and renal cell carcinoma [5]. Sunitinib can improve the prognosis for patients with GIST and renal cell carcinoma [6]. Fudan University Zhongshan Hospital reported a rare case of synchronous wild-type GIST and renal cell carcinoma caused by *SDHA* germline mutation [7].

The patient in this case was diagnosed with both renal carcinoma and GIST. Both tumors shared different origins which require swift intervention. At present, preoperative imatinib treatment for GIST is common, and is recommended by almost all GIST treatment guidelines. According to both international and domestic consensus and guidelines on the diagnosis and treatment of GIST, the recommended time for preoperative treatment to achieve maximum remission, where the tumor volume remains stable after two reviews, generally requires 6–12 months. In addition, the existing evidence shows that for GIST sensitive to imatinib, the therapeutic effect can be observed by imaging studies after only 1 week of treatment [8]. A retrospective study of preoperative treatment in West China Hospital demonstrated that most patients achieved the maximum effect after approximately 3 months of treatment [9]. It should be noted that the preoperative treatment for GIST is different from the neoadjuvant treatment of gastric and colorectal cancer. There is no evidence that preoperative treatment can improve the overall prognosis of patients; instead, the purpose is to reduce the surgical risk, avoid multi-visceral resection, and preserve organ function [10]. Therefore, pursuing the maximum tumor reduction or exceeding 6 months preoperative treatment time should not be the treatment goal. In the case of synchronous renal tumor and giant abdominopelvic GIST, the risk of GIST rupture and implantation is high in a single stage operation. On the other hand, if preoperative imatinib therapy for GIST is administered only to reach maximum effect in tumor volume reduction, the renal tumor may progress leading to a two-staged operation. Thus, we have learned that in the process of diagnosis and treatment of GIST, the maximum benefit is warranted by formulating individualized treatment strategies for each patient under different scenarios, including drug treatment and surgical timing.

Sunitinib is recommended by the treatment guidelines for both renal cell carcinoma and GIST treatment. Although the targets of sunitinib in GIST and renal cell carcinoma are different, sunitinib still has treatment value in patients with these synchronous tumors. A case report from the department of urology, West China Hospital, described a patient who was diagnosed with gastric GIST and renal clear cell carcinoma. Metastatic invasion of the hepatic portal vein was found at the time of first diagnosis. After surgical resection of the two primary tumors, the patient took sunitinib orally leading to the complete remission of the portal vein metastasis. If patients with renal cell carcinoma have GIST progression, imatinib or sunitinib should be considered as the targeted therapy.

19.2 Expert Comments

Yong Li

Prostate cancer is the most common genitourinary tumor found synchronously with GIST, as opposed to renal tumors which are rare. Synchronous malignant tumors, especially ones which have developed to a later stage, bring great difficulty to clinical treatment. Different from GIST with gastrointestinal cancer, where both tumors originate from adjacent tissues, renal cell carcinoma and GIST not only originate from different tissues, but also have large differences in potential carcinogenic factors. For such patients, there should be a complete pathological diagnosis before operation, and it is appropriate to conduct an MDT discussion to determine appropriate treatment. After the operation, with complete pathological report and genetic testing results, another MDT meeting should be held to discuss adjuvant therapy.

Sunitinib has a distinct indication for the treatment of advanced GIST and renal cell carcinoma. At present, sunitinib has not been indicated for preoperative treatment or adjuvant treatment for renal cell carcinoma. It is worth exploring in this regard as this may benefit some patients. In this case, both tumors could be radically resected as the initial treatment. Advice for surgical intervention was thus appropriate. Sunitinib, a multi-targeted drug, can be used in the treatment of two tumors at the same time, which also suggests the possible existence of common pathogenesis. If sunitinib is used for preoperative treatment and adjuvant treatment is indicated for both tumors, sunitinib is an option which is expected to benefit patients.

References

1. Murphy JD, Ma GL, Baumgartner JM, Madlensky L, Burgoyne AM, Tang CM, Martinez ME, Sicklick JK. Increased risk of additional cancers among patients with gastrointestinal stromal tumors: a population-based study. Cancer. 2015;121(17):2960–7. https://doi.org/10.1002/cncr.29434.
2. Kramer K, Wolf S, Mayer B, Schmidt SA, Agaimy A, Henne-Bruns D, Knippschild U, Schwab M, Schmiede M. Frequence, spectrum and prognostic impact of additional malignancies in patients with gastrointestinal stromal tumors. Neoplasia. 2015;17(1):134–40. https://doi.org/10.1016/j.neo.2014.12.001.
3. Vassos N, Agaimy A, Hohenberger W, Croner RS. Coexistence of gastrointestinal stromal tumours (GIST) and malignant neoplasms of different origin: prognostic implications. Int J Surg. 2014;12(5):371–7. https://doi.org/10.1016/j.ijsu.2014.03.004.
4. Mao G, Wang T, Yang WC, Shen Q, Jiang Q, Lyu JB, Zeng XY, Jia J, Liu WZ, Zeng XY, Tao KX, Zhang P. Clinicopathological features and prognosis analysis of patients with gastric gastrointestinal stromal tumor combined with digestive tract cancer. Zhonghua Xiao Hua Wai Ke Za Zhi. 2022;21(8):1071–7. Chinese. https://doi.org/10.3760/cma.j.cn115610-20220622-00363.
5. Mendonca SJ, Sanchez A, Blum KA, Ghanaat M, Kashan MY, Benfante N, Russo P, Coleman JA, Crago AM, Hakimi AA. The association of renal cell carcinoma with gastrointestinal stromal tumors. J Surg Oncol. 2018;117(8):1716–20. https://doi.org/10.1002/jso.25080.
6. Motzer RJ, Escudier B, Gannon A, Figlin RA. Sunitinib: ten years of successful clinical use and study in advanced renal cell carcinoma. Oncologist. 2017;22(1):41–52. https://doi.org/10.1634/theoncologist.2016-019.
7. Jiang Q, Zhang Y, Zhou YH, Hou YY, Wang JY, Li JL, Li M, Tong HX, Lu WQ. A novel germline mutation in SDHA identified in a rare case of gastrointestinal stromal tumor complicated with renal cell carcinoma. Int J Clin Exp Pathol. 2015;8(10):12188–97. https://www.ncbi.nlm.nih.gov/pmc/articles/PMC4680348
8. Li J, Ye YJ, Wang J, Zhang B, Qin SK, Shi YQ, He YL, Liang XB, Liu XF, Zhou Y, Wu X, Zhang XH, Wang M, Gao ZD, Lin TL, Cao H, Shen L, Chinese Society of Clinical Oncology (CSCO) Expert Committee on Gastrointestinal Stromal Tumor. Chinese consensus guidelines for diagnosis and management of gastrointestinal stromal tumor. Chin J Cancer Res. 2017;29(4):281–93. https://doi.org/10.21147/j.issn.1000-9604.2017.04.01.
9. Tao J, Ni C, Jin Y, Zhu YC, Zhang P, Yang YY, Zeng H. The coexistence of clear cell renal cell carcinoma and gastrointestinal stromal tumor with portal vein metastasis, and its favorable response to sunitinib. Expert Rev Anticancer Ther. 2013;13(2):131–6. https://doi.org/10.1586/era.12.162.
10. Tang S, Yin Y, Shen CY, Chen JJ, Yin XN, Zhang B, Yao YQ, Yang JL, Chen ZX. Preoperative imatinib mesylate (IM) for huge gastrointestinal stromal tumors (GIST). World J Surg Oncol. 2017;15(1):79–86. https://doi.org/10.1186/s12957-017-1143-2.

Part V

Targeted Therapy for Gastrointestinal Stromal Tumors

Gastrointestinal Stromal Tumors Progression During Adjuvant Therapy

20

Tianlong Ling, Ming Wang, and Xianfa Wang

Keywords

Gastrointestinal stromal tumors · Adjuvant therapy · Recurrence

20.1 Case 27 A 74-Year-Old Man with Recurrence During GIST Adjuvant Therapy

Tianlong Ling and Ming Wang

20.1.1 Introduction

After radical surgical resection of primary GIST, pathology evaluates the risk of postoperative recurrence according to the corresponding criteria based on the size, mitotic count, site of the primary tumor, and presence of preoperative or intraoperative rupture. The consensus guidelines suggest that patients with primary GIST with intermediate or high risk of recurrence should receive imatinib adjuvant therapy for 1 or 3 years, respectively. The probability of tumor recurrence and metastasis during adjuvant therapy is believed to be as low as 10%. Therefore, recurrence during the adjuvant treatment period requires further research.

20.1.2 Case Background

A 74-year-old man received gastric GIST resection 5 years ago and multiple metastases were identified 1 month previously, leading to a visit to Renji Hospital, Shanghai Jiao Tong University School of Medicine. The patient underwent gastric wedge resection in a local hospital to treat a tumor at the lesser curvature in August 2013 and recovered well after surgery. Postoperative pathology revealed gastric GIST, 5 cm × 4 cm × 4 cm in size, with mitotic count >10/50 HPF, and genetic testing was not performed. Adjuvant therapy with 400 mg/d imatinib was initiated by the local hospital. In August 2015, a mass in the hepatogastric space was found, which was considered to be a recurrent tumor, and the patient underwent surgery again at another hospital. The postoperative pathology revealed a recurrence of gastric GIST, 4 cm × 3 cm × 2 cm in size, with mitotic count >10/50 HPF. The genetic testing of the resected tumor revealed a heterozygous mutation in exon 11 of *KIT*, 576CTT>CCT, which caused the encoded amino acid to be converted from leucine to proline. The patient was treated with 400 mg/d imatinib in the outpatient clinic and followed up regularly with enhanced CT scans. On May 9, 2017, the abdominal CT showed new nodules in the capsule of the left lobe of the liver, considered to be metastasis (Fig. 20.1). On June 2, 2017, the patient underwent abdominal tumor resection in Renji Hospital. Intraoperatively, liver metastases were not found. The tumor was located at the right diaphragmatic dome, compressing the liver (Fig. 20.2).

Postoperative pathology at that time revealed that the abdominal tumor was consistent with GIST recurrence, 3.5 cm × 3 cm × 2 cm in size, mitotic count >10/50 HPF. Genetic testing again revealed a heterozygous mutation in exon 11 of *KIT*, 576CTT>CCT. Two weeks after surgery, the patient resumed imatinib therapy at a dose of 600 mg/d. Abdominal CT on May 4, 2018 revealed further possible tumor recurrence (Fig. 20.3). On June 5, 2018, the patient was admitted to the Department of Interventional Oncology

T. Ling · M. Wang (✉)
Department of Gastrointestinal Surgery, Renji Hospital, Shanghai Jiaotong University School of Medicine, Shanghai, China

X. Wang
Department of General Surgery, Sir Run Run Shaw Hospital, affiliated with the Zhejiang University School of Medicine, Hangzhou, China
e-mail: 3195011@zju.edu.cn

K. Tao, H. Cao (eds.), *Clinical Management of Gastrointestinal Stromal Tumor*, https://doi.org/10.1007/978-981-99-9392-5_20

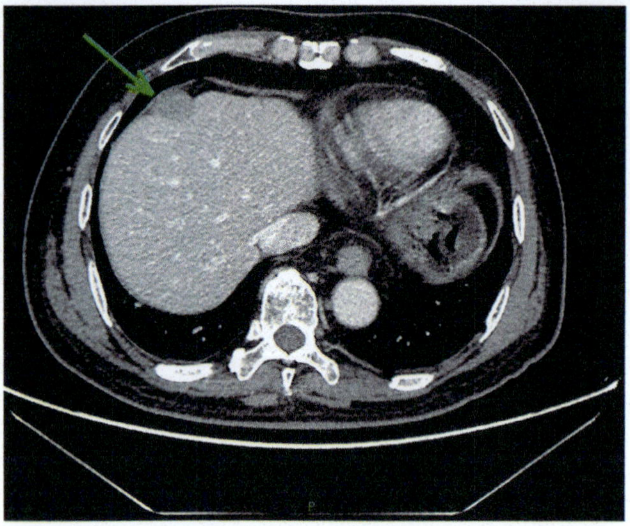

Fig. 20.1 CT revealed a new nodule in the capsule of the left lobe of the liver, considered to be GIST metastasis

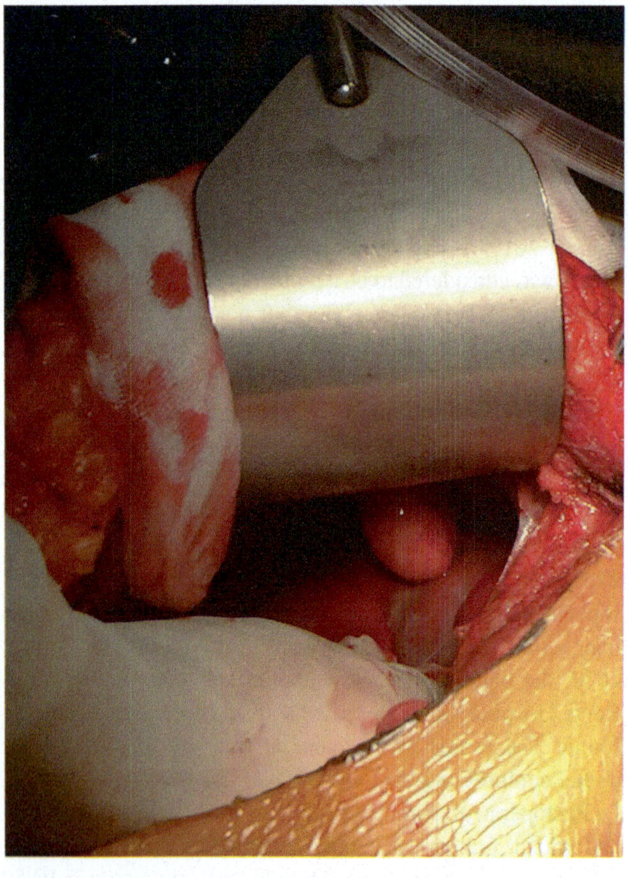

Fig. 20.2 Intraoperative finding of recurrent tumor located in the right diaphragmatic dome, there were no tumors on the liver

of Renji Hospital, Shanghai Jiao Tong University School of Medicine for ultrasound-guided radiofrequency ablation of liver tumors under general anesthesia. However, intraoperative contrast-enhanced ultrasound showed no significant

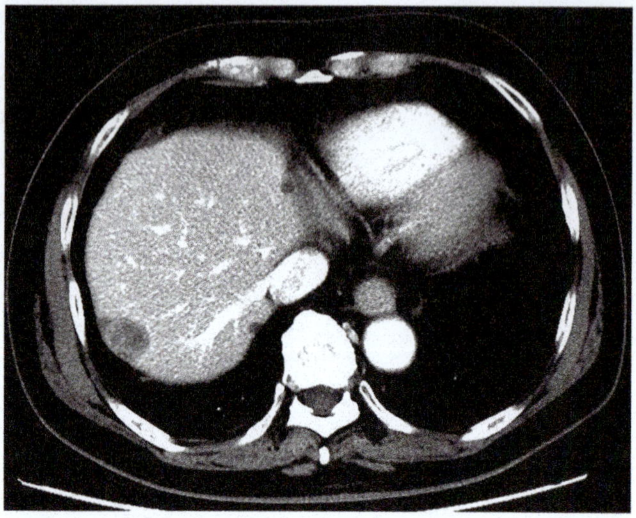

Fig. 20.3 CT from May 2018 showed new nodules in the right lobe of the liver, considered to be possible GIST metastasis

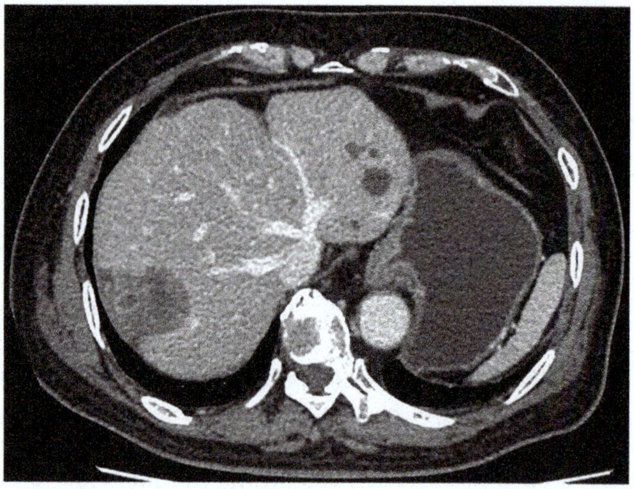

Fig. 20.4 CT from October 2018 found that the extracapsular low-density lesions in the right lobe of the liver were significantly larger than before

tumor staining. Further MRI examination or continued follow-up was recommended. An enhanced CT on October 16, 2018, revealed that the extracapsular low-density lesion in the right lobe of the liver was significantly larger than before, which was considered to be diaphragmatic metastasis. Additionally, a new subperitoneal metastatic nodule was visible in the upper abdomen (Figs. 20.4 and 20.5). During the course of the disease, the patient had occasional discomfort in the right upper abdomen, without hematemesis, melena, cough, expectoration, chills, high fever, abdominal distension, or diarrhea. The patient sought further treatment at the Department of Gastrointestinal Surgery, Renji Hospital, Shanghai Jiao Tong University School of Medicine.

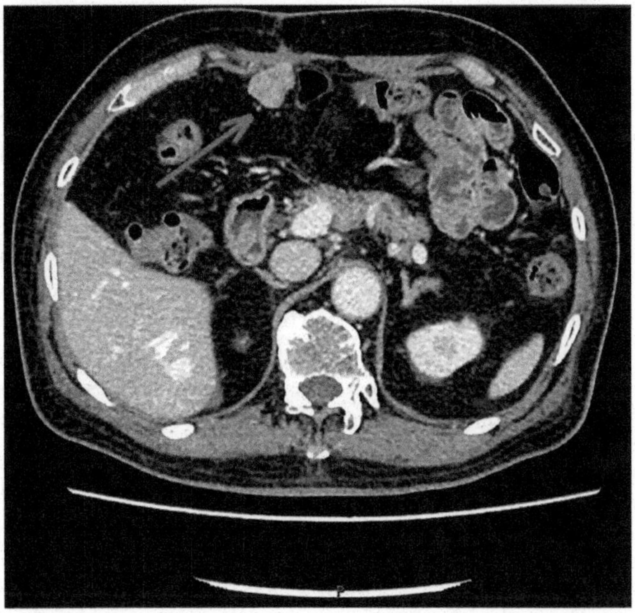

Fig. 20.5 CT revealed new subperitoneal metastatic nodules in the upper abdomen

20.1.2.1 Past History and Family History

The patient was otherwise healthy and reported no history of drug allergies. There was no similar medical history in the family.

20.1.2.2 Physical Examination

The patient's vital signs were stable, and the skin and sclera were not yellowish or pale. The abdomen was flat and showed no gastrointestinal or peristaltic waves. A surgical scar was noted on the abdomen. The abdomen was soft without tenderness or rebound tenderness. The bowel sounds were normal.

20.1.2.3 Auxiliary Examination

Enhanced Abdominal CT, October 2018 Appearing after gastric GIST surgery and liver surgery, the low-density lesions outside the capsule of the right lobe of the liver were significantly larger than before, suggestive of diaphragmatic metastases, and subperitoneal metastatic nodules in the upper abdomen were now apparent. Multiple cysts and small calcifications were observed in the liver, and a hemangioma was observed in the right lobe of the liver. A gallstone and multiple small cysts in both kidneys were also observed.

20.1.2.4 Preliminary Diagnosis

1. Abdominal recurrence after gastric GIST surgery
2. Metastatic tumor progression after surgery

20.1.3 Therapy

20.1.3.1 Case Analysis

The patient was an elderly man. After gastric GIST surgery, he was treated with the standard dose of imatinib until abdominal metastasis progressed. After resection of the abdominal metastatic lesions, the disease progressed again while the patient received treatment with an increased dose of imatinib. The abdominal metastasis was evaluated to be resectable. The surgical treatment was assessed to be feasible, and subsequent targeted therapy was to be determined by pathology and genetic testing results.

20.1.3.2 Treatment

On November 5, 2018, the patient underwent diaphragmatic tumor resection, abdominal lesion resection, and intestinal adhesiolysis under general anesthesia. During the operation, the original surgical incision in the abdomen was reopened, and severe intra-abdominal adhesions were observed. Following adhesiolysis, a tumor, 4 cm in size, was found below the original abdominal incision which formed strong adhesion with the greater omentum. No liver mass was found. Additionally, a right diaphragmatic tumor, approximately 5 cm in diameter, compressed the right lobe of the liver. After partial resection of the right diaphragm, diaphragmatic repair was performed (Fig. 20.6). Exploration of other parts of the abdomen revealed no metastases or ascites. The patient recovered well after the surgery and was discharged on postoperative day 6.

20.1.3.3 Postoperative Pathology and Genetic Testing

Pathological Diagnosis The diaphragmatic tumor, 5.0 cm × 4.0 cm × 2.0 cm in size, and abdominal tumor, 4.0 cm × 2.0 cm × 2.0 cm in size, were consistent with GIST recurrence, mitotic count >10/50 HPF.

Immunohistochemically CD117 (+), DOG-1 (+), CD34 (+), P53 (+ +), Ki-67 (LI>50%), SMA (−), desmin (−), S100 (−).

Genetic Testing The abdominal tumor was consistent with GIST recurrence. The sequencing analysis revealed heterozygous mutation in exon 11 of *KIT*, 576CTT>CCT, which caused the encoded amino acid to be converted from leucine to proline. An additional heterozygous mutation was found at codon 654 in exon 13 of *KIT*, 654GTG>GCG, which caused the encoded amino acid to be converted from valine to alanine. Exons 9 and 17 of *KIT* and exons 12 and 18 of *PDGFRA* were wild type.

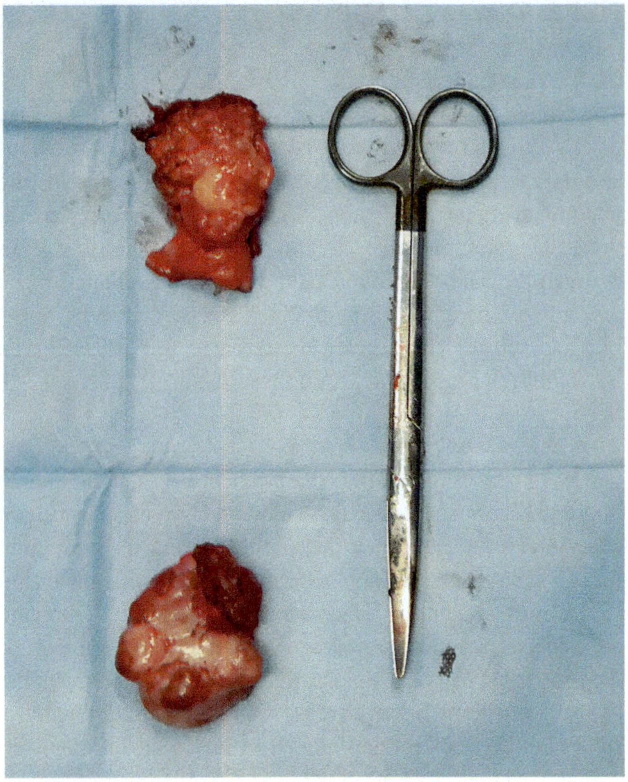

Fig. 20.6 The gross specimen

20.1.4 Prognosis

The patient was discharged on postoperative day 6 and began 37.5 mg/d sunitinib treatment 2 weeks after the surgery. There were no signs of side effects or toxicity. In September 2020, 2 years after the surgery, advanced abdominal tumor progression was detected. Due to his poor conditions, palliative imatinib was administered until the patient passed away in March 2021.

20.1.5 Experience of Diagnosis and Therapy

20.1.5.1 Second-Line Treatment Options After Failure of Adjuvant Therapy

Choosing second-line treatment for patients with GIST with primary mutation in *KIT* who have disease progression during adjuvant therapy is complex. Treatment options for these patients include increasing the imatinib dosage or changing to sunitinib [1]. Since mutation in exon 9 of *KIT* is less likely to have secondary mutations than mutations in exon 11, it is generally believed that second-line treatment, after failure of first-line treatment, for recurrent metastatic GIST with primary mutation in exon 9 of *KIT* will be more effective than that for patients with mutations in exon 11, regardless of whether second-line therapy involves increasing imatinib dosage or switching to sunitinib [2, 3]. The results of Professor Jian Li's research at Peking University Cancer Hospital suggest that if the second-line treatment regimen is 600 mg/d imatinib, patients with primary mutation in exon 9 could obtain 47-week median progression free survival (PFS), which is better than that for mutation in exon 11 or wild-type [4]. It is rather 17-week for the whole GIST population. If sunitinib is the second-line treatment, patients with GIST can obtain 35-week median PFS, in which primary mutation in exon 9 could obtain 60-week median PFS, which is also better than patients with mutations in exon 11 or wild-type *KIT*. Clinically, second-line treatment of GIST with primary mutation in exon 9 of *KIT* can achieve better treatment results [5].

Although a small number of studies have investigated which second-line treatment regimen yields better results, the results are not convincing because of the limited number of included patients and the retrospective nature of the studies. Currently, it has been recognized that increasing imatinib dosage can benefit patients with a mutation in exon 9 whose original dosage provided insufficient drug concentration or who require more effective treatment. On the other hand, increasing the dosage cannot benefit patients who have had sufficient drug concentration.

The genetic testing of the specimen obtained at the final operation showed a new V654A point mutation in exon 13 of *KIT* in addition to the original mutation in exon 11. Secondary mutations, such as mutations in exons 13 and 17 of *KIT*, can lower imatinib binding by altering the ATP-binding and activation loop domain of KIT protein, respectively, leading to drug resistance. Other rare types of mutations, such as the T670 mutation in exon 14 of *KIT*, affect the binding of imatinib by altering the threonine, gatekeeper amino acid, of the ATP-binding domain [6]. Sunitinib is the preferred second-line treatment after imatinib failure. Sunitinib may benefit GIST patients with mutation in exon 9 of *KIT*, wild-type, and GIST with secondary mutations in V654A and T670I. Thus, based on the genetic test, patients received sunitinib treatment after surgery.

20.1.5.2 The Value of Surgery for Locally Advanced GIST

Compared to advanced gastric or intestinal cancer, the progress of most recurrent and metastatic GIST is relatively slow under targeted therapy, and only a small proportion of patients will show multifocal progression in a short time. During the slow development phase of the disease, it is often manifested as partial progression, known as treatment resistance, while others remain stable, known as responding to treatments. In addition to second-line therapy, surgery is another option. At present, for the surgical treatment of recurrent metastatic GIST, the timing and the resection range are the focus of the intervention [7]. According to the guideline and consensus, for late-staged GIST, the appropriate time to perform surgery is when targeted drugs are effective or localized progression happens. The goal of surgery is to remove all recurrent and metastatic lesions that can be detected on imaging studies as much as possible. In this patient, the metastatic recurrence was more localized with good general conditions. The surgery could achieve satisfactory cytoreduction. Surgical resection of metastatic lesions allows patients to achieve a longer response time for targeted drugs, which in turn prolongs patients' survival. Although the value of surgery in late GIST remains to be explored, it does benefit patients who receive surgical intervention under localized progression [8].

20.2 Expert Comments

Xianfa Wang

Primary GIST have now entered an era where surgical treatment and targeted therapy have the same value due to the emergence of targeted drugs. It is even difficult to determine which therapy dominates over the other. For high-risk primary GIST, conservative surgical procedure plus postoperative targeted therapy is mostly applied in clinical practice, which not only ensures long-term survival but also quality of life. However, there is still room for discussion on the timing of adjuvant targeted therapy, whether the therapy can benefit patients with non-exon 11 mutations, and whether high-dose adjuvant therapy is required for exon 9 mutations.

We can learn the following from this case:

1. Whether the so-called primary GIST are truly primary is debatable. In this case, the recurrence was presented through a series of intra-abdominal metastases, which occurred during the adjuvant therapy about 2 years after surgery which is in line with the median PFS with imatinib as first-line therapy. It was impossible to determine whether micro-metastasis was present during the initial surgery at the local hospital. The mitotic count of the original histopathological report revealed poor prognosis. For this type of patients, it is rather important to have adjuvant therapy after surgery without any hesitation and to comply with closer imaging follow-up periods. This patient benefited from series of close follow-up with enhanced CT and MDT for assessment in his diagnosis and treatment. An effective intervention was taken during two instances of localized tumor progression. This thus prolonged the patient survival to 4 years.
2. Whether adjuvant imatinib treatment reduces the recurrence rate of GIST or delays the recurrence of GIST is the most critical issue for postoperative medical treatment of primary GIST in the future. As a role model in targeted drugs, imatinib has two characteristics: high efficacy and low side effects and has also been proved to be safe and reliable in the long-term treatment for late-staged patients. Therefore, for patients with primary GIST and ultra-high risk of recurrence, it is also acceptable for patients to continue to take imatinib for a long time as the principle treatment for patients, which is already accepted by some doctors and patients. More clinical data are needed to determine which groups of patients require such radical adjuvant therapy.

References

1. Vincenzi B, Nannini M, Fumagalli E, Bronte G, Frezza AM, Lisi DD, Ceruso MS, Santini D, Badalamenti G, Pantaleo MA, Russo A, Dei Tos AP, Casali P, Tonini G. Imatinib dose escalation versus sunitinib as a second line treatment in KIT exon 11 mutated GIST: a retrospective analysis. Oncotarget. 2016;7(43):69412–9. https://doi.org/10.18632/oncotarget.5136.
2. Kelly CM, Sainz LG, Chi P. The management of metastatic GIST: current standard and investigational therapeutics. J Hematol Oncol. 2021;14(1):2–14. https://doi.org/10.1186/s13045-020-01026-6.
3. Joensuu H, Wardelmann E, Sihto H, Eriksson M, Hall KS, Reichardt A, Hartmann JT, Pink D, Cameron S, Hohenberger P, Al-Batran SE, Schlemmer M, Bauer S, Nilsson B, Kallio R, Junnila J, Vehtari A, Reichardt P. Effect of *KIT* and *PDGFRA* mutations on survival in patients with gastrointestinal stromal tumors treated with adjuvant imatinib: an exploratory analysis of a randomized clinical trial. JAMA Oncol. 2017;3(5):602–9. https://doi.org/10.1001/jamaoncol.2016.5751.
4. Li J, Gong JF, Li J, Gao J, Sun NP, Shen L. Efficacy of imatinib dose escalation in Chinese gastrointestinal stromal tumor patients. World J Gastroenterol. 2012;18(7):698–703. https://doi.org/10.3748/wjg.v18.i7.698.
5. Li J, Gao J, Hong J, Shen L. Efficacy and safety of sunitinib in Chinese patients with imatinib-resistant or -intolerant gastrointestinal stromal tumors. Future Oncol. 2012;8(5):617–24. https://doi.org/10.2217/fon.12.29.
6. Li GZ, Raut CP. Targeted therapy and personalized medicine in gastrointestinal stromal tumors: drug resistance, mechanisms, and treatment strategies. Onco Targets Ther. 2019;12:5123–33. https://doi.org/10.2147/OTT.S180763.
7. Mussi C, Ronellenfitsch U, Jakob J, Tamborini E, Reichardt P, Casali PG, Fiore M, Hohenberger P, Gronchi A. Post-imatinib surgery in advanced/metastatic GIST: is it worthwhile in all patients? Ann Oncol. 2010;21(2):403–8. https://doi.org/10.1093/annonc/mdp310.
8. Ford JF, Gronchi A. Indications for surgery in advanced/metastatic GIST. Eur J Cancer. 2016;63:154–67. https://doi.org/10.1016/j.ejca.2016.05.019.

Gastrointestinal Stromal Tumors Recurrence After Stopping Adjuvant Therapy

21

Xiaoqi Li, Wenze Wan, and Han Liang

Keywords

Gastrointestinal stromal tumor · Adjuvant therapy · Recurrence

21.1 Case 28 A 58-Year-Old Man with High-Risk GIST Suffered from Recurrence After Stopping Adjuvant Therapy

Xiaoqi Li and Wenze Wan

21.1.1 Introduction

Imatinib, as the first-choice drug for the treatment of GIST, has become a classic of targeted drug therapy. In the past 10 years, imatinib has been used as postoperative adjuvant treatment for GIST to prevent recurrence and metastasis and has obtained a good effect. However, two clinical studies, the Z9001 and SSGXVIII trials, suggested that recurrence and metastasis still occurred for some patients after cessation of adjuvant therapy. As the number of patients with primary GIST who receive adjuvant imatinib treatment increases year by year, the number of patients who experience tumor recurrence after imatinib discontinuation will increase too, and relapse after discontinuation will become a hotspot in the diagnosis and treatment of GIST. However, the cause of relapse after drug withdrawal is currently unclear, and the treatment strategies for patients who relapse after drug withdrawal remain controversial. The diagnosis and treatment of this subgroup of patients with GIST needs further exploration. Here we describe the diagnosis and treatment for 1 patient with relapse after discontinuation of imatinib adjuvant therapy for reference.

21.1.2 Case Background

The patient, a 58-year-old man, presented to the local hospital for investigation of 1 week of upper GI hemorrhage in September 2010. Gastric endoscopy showed a mass in the gastric antrum, which was diagnosed as GIST. The patient was admitted to Union Hospital, Tongji Medical College, Huazhong University of Science and Technology for further treatment.

21.1.2.1 Past History and Family History

The patient was previously healthy and had a history of appendicectomy for appendicitis more than 30 years previously. The patient reported no history of drug allergy and his parents were deceased.

21.1.2.2 Physical Examination

The patient's vital signs were stable, and the skin and mucous membranes were not yellowish or pale. The abdomen was flat, and no gastrointestinal or peristaltic wave was observed. The abdomen was soft, with no tenderness, rebound tenderness, or palpable mass. The bowel sounds were normal.

X. Li
Department of Gastrointestinal Surgery, Renji Hospital, Shanghai Jiaotong University School of Medicine, Shanghai, China

W. Wan (✉)
Department of Gastrointestinal Surgery, Union Hospital, Tongji Medical College, Huazhong University of Science and Technology, Wuhan, China
e-mail: wanwenze@hust.edu.cn

H. Liang
Department of Gastric Surgery, Tianjin Medical University Cancer Institute & Hospital, Tianjin, China

K. Tao, H. Cao (eds.), *Clinical Management of Gastrointestinal Stromal Tumor*, https://doi.org/10.1007/978-981-99-9392-5_21

21.1.2.3 Auxiliary Examination

Blood Routine WBC 6.16 × 10^9/L, RBC 3.51 × 10^{12}/L, Hb 97 g/L, PLT 333 × 10^9/L, NEUT% 62.4%, LY% 23.5%.

Blood Biochemistry No obvious abnormalities.

Abdominal CT, Plain and Enhanced Scans The images showed localized thickening in the wall of the gastric fundus, approximately 3.7 cm × 3.2 cm in size, and the boundary was unclear. The enhanced scan showed that the degree of enhancement was slightly lower than that of the surrounding stomach wall (Fig. 21.1).

Ultrasound Gastroscopy The mucosa on the lesser curvature of the anterior pylorus showed swelling and erosion. A new nodular neoplasm was found in the fundus of the stomach under the cardia with an uneven surface. The neoplasm originated from the muscularis propria, demonstrated uneven hypoechoic changes, was irregular in shape, and close to the cardia, and the most likely diagnosis was a GIST.

21.1.2.4 Preliminary Diagnosis

1. Gastric GIST
2. History of appendectomy

21.1.3 Therapy

21.1.3.1 Case Analysis

The patient was an elderly man, who consulted a doctor for investigation of upper GI bleeding. The patient was generally in good condition, and gastroscopy performed in the local hospital suggested the possibility of GIST. The tumor was assessed to be resectable, no metastasis was found, and surgery was recommended. Since the gastric tumor derived from the muscularis propria was 3.7 cm × 3.2 cm in size, it was suitable for elective surgical treatment. Follow-up treatment was recommended based on the results of pathological examination.

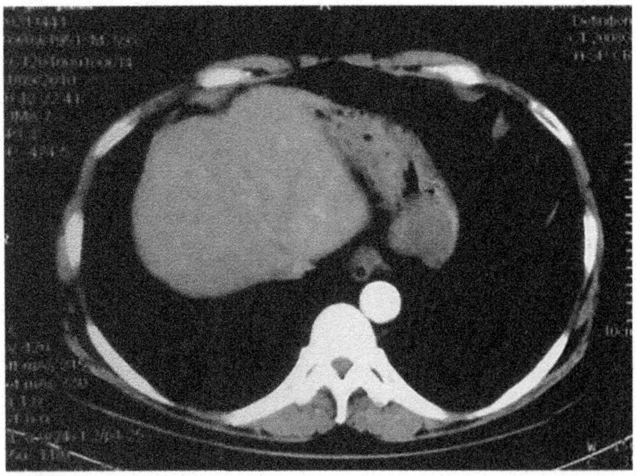

Fig. 21.1 Abdominal CT from September 2010 showed limited thickening of the stomach wall at the fundus of the stomach

21.1.3.2 Treatment

An exploratory laparotomy was performed on September 14, 2010. During the operation, a 5.0 cm × 5.0 cm mass was palpable near the cardia of the greater curvature of the stomach, which was of medium firmness, mobile, and adhered to the greater omentum. The tumor was found to be larger than indicated by the imaging evaluation and was close to the cardia. Since it was difficult to perform local resection or wedge resection, proximal gastrectomy was performed. The surgical procedure went well. Approximately 200 mL of blood was lost during the operation and the surgical time was 120 min.

21.1.3.3 Postoperative Pathology

Pathological Diagnosis Gastric GIST, no tumor metastasis on the sections of the lesser curvature or greater curvature lymph nodes, and no tumor involvement was seen on the surgical margin sections. The mass was 6.0 cm × 5.5 cm in size, with mitotic count 7 ~ 8/50 HPF, was diagnosed as high risk according to the modified NIH classification.

Immunohistochemistry CD117 (+), CD34 (+), DOG-1 (+), SMA (−), S-100 (partial+), Ki-67 (Li <5%).

21.1.4 Prognosis

The patient was discharged 11 days after surgery. He took imatinib 400 mg/d and was reviewed regularly. In September 2011, a CT scan of the abdomen at a local hospital did not find tumor recurrence or metastasis, and imatinib treatment drug was discontinued. A CT re-examination in June 2012 showed no obvious abnormalities.

In July 2013, an MRI revealed multiple nodules in the liver, which indicated possible GIST metastasis (Fig. 21.2). The patient was recommended to restart imatinib 400 mg/d, and attend regular follow-up appointments for observation. In October 2013, after taking 3 months of imatinib treatment, the liver MRI was reexamined. The images showed that the lesion in the left lobe of the liver was smaller than in the previous scan, with a diameter of approximately 1 cm. The larger lesion in right lobe of the liver was also slightly smaller than in the previous scan, and the enhancement was not obvious. According to the imaging assessment, the patient achieved partial remission, and continued to take imatinib 400 mg/d. After that, the patient's liver MRI was reviewed every 6 months, results showed no significant change in the size of the lesions, and the disease was considered stable (Fig. 21.3).

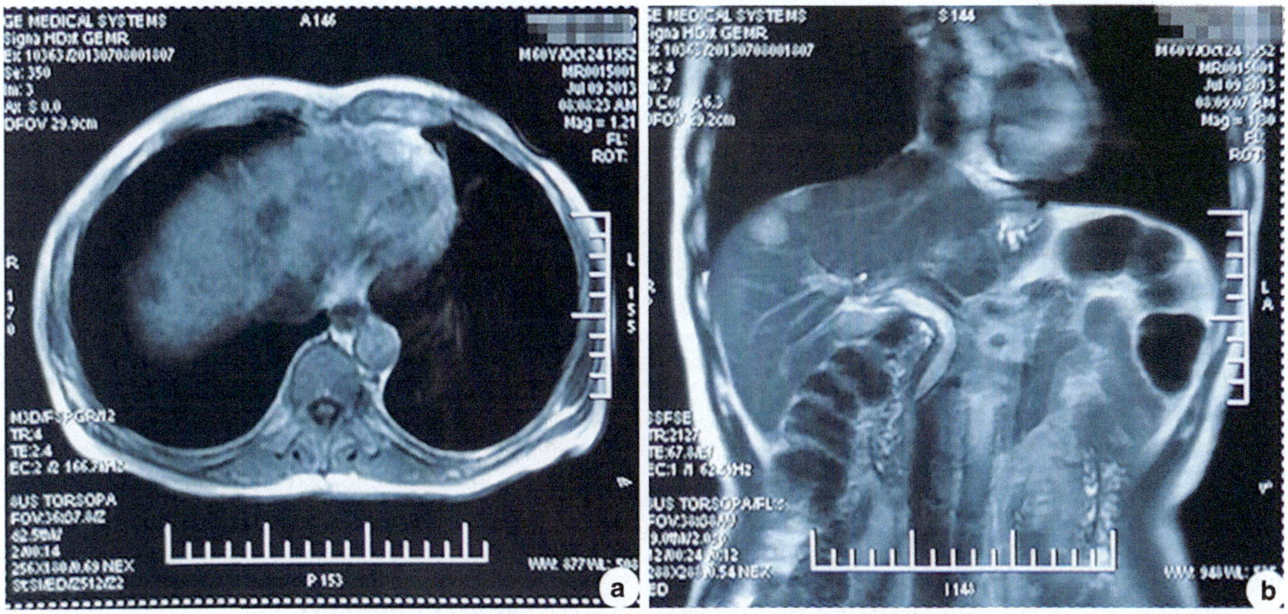

Fig. 21.2 MRI indicated multiple GIST metastases in the liver in July 2013. (**a**) Transverse plane; (**b**) Coronal plane

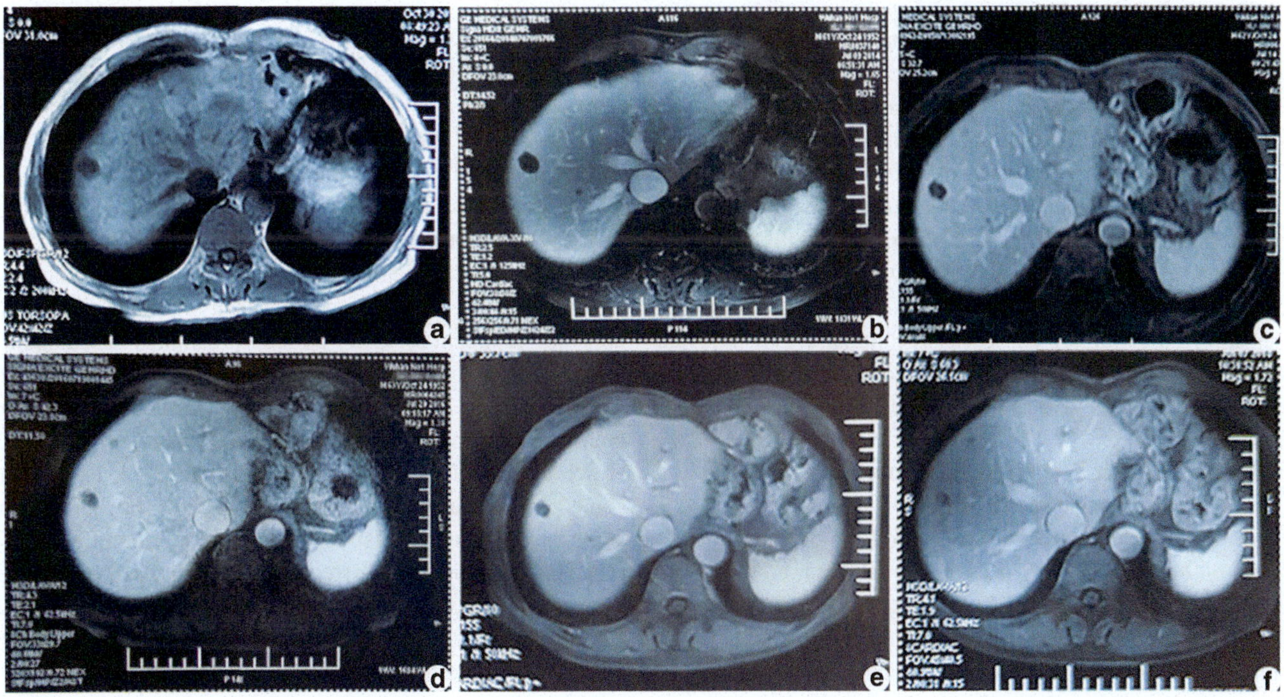

Fig. 21.3 The changes of large lesions in the right lobe of liver. **a** October 2013; **b** July 2014; **c** July 2015; **d** March 2016; **e** May 2017; **f** March 2018

21.1.5 Experience of Diagnosis and Therapy

It is not uncommon for patients with GIST to present with tumor metastasis after ceasing adjuvant therapy. A randomized, multi-center phase III clinical study conducted by the European Cancer Research and Treatment Organization showed that the average annual recurrence rate for patients receiving adjuvant therapy was 6%, which rose to 14% after ceasing adjuvant therapy [1]. The average annual recurrence rate of patients in the SSG XVIII study was 4%, and after stopping adjuvant therapy, it was 8%. A study conducted by Professor Hui Cao's team from Renji Hospital affiliated to Shanghai Jiaotong University School of Medicine included 138 patients with GIST who had received adjuvant therapy for more than 1 year [2]. The study found that the median follow-up after drug withdrawal was 27 months, and the total recurrence rate was 25.4%. The median time to relapse was 17 months. A study by Professor Kaixiong Tao's team from Union Hospital, Tongji Medical College, Huazhong University of Science and Technology included 80 patients with GIST who discontinued adjuvant treatment after more than 1 year [3]. This study showed that the median follow-up time after discontinuation was 39 months, and the total recurrence rate was 21.3%. Patients with recurrence and metastasis had no specific clinical manifestations, all were found by enhanced CT during follow-up review, and recurrence or metastasis occurred more often 1–2 years after treatment cessation. This suggests that for patients with GIST who stop adjuvant therapy, the frequency of follow-up should be increased within 2 years after imatinib therapy is stopped, and enhanced CT or MRI should be performed as part of routine review to detect tumor recurrence earlier.

It can be seen from the above reports that the recurrence rate of GIST after stopping adjuvant treatment of imatinib is worthy of concern. Therefore, it is necessary to screen groups with a high risk of recurrence and metastasis after ceasing adjuvant treatment for GIST, and an individualized diagnosis and treatment plan should be provided. The research of Professor Hui Cao's team showed that the Ki-67 expression index and local tumor invasion are independent risk factors for the recurrence of GIST after discontinuation of imatinib, while Professor Kaixiong Tao's team found that non-gastric-derived GIST has a higher risk of recurrence after adjuvant treatment is stopped than gastric-derived GIST. At the same time, both the NCCN guidelines and Chinese gastrointestinal stromal tumor expert consensus recommend that adjuvant therapy be appropriately extended beyond the standard 3-year course for patients who present with tumor rupture [4].

21.1.5.1 Basic Principles of Laparoscopic Surgery for GIST

Laparoscopic surgery for GIST also follows the basic principles of open surgery. The principle of "non-contact, less squeezing" should be followed during surgery, and attention should be paid to avoid tumor ulceration and spreading, leading to abdominal implantation or blood metastasis. A retrieval bag must be used, and the pursuit of minimally invasive and small incisions should be avoided. Removal of the tumor will affect the pathological evaluation after surgery.

In addition, there is still a lack of high-level evidence-based medical research regarding whether patients who relapse after stopping adjuvant therapy should be treated with re-administration of standard dose imatinib, an increased dose of imatinib or with second-line sunitinib therapy. A report by Reichardt et al. based on the SSG XVIII/AIO study showed that the clinical benefit rate of imatinib retreatment in patients who discontinued and relapsed was 84.8% [5]. Professor Jian Li from Peking University Cancer Hospital reported that when 24 patients who relapsed after stopping the drug were treated with the standard dose of imatinib again, eleven patients (45.8%) achieved partial remission, 12 patients (50.0%) had stable tumors, and 1 had tumor progression [6]. This suggests that most patients with tumor recurrence after the discontinuation of imatinib adjuvant therapy did not develop resistance to imatinib, and the standard dose of imatinib can be used again to obtain an objective effect similar to the initial treatment. This patient was treated with imatinib 400 mg/d again after recurrence, and the tumors shrank to a certain extent. Therefore, repeating the standard dose of imatinib can be considered for patients who relapse after stopping therapy, but close follow-up is required to observe the treatment effect. If the tumor progresses, the treatment plan needs to be adjusted appropriately.

21.2 Expert Comments

Han Liang

At present, NCCN and ESMO guidelines both recommend that patients with high recurrence risk need to receive imatinib adjuvant treatment for at least 3 years after complete resection, while the Chinese Guidelines on Diagnosis and Treatment of GIST recommends 3 years of adjuvant treatment for high-risk and intermediate-risk patients with tumors of non-gastric origin, and 1 year of adjuvant treatment for intermediate-risk patients of gastric origin. Recommendations from the above guidelines and consensus on the time limit of adjuvant treatment for GIST patients are mainly based on the Z9001 trial which compared taking a placebo with 1 year of imatinib and the SSG XVIII trial which compared a one-year course of imatinib with a 3-year course of imatinib [5, 7]. However, in real clinical situations, it is often observed that some patients relapsed after stopping adjuvant therapy. In addition, studies have also reported an increase in the recurrence rate of patients after stopping the drug, so the best time limit for adjuvant treatment remains to be discussed. Currently, some scholars advocate extension of adjuvant treatment time, and PERSIST-5 verified that 5 years of adjuvant therapy is safe and effective [8], but whether 5 years vs. 3 years of treatment can further improve the prognosis of GIST patients remains to be discussed after the end of the FAITH study.

In the era of precision and individualized medical care, we need to screen patients rationally and scientifically to make targeted adjuvant treatment plans which avoid over-treatment and under-treatment. Currently, commonly used GIST risk assessment standards mainly consider factors, such as tumor location, size, mitotic count, and tumor rupture, which have certain limitations. In the future, it is necessary to incorporate indicators, such as cell atypia, neurovascular infiltration, Ki-67, tumor necrosis, gene mutation type, and neutrophil/lymphocyte ratio. Additionally, new methods, such as artificial intelligence machine learning, can be used to develop more detailed evaluation criteria for patients with GIST and provide reference for individualized treatment. Laparoscopic surgery has the advantages of smaller incisions, better vision, less bleeding, and less pain. However, because GIST is brittle and prone to ulceration and bleeding, once it ruptures, the risk of postoperative recurrence is greatly increased, as is the risk of metastasis. Therefore, surgeons who have undergone rigorous training in laparoscopic techniques must not focus only on providing minimally invasive surgery.

This patient was diagnosed with a high recurrence risk GIST. The diameter of the tumor during the operation was significantly larger than that indicated by preoperative CT diagnosis. For special gastric GIST, the preoperative impact assessment should include gastroscopy, ultrasound gastroscopy, and CT. Gastroscopy can show the distance of the tumor from the dentate line of the esophagus and stomach. If the edge of the tumor is more than 2 cm from the dentate line, local resection can be attempted to preserve complete gastric function. The patient discontinued adjuvant imatinib treatment 1 year after the operation. It is unknown whether the drug was discontinued due to postoperative digestive dysfunction, economic reasons, drug side effects, or unclear awareness of the possibility of tumor recurrence. The vast majority of patients with GIST can survive long-term after receiving standard treatment. Therefore, the quality of life after surgery should be fully considered on the premise of ensuring radical surgery. For patients with a high risk of recurrence, it is particularly important to give adequate patient education and postoperative adjuvant targeted therapy. Approximately 30% of patients in the SSG XVIII study could not complete the postoperative adjuvant treatment plan, and a considerable number of patients believed that they would not relapse even if the drug was stopped. Therefore, radical treatment physicians are obliged to strengthen patient education and adherence to strict follow-up to ensure patient compliance with treatment, thereby increasing the completion rate of postoperative adjuvant therapy.

References

1. Benjamin RS, Casali PG. Adjuvant imatinib for GI stromal tumors: when and for how long? J Clin Oncol. 2016;34(3):215–8. https://doi.org/10.1200/JCO.2015.64.0102.
2. Xu J, Zhao WY, Zhuang C, Wang M, Zhang ZZ, Zhao G, Cao H. Risk factors related to gastrointestinal stromal tumor recurrence after discontinuing postoperative adjuvant imatinib treatment. Zhonghua Pu Tong Wai Ke Za Zhi. 2016;31(2):104–7. Chinese. https://doi.org/10.3760/cma.j.issn.1007-631X.2016.02.006.
3. Wan WZ, Tao KX, Zhang RZ, Li CG, Yang WC, Wang T, Zeng XY, Cai M, Wang GB, Zhang P. Analysis of diagnosis and treatment of gastrointestinal stromal tumor recurrence and metastasis after postoperative adjuvant imatinib treatment. J Int Oncol. 2018;45(11):665–9. Chinese. https://doi.org/10.3760/cma.j.issn.1673-422X.2018.11.006.
4. Li J, Ye Y, Wang J, Zhang B, Qin S, Shi Y, He Y, Liang X, Liu X, Zhou Y, Wu X, Zhang X, Wang M, Gao Z, Lin T, Cao H, Shen L, Chinese Society Of Clinical Oncology (CSCO) Expert Committee On Gastrointestinal Stromal Tumor. Chinese consensus guidelines for diagnosis and management of gastrointestinal stromal tumor. Chin J Cancer Res. 2017;29(4):281–93. https://doi.org/10.21147/j.issn.1000-9604.2017.04.01.
5. Reichardt P, Hartmann JT, Hall KS, Eriksson M, Joensuu H. Response to imatinib rechallenge of GIST that recurs following completion of adjuvant imatinib treatment-the first analysis in the SSGX VIII/AIO trail patient population. Eur J Cancer. 2011;47(1):81–90. https://doi.org/10.1016/S0959-8049(11)70130-7.
6. Dong Z, Gao J, Gong JF, Li J, Li Y, Wang XC, Li YY, Shen L, Li J. Efficacy observation on imatinib reintroduction in gastrointestinal stromal tumor with high recurrence risk after imatinib adjuvant therapy failure. Zhonghua Wei Chang Wai Ke Za Zhi. 2016;19(11):1286–9. Chinese. https://doi.org/10.3760/cma.j.issn.1671-0274.2016.11.017.
7. Dematteo RP, Ballman KV, Antonescu CR, Maki RG, Pisters PW, Demetri GD, Blackstein ME, Blanke CD, Von Mehren M, Brennan MF, Patel S, McCarter MD, Polikoff JA, Tan BR, Owzar K, American College of Surgeons Oncology Group (ACOSOG) Intergroup Adjuvant GIST Study Team. Adjuvant imatinib mesylate after resection of localised, primary gastrointestinal stromal tumour: a randomised, double-blind, placebo- controlled trial. Lancet. 2009;373(9669):1097–104. https://doi.org/10.1016/S0140-6736(09)60500-6.
8. Raut CP, Espat NJ, Maki RG, Araujo DM, Trent J, Williams TF, Purkayastha DD, DeMatteo RP. Efficacy and tolerability of 5-year adjuvant imatinib treatment for patients with resected intermediate or high-risk primary gastrointestinal stromal tumor: the PERSIST-5 clinical trial. JAMA Oncol. 2018;4(12):e184060. https://doi.org/10.1001/jamaoncol.2018.4060.

22

Low Risk Rectal Gastrointestinal Stromal Tumors Recurrence 12 Years After Surgery

Xiaoqi Li, Cong Li, and Zekuan Xu

Keywords

Gastrointestinal stromal tumor · Rectum · Low risk · Metastasis · Imatinib

22.1 Case 29 A 64-Year-Old Woman with Recurrence of a Low-Risk Rectal GIST 12 Years After Surgery

Xiaoqi Li and Cong Li

22.1.1 Introduction

The modified NIH classification categorizes GIST into four risk grades according to tumor size, location, mitotic count, and tumor rupture, namely: very low risk, low risk, intermediate risk, and high risk. A higher risk grade indicates a higher risk of tumor recurrence and metastasis. Low-risk GIST refer to GIST with a tumor size of 2–5 cm, mitotic count <5/50 HPF, and without rupture. Unlike the grades of medium and high-risk GIST, low-risk GIST does not take the primary site of tumor into consideration. The possibility of recurrence and metastasis still exists for low-risk GIST in special sites even more than 10 years after surgery.

X. Li
Department of Gastrointestinal Surgery, Renji Hospital, Shanghai Jiaotong University School of Medicine, Shanghai, China

C. Li (✉)
Department of Colorectal Surgery, Sun Yat-sen University Cancer Center, Guangzhou, China
e-mail: congli@mail.sysu.edu.cn

Z. Xu
Department of Gastric Surgery, The First Affiliated Hospital with Nanjing Medical University, Nanjing, China
e-mail: xuzekuan@njmu.edu.cn

22.1.2 Case Background

The patient, a 64-year-old woman, presented to the local hospital for investigation of a two-year history of changes in stool nature and 3 months of diffcult defecation. The patient reported no history of chronic diseases, such as hypertension or diabetes, and no history of surgery or blood transfusion. A digital rectal examination revealed a 3 cm × 3 cm soft submucosal lesion on the back wall of the rectum 2 cm away from anus, and approximately one third of the intestinal lumen was obstructed. The lesion was smooth with poor mobility. The outpatient primary diagnosis was a huge bulge under the mucosa of the rectum, possibly a leiomyoma or GIST.

22.1.2.1 Past History and Family History

The patient was previously healthy and reported no history of drug allergies. The patient's parents were alive, and there was no similar medical history in the family.

22.1.2.2 Physical Examination

The patient's vital signs were stable, and the skin and mucous membranes were not yellowish or pale. The abdomen was flat, and no gastrointestinal or peristaltic wave was observed. The abdomen was soft, with no tenderness, rebound tenderness, or palpable masses. The bowel sounds were normal.

22.1.2.3 Auxiliary Examination

Blood Routine WBC 4.6×10^9/L, RBC 4.05×10^{12}/L, Hb 129 g/L, PLT 137×10^9/L, NEUT% 52.7%, LY% 36.9%.

Ultrasound Colonoscopy A submucosal bulge on the posterior wall of the rectum was observed. A hypoechoic mass derived from the muscularis mucosa was seen under ultra-

K. Tao, H. Cao (eds.), *Clinical Management of Gastrointestinal Stromal Tumor*, https://doi.org/10.1007/978-981-99-9392-5_22

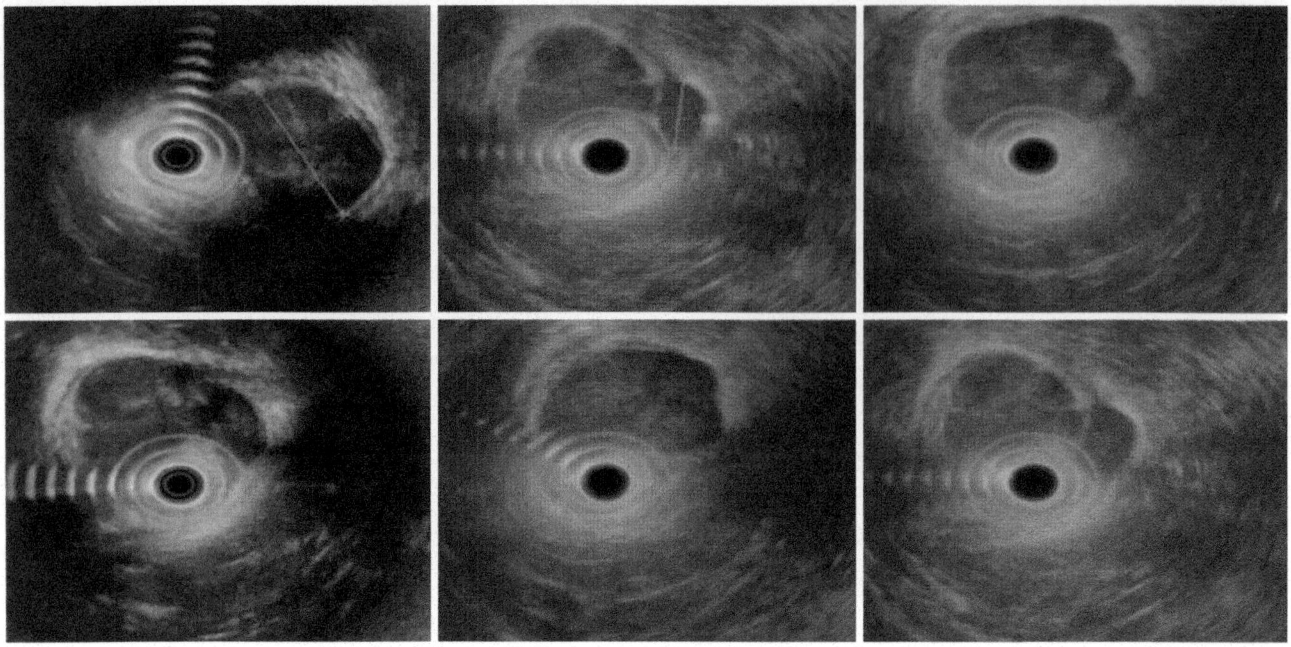

Fig. 22.1 Color Doppler ultrasound showed a submucosal mass on the posterior wall of the rectum

sound, which was inhomogeneous, with a maximum cross section of 31.7 mm × 22.9 mm (Fig. 22.1).

Abdominal and Pelvic Color Doppler Ultrasound A solid mass was observed behind the vagina, which was considered to originate from the lower rectum. No obvious abnormality was observed in the hepatobiliary system, pancreas, or spleen.

22.1.2.4 Preliminary Diagnosis

1. Rectal mass, possible leiomyoma or GIST

22.1.3 Therapy

22.1.3.1 Case Analysis

The patient was an elderly woman, who consulted a doctor because of changes in stool nature and difficulty defecating. The initial diagnosis was of a huge bulge under the mucosa of rectum, considered to be a possible leiomyoma or GIST. The patient was generally in good condition, the tumor was assessed as resectable, no metastasis was found, and surgery was deemed appropriate. Postoperative treatment was to be guided by the results of pathology.

22.1.3.2 Treatment

A transanal mass resection was performed on October 16, 2004. A mass located on the posterior wall of the rectum was found during operation. The mass was of moderate hardness, displayed clear borders, and was mobile. The tumor was completely removed without rupture, and the operation process went smoothly.

22.1.3.3 Postoperative Pathology

Pathological Diagnosis Rectal nodular mass with a diameter of 3 cm, the cut surface was gray, the tumor cells were spindle-shaped, arranged in bundles, and the cells displayed mildly atypia, consistent with a diagnosis of GIST, mitotic count 2/50 HPF, and there was no obvious necrosis, bleeding, or mucoid degeneration.

Immunohistochemistry CD117 (+), CD34 (+), CK (−), VIM (+), S-100 (−), HHF 35 (−), desmin (−), Ki-67 (Li: 5%).

22.1.4 Prognosis

The patient did not take imatinib after the operation and was followed up regularly in the first 5 years postoperative, as instructed, but did not have regular follow-up after that time. Twelve years after surgery, in January 2016, she developed right iliac crest and lower back pain. Both MRI and PET-CT showed that there was no tumor recurrence at the original surgical site, but the bilateral iliac bones, multiple thoracic vertebrae, and lumbar vertebrae were damaged, indicative of possible tumor metastasis. Additionally, liver nodules were detected at segments S6 and S8, and these were also considered possible metastases (Fig. 22.2).

The results of a needle biopsy of the right iliac bone revealed a few spindle cells, CD 117 (+), CD34 (+), DOG-1 (+), S-100 (−), desmin (−), SMA (−), Ki-67 (Li: 3%), consistent with GIST recurrence and metastasis. Genetic testing revealed an exon 11 insertion mutation. The presence of mul-

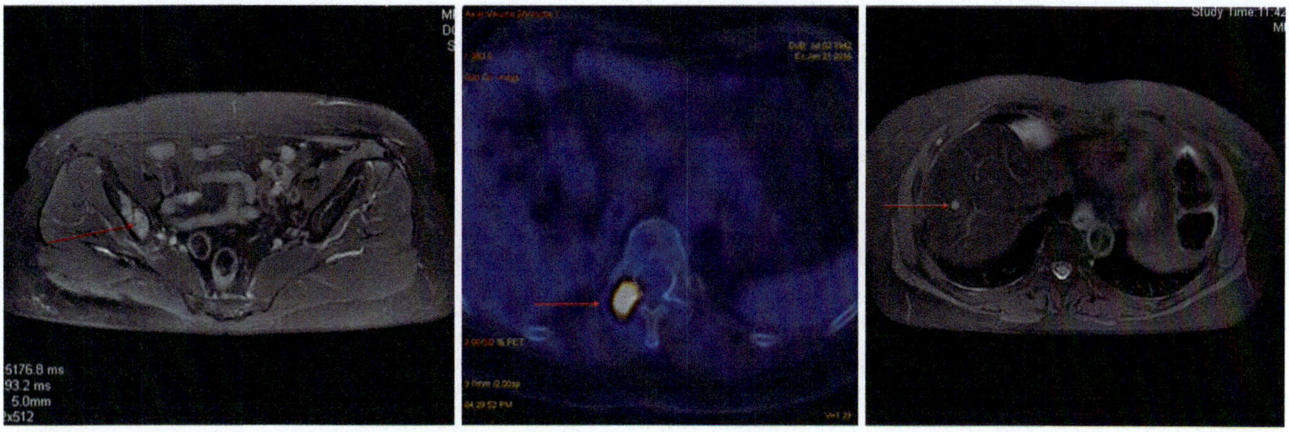

Fig. 22.2 MRI and PET-CT showed multiple metastases in ilium, lumbar spine and liver

tiple GIST metastases in the bone and liver was confirmed. After imatinib 400 mg/d treatment, the bone pain symptoms improved significantly after 3 days. A re-examination of the abdominal and pelvic MRI showed that the lesions in liver segments S6 and S8 were smaller than before, and the thoracic and lumbar spine lesions had no significant changes. The curative effect was evaluated as PR.

22.1.5 Experience of Diagnosis and Therapy

22.1.5.1 Choosing a Preoperative Biopsy Method for Rectal Gastrointestinal Stromal Tumor

The published guidelines and expert consensus pointed out that for rectal GIST, if the preoperative assessment determines that the mass can be completely resected, direct surgery without biopsy can be performed to avoid tumor dissemination due to biopsy [1, 2]. However, if neoadjuvant treatment is required, endoscopic ultrasound or rectal ultrasound guidance can be used to perform transmucosal biopsy. It is recommended to use a core needle to puncture, collect material from multiple points, and obtain enough tissue for genetic testing, which can eliminate the presence of any drug resistance, and can also avoid the possibility of being unable to obtain sufficient samples for pathological and genetic analysis because of tumor necrosis after preoperative treatment. It is unfortunate that for this patient, the specimens from the first operation in 2004 were not genetically tested, and the recurrence could not be compared to confirm whether there were secondary mutations in the metastatic tumors.

22.1.5.2 The Choice of Surgery for Rectal GIST

GIST mostly exhibit extroverted growth, and an obvious capsule. In theory, ensuring a negative margin is enough to reduce the incidence of recurrence and metastasis. Due to the special location of the rectum, resection involves the problem of preserving anal function. Radical surgery, such as Dixon or Miles surgery, or combined organ resection may affect the quality of life of patients after surgery [3]. Partial resection can be used on the premise of ensuring negative margins [4]. Therefore, for rectal GIST which cannot adopt local excision, preoperative treatment is recommended, provided a drug-resistant genotype is ruled out and the patient tolerates treatment well. As for the specific surgical procedure and approach, the choice should be individualized according to the actual situation.

22.1.5.3 Postoperative Follow-up for Low-Risk Gastrointestinal Stromal Tumors

The Chinese Guidelines on Diagnosis and Treatment of Gastrointestinal Stromal Tumors recommends that low-risk patients should be followed up for 5 years after surgery; The NCCN recommends close follow-up within 5 years, and once a year after 5 years. At present, no guideline plainly states that follow-up to the first few years after surgery without recurrence can be considered as a permanent cure. However, in clinical work, a considerable number of low risk patients have recurrence or metastasis more than 5 years after surgery, so lifelong follow-up is recommended for all risk-grade GIST patients. This is especially important for this kind of low-risk patient who has no recurrence in the original surgical area but have distant metastases. A method of predicting the recurrence and metastasis risk needs further basic and clinical research.

22.2 Expert Comments

Zekuan Xu

Along with further deep understanding of GIST, our clinical thinking on GIST diagnosis and treatment is also changing. In combination with this case, the current risk classification for rectal GIST refers to the 2008 modified NIH criteria, which only classifies the primary location as stomach and non-gastric, and has not been further refined into duodenum, small intestine, and colorectum. Although the National Defense Pathology Institute (AFIP) standards have classified the risk of rectal GIST, the categories are only low-risk and high-risk [5, 6]. Therefore, the accuracy of the current risk classification for rectal GIST needs to be further improved [7]. Secondly, the current 2008 modified NIH criteria only use tumor location, size, and mitosis as factors for risk classification, and other pathological features of tumors, such as depth of invasion, and various markers of immunohistochemistry, such as the Ki-67 index, are not included. Some scholars believe that a Ki-67 index greater than 4% is indicative of poor prognosis [8], in which case a Ki-67 index of 4% in this patient indicates that the patient has a higher risk of recurrence. In addition, from clinical experience, GIST for special sites, such as the rectum and duodenum, have a higher risk of recurrence [7], so the frequency of follow-up should be appropriately increased after surgery. At present, the treatment and follow-up time for GIST have been adjusted, and corresponding clinical research is also being conducted. It is believed that with the continuous accumulation of clinical experience and enrichment of clinical trial data, the treatment and follow-up strategies for patients with GIST will be made on the basis of relatively sufficient clinical proof.

References

1. Li J, Ye Y, Wang J, Zhang B, Qin S, Shi Y, He Y, Liang X, Liu X, Zhou Y, Wu X, Zhang X, Wang M, Gao Z, Lin T, Cao H, Shen L, Chinese Society of Clinical Oncology (CSCO) Expert Committee on Gastrointestinal Stromal Tumor. Chinese consensus guidelines for diagnosis and management of gastrointestinal stromal tumor. Chin J Cancer Res. 2017;29(4):281–93. https://doi.org/10.21147/j.issn.1000-9604.2017.04.01.
2. von Mehren M, Randall RL, Benjamin RS, Boles S, Bui MM, Ganjoo KN, George S, Gonzalez RJ, Heslin MJ, Kane JM, Keedy V, Kim E, Koon H, Mayerson J, McCarter M, McGarry SV, Meyer C, Morris ZS, O'Donnell RJ, Pappo AS, Paz IB, Petersen IA, Pfeifer JD, Riedel RF, Ruo B, Schuetze S, Tap WD, Wayne JD, Bergman MA, Scavone JL. Soft tissue sarcoma, version 2.2018, NCCN clinical practice guidelines in oncology. J Natl Compr Cancer Netw. 2018;16(5):536–63. https://doi.org/10.6004/jnccn.2018.0025.
3. Shu P, Sun XF, Fang Y, Gao XD, Hou YY, Shen KT, Qin J, Sun YH, Qin XY, Xue AW, Fu M. Clinical outcomes of different therapeutic modalities for rectal gastrointestinal stromal tumor: summary of 14-year clinical experience in a single center. Int J Surg. 2020;77:1–7. https://doi.org/10.1016/j.ijsu.2020.03.007.
4. IJzerman NS, Mohammadi M, Tzanis D, Gelderblom H, Fiore M, Fumagalli E, Rutkowski P, Bylina E, Zavrakidis I, Steeghs N, Bonenkamp HJ, van Etten B, Grünhagen DJ, Rasheed S, Tekkis P, Honoré C, van Houdt W, van der Hage J, Bonvalot S, Schrage Y, Smith M. Quality of treatment and surgical approach for rectal gastrointestinal stromal tumour (GIST) in a large European cohort. Eur J Surg Oncol. 2020;46(6):1124–30. https://doi.org/10.1016/j.ejso.2020.02.033.
5. Joensuu H, Vehtari A, Riihimäki J, Nishida T, Steigen SE, Brabec P, Plank L, Nilsson B, Cirilli C, Braconi C, Bordoni A, Magnusson MK, Linke Z, Sufliarsky J, Federico M, Jonasson JG, Dei Tos AP, Rutkowski P. Risk of recurrence of gastrointestinal stromal tumour after surgery: an analysis of pooled population-based cohorts. Lancet Oncol. 2012;13(3):265–74. https://doi.org/10.1016/S1470-2045(11)70299-6.
6. Miettinen M, Lasota J. Gastrointestinal stromal tumors: pathology and prognosis at different sites. Semin Diagn Pathol. 2006;23(2):70–83. https://doi.org/10.1053/j.semdp.2006.09.001.
7. Hawkins AT, Wells KO, Krishnamurty DM, Hunt SR, Mutch MG, Glasgow SC, Wise PE, Silviera ML. Preoperative chemotherapy and survival for large anorectal gastrointestinal stromal tumors: a National Analysis of 333 cases. Ann Surg Oncol. 2017;24(5):1195–201. https://doi.org/10.1245/s10434-016-5706-1.
8. Liu X, Qiu H, Zhang P, Feng X, Chen T, Li Y, Tao K, Li G, Sun X, Zhou Z, China Gastrointestinal Stromal Tumor Study Group (CN-GIST). Ki-67 labeling index may be a promising indicator to identify "very high-risk" gastrointestinal stromal tumor: a multicenter retrospective study of 1022 patients. Hum Pathol. 2018;74:17–24. https://doi.org/10.1016/j.humpath.2017.09.003.

23 Surgery Combined with Targeted Therapy in Advanced Gastrointestinal Stromal Tumors

Chun Zhuang, Ming Wang, Haibo Qiu, and Ye Zhou

Keywords

Gastrointestinal stromal tumor · Palliative surgery · Targeted therapy · Liver metastasis · Spleen metastasis · Combination · PD-1

23.1 Case 30 A 54-Year-Old Man with Advanced GIST Received Palliative Surgery and Second- and Third-Line Drug Therapy

Chun Zhuang and Ming Wang

23.1.1 Introduction

It is helpless that surgery is used to treat patients with advanced GIST in order to prolong their survival. In addition, surgery is the only option when patients with advanced tumors experience complications, such as bleeding, perforation, and obstruction. However, the results of surgery alone for this group of patients with GIST are not satisfactory. The identification of a series of tyrosine kinase receptor inhibitors has greatly prolonged the survival time for patients with advanced GIST. In the era of targeted therapy, surgery has become the second-line treatment for advanced GIST, but still plays a very important role, especially when the drug treatments provided by oncology physicians are ineffective. The timing of surgical intervention during targeted drug therapy for advanced GIST remains controversial and warrants further research.

23.1.2 Case Background

The patient, a 54-year-old man, underwent surgery 13 years previously for malignant gastric GIST, and subsequently had recurrence and metastasis for more than 6 years. In September 2004, the patient underwent proximal gastrectomy for a gastric mass (14 cm in size), and postoperative pathology suggested malignant GIST. No adjuvant therapy was administered. On March 14, 2011, A large mass was found in the left upper abdomen according to the CT reexamination at another hospital, which was considered to represent a recurrence of GIST (Fig. 23.1).

The patient visited our hospital, and PET-CT showed a metal shadow in the anastomotic area, and a soft tissue mass, 11.0 cm × 8.0 cm × 8.0 cm was observed in the operative area, with uneven internal density and a patchy irregular, calcification shadow. Increased FDG metabolism was seen in the lesion, and the boundary between the lesion and the left lobe of the liver was unclear. Another irregular mass, 17.5 cm × 15 cm × 11 cm, was seen in the upper left abdominal cavity, with uneven internal density and cystic solid mixed density. Increased metabolic heterogeneity of FDG and compression of adjacent organs of the lesion were also observed. After departmental discussion, an ultrasound-guided puncture biopsy of the intraperitoneal mass was performed on March 24, 2011. Pathology showed that the intraperitoneal mass was recurrent GIST. Immunohistochemistry of tumor cells showed CD117, CD34 and DOG-1 were positive. Genetic analysis showed a heterozygous mutation at codon 558 and the loss of heterozygosity at codon 559–565 of exon

C. Zhuang · M. Wang (✉)
Department of Gastrointestinal Surgery, Renji Hospital, Shanghai Jiaotong University School of Medicine, Shanghai, China

H. Qiu (✉)
Department of Gastric Surgery, Sun Yat-sen University Cancer Center, Guangzhou, China
e-mail: qiuhb@sysucc.org.cn

Y. Zhou
Department of Gastric Surgery, Fudan University Cancer Hospital, Shanghai, China

K. Tao, H. Cao (eds.), *Clinical Management of Gastrointestinal Stromal Tumor*, https://doi.org/10.1007/978-981-99-9392-5_23

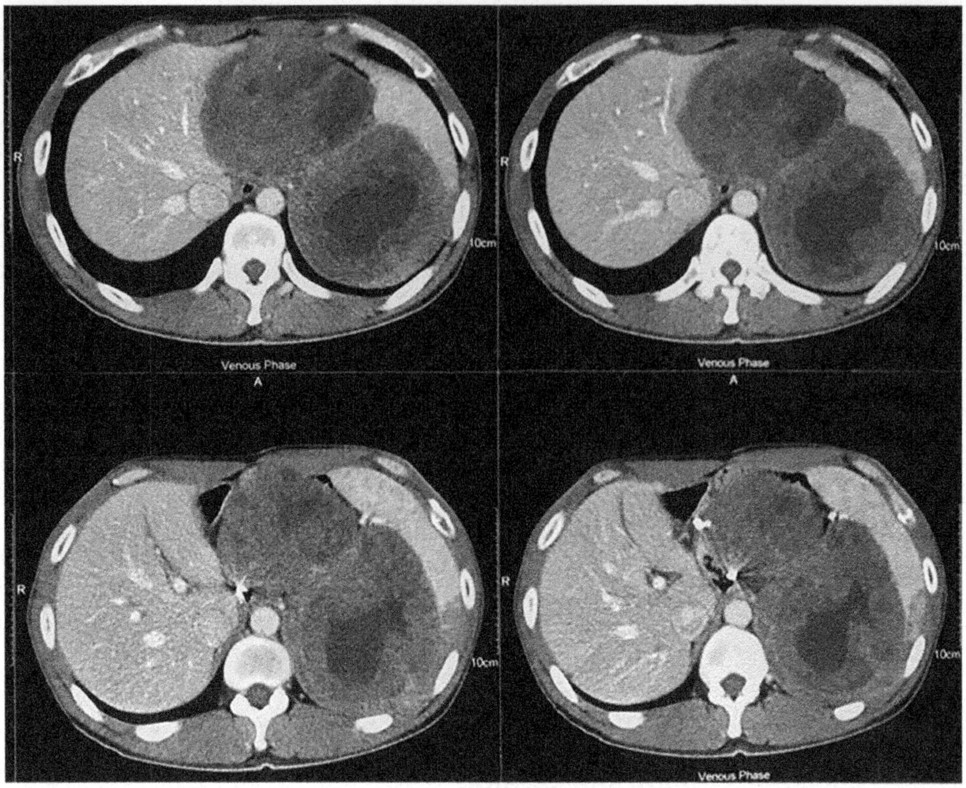

Fig. 23.1 CT showed metastases

11 of *KIT*. The patient took imatinib 400 mg/d orally from April 2011. A CT scan in December 2012 showed that the maximum diameter of the tumor was reduced to 8.2 cm × 6.3 cm × 6.0 cm and 8.5 cm × 7.4 cm × 7 cm (Fig. 23.2).

The patient was classified as stable disease (SD) with several CT assessments. However, CT reexamination in April 2015 suggested progression of the disease (Fig. 23.3).

After switching to sunitinib at 37.5 mg/d, the patient's 6-month follow-up enhanced CT showed stable disease (SD). However, a CT scan in June 2017 indicated disease progression (Fig. 23.4).

The patient had difficulty eating and had a strong willingness for surgery and was admitted to hospital for palliative surgery to relieve gastrointestinal obstruction.

23.1.2.1 Past History and Family History

The patient was previously healthy and reported no history of drug allergies. The patient's parents were alive and there was no similar medical history in the family.

23.1.2.2 Physical Examination

The patient's vital signs were stable, and the skin and mucous membranes were not yellowish or pale. The abdomen was swollen, and no gastrointestinal or peristaltic waves were seen. Old surgical scars were seen in the middle of the abdomen. A hard mass was found in the abdomen. The bowel sounds were normal.

23.1.2.3 Auxiliary Examination

Enhanced CT of the whole abdomen: (1) Post-gastric GIST surgery, the mass lesions near the anastomosis are accompanied by multi-windows and sheet-like dense shadows. (2) Multiple liver metastases with abnormal liver tissue perfusion around the lesion; splenomegaly with multiple metastases; abdominal and pelvic effusion. (3) Several small cysts in the left kidney. A scan of the left lung lingual section revealed strip foci in the lower lobes of both lungs, and a small amount effusion in the right thoracic cavity (Fig. 23.5).

23.1.2.4 Preliminary Diagnosis

Postoperative recurrence of GIST with liver and spleen metastases.

23.1.3 Therapy

23.1.3.1 Case Analysis

The patient was a middle-aged man with advanced GIST. Although the extensive progress of the disease under the second-line drug treatment led to limited surgical significance, considering the patient's eating difficulties, palliative surgery to relieve gastrointestinal obstruction or directly switch to the third-line drug treatment was feasible. After full communication with the patient and his family, the patient had a strong desire for surgery, so he underwent surgical exploration on August 31, 2017.

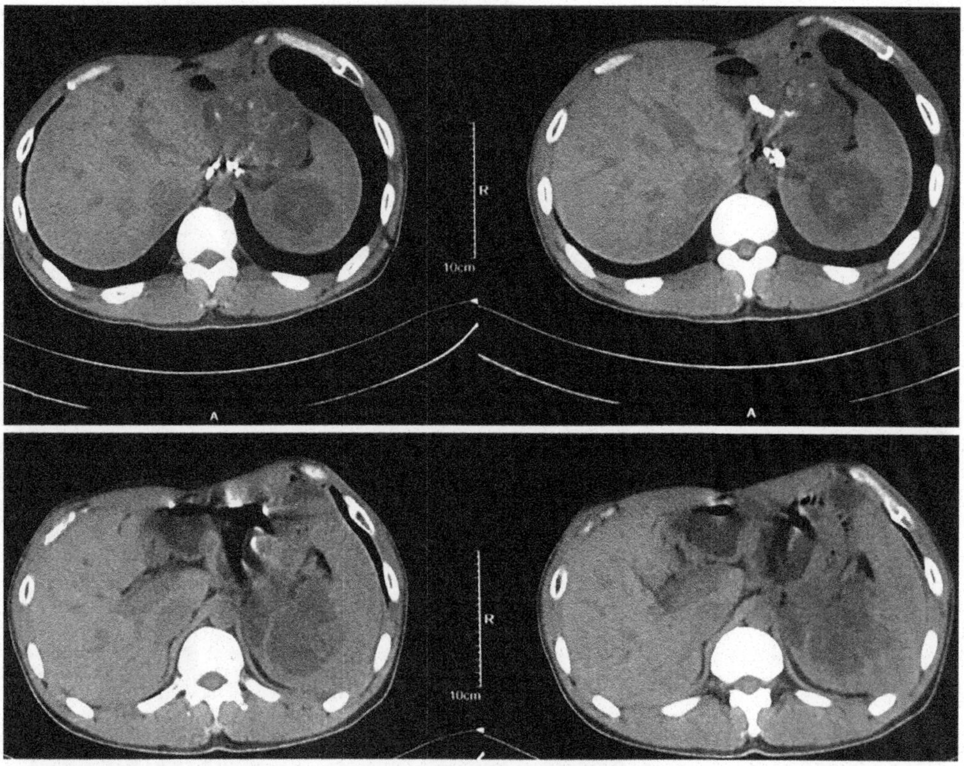

Fig. 23.2 CT Reexamination in December 2012

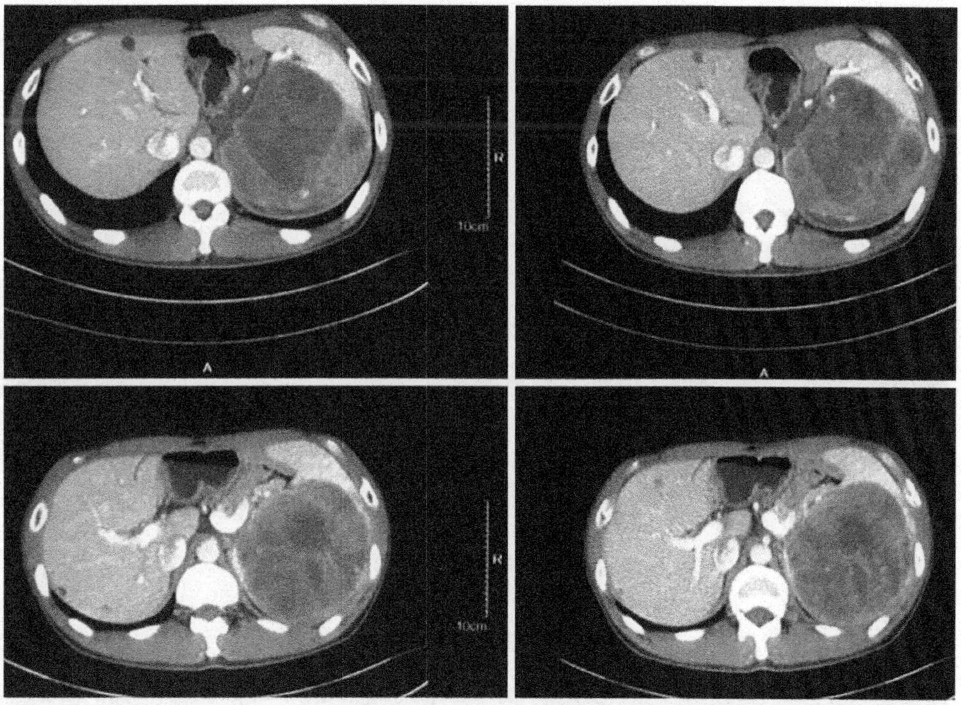

Fig. 23.3 CT Reexamination in April 2015

23.1.3.2 Treatment

The patient underwent splenic massive tumor resection (splenectomy) with resection of multiple metastatic tumors in the liver and diaphragmatic lump resection in our hospital in August 2017. During the operation, severe adhesions were seen at the original surgical site in the upper abdomen. The tumor on the spleen was huge, and occupied the entire upper left quadrant, approximately 30 cm × 20 cm × 10 cm in size. The tumor capsule was densely attached to the posterior peritoneum, and the left diaphragm muscle, leading to partial diaphragm resection with the tumor. There were multiple

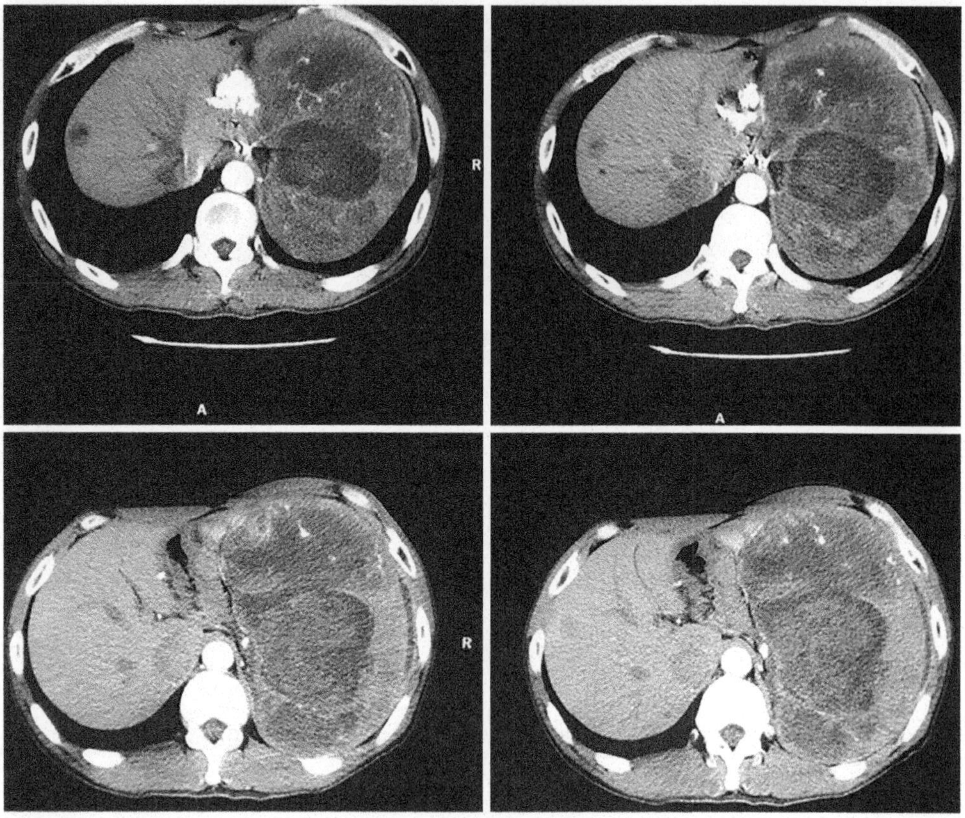

Fig. 23.4 CT Reexamination in July 2017

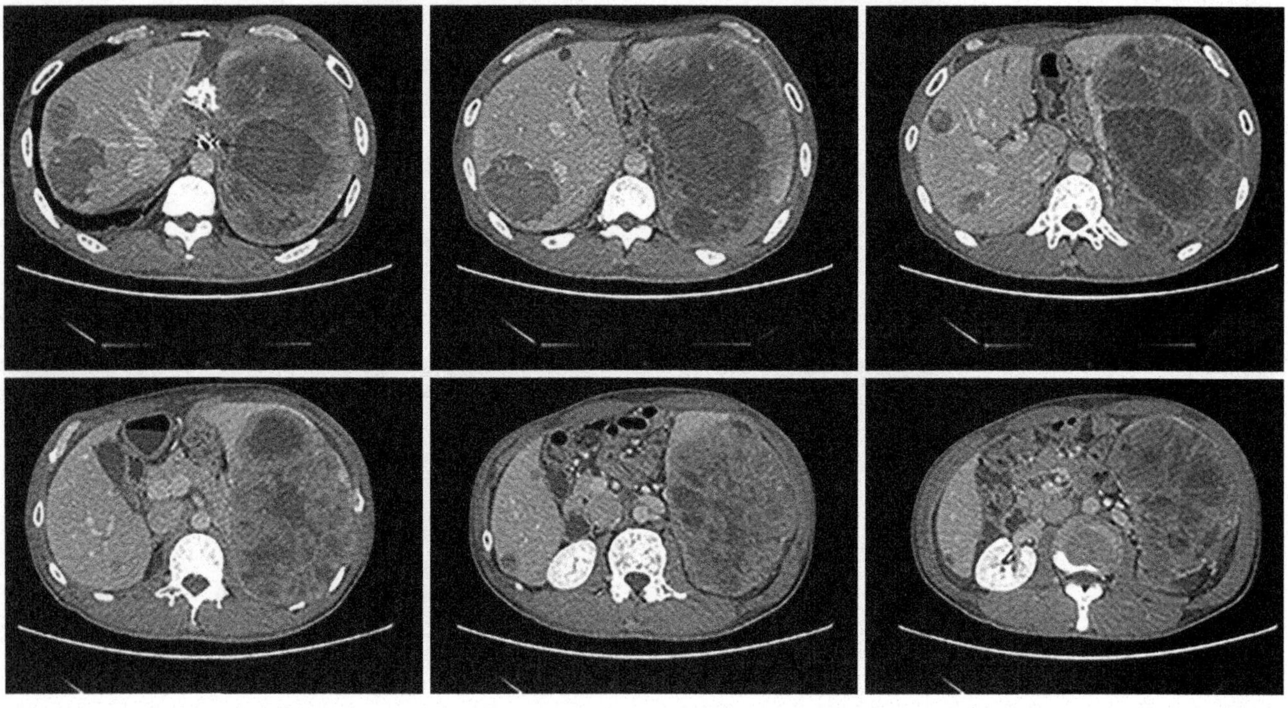

Fig. 23.5 Preoperative CT assessment in August 2017

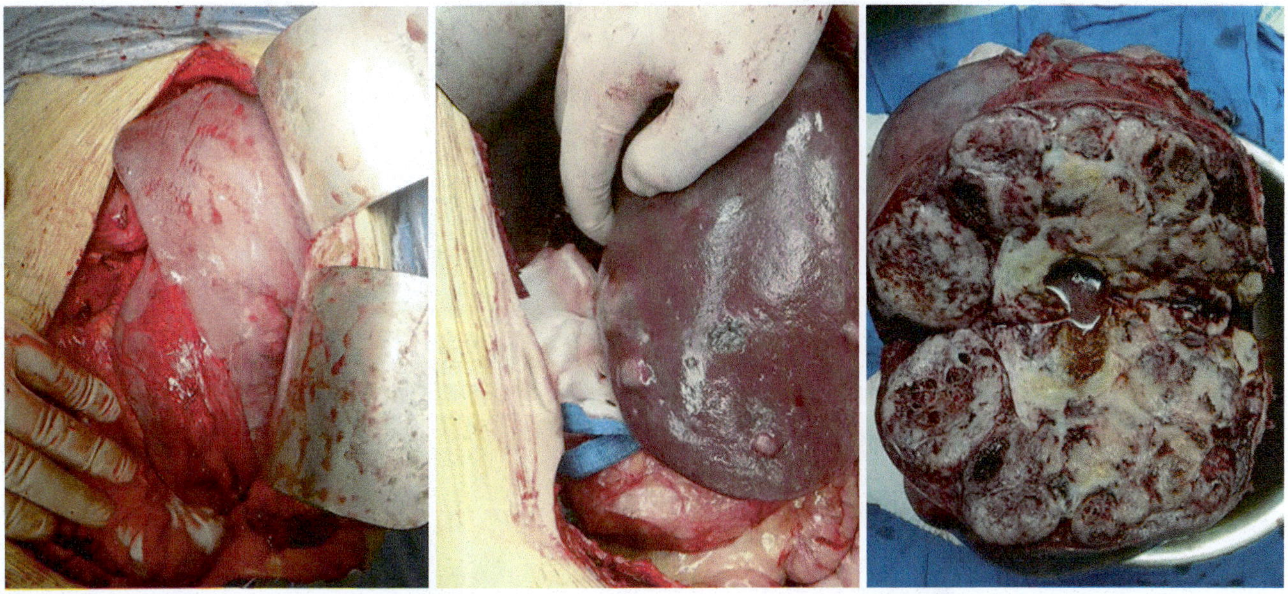

Fig. 23.6 Findings during the second surgery

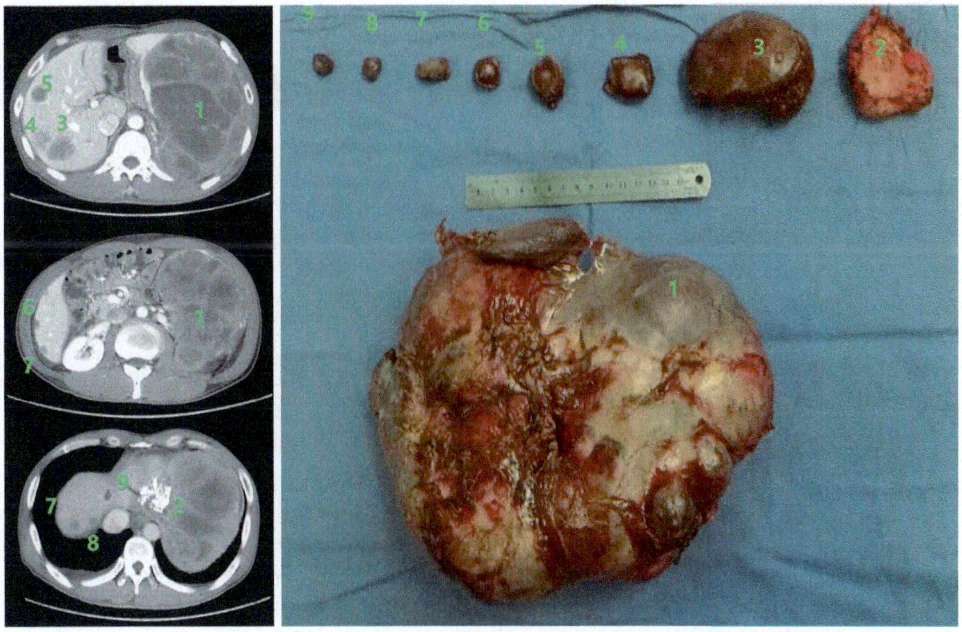

Fig. 23.7 The gross specimen in the second surgery

metastases in the liver, ranging in size from 0.5 to 8 cm. A hard mass, 3 cm × 4 cm in size, was found on the surface of the diaphragm at the original anastomosis site, which was completely resected. No metastases were found in the small intestine, colon, peritoneum, or pelvis. No ascites was observed during the operation. The surgery was challenging, with an intraoperative blood loss of approximately 600 mL, requiring transfusion of 4 units of red blood cells and 400 mL of plasma (Figs. 23.6 and 23.7).

23.1.3.3 Postoperative Pathology and Genetic Testing

Pathological Diagnosis There were multiple nodules in the spleen, with a maximum diameter of 1.0–12.0 cm, mitotic count >10/50 HPF, accompanied by necrosis. Combined with the patient history, the tumors were consistent with metastatic GIST. The liver metastatic nodules 1–7 were also metastatic GISTs. The mass near the anastomosis was determined to be fibrotic calcified nodules.

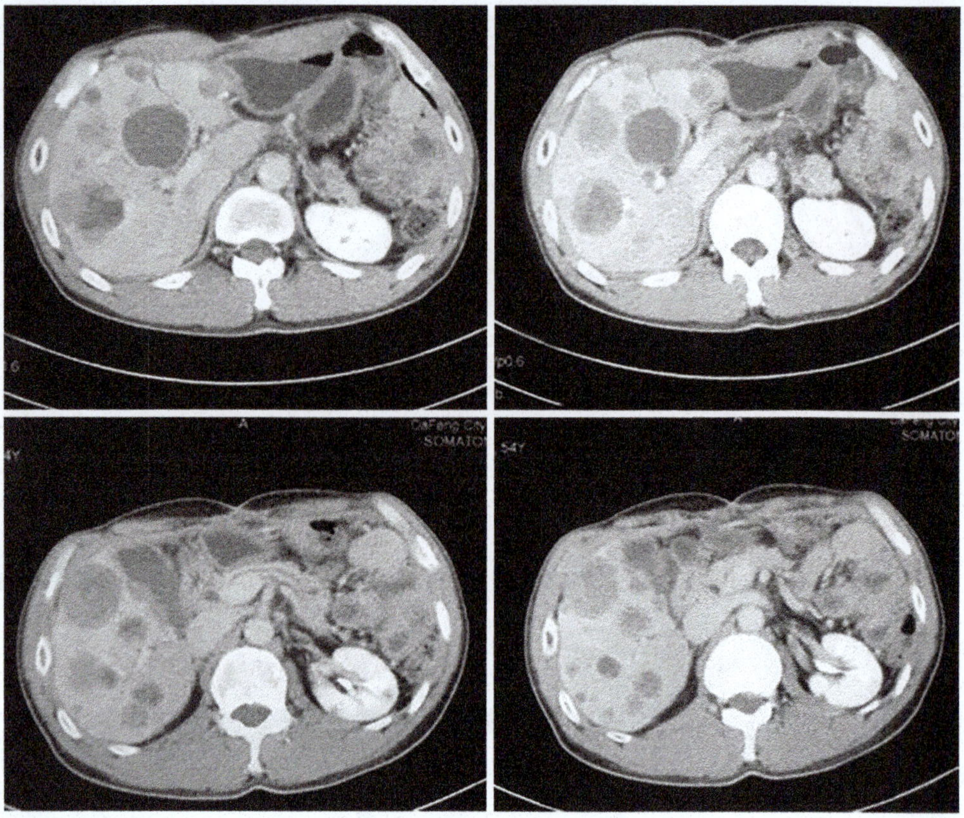

Fig. 23.8 CT results in January 2018

Immunohistochemistry CD117 (+), DOG-1 (+), CD34 (local+), SDHB (+), p53 (+), EMA (−), SMA (−), desmin (−), Ki-67 (Li: 40%).

Genetic Testing The mass in the spleen was found to have a heterozygous mutation, 558AAG>AGA, in *KIT* exon 11, codon 558, resulting in the change of coding amino acid from lysine to arginine, and a heterozygous deletion of codons 559–565. There was an additional heterozygous mutation of codon 654 in exon 13 of *KIT*, 654GTG>GCG.

Liver metastasis nodule 1 was found to have a heterozygous mutation of codon 558 in exon 11 of *KIT*, 558AAG>AGA, and a heterozygous deletion of codons 559–565.

Liver metastasis nodules 2–4 were found to have a heterozygous mutation, 558AAG>AGA in exon 11 of *KIT*, and a heterozygous deletion of codons 559–565. There was an additional heterozygous mutation of codon 654 in exon 13 of *KIT*, 654GTG>GCG.

Liver metastasis nodules 5–7 were found to have a heterozygous mutation, 558AAG>AGA, in exon 11 of *KIT*, and a heterozygous deletion of codons 559–565. An additional heterozygous mutation of codon 823 in exon 17 of *KIT*, 823TAT>GAT, was also found.

23.1.4 Prognosis

The patient resumed sunitinib treatment 2 weeks after surgery, and the findings of an enhanced CT reexamination in January 2018 were suggestive of multiple new metastases in the liver (Fig. 23.8).

Third-line treatment with regorafenib was suggested, but the patient refused the treatment for economic reasons, so he commenced treatment with a combination of first-line and second-line targeted drugs (imatinib 300 mg/d and sunitinib 25 mg/d). The side effects of the drugs were tolerable. The reexamination of liver MR in March 2018 showed that the size and number of intrahepatic metastases were similar to the previous scan, and some lesions were obviously liquefied (Fig. 23.9).

In August 2018, 14 years after the initial diagnosis of high-risk GIST, 7 years after discovery of recurrence and metastasis, and 1 year after reoperation, the patient died due to rapid progression of the disease.

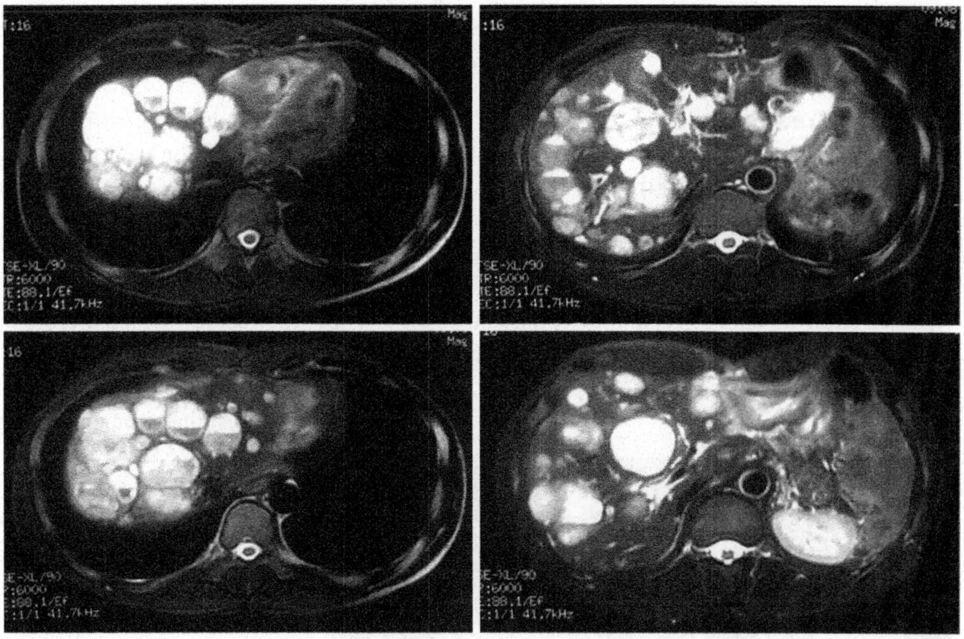

Fig. 23.9 Liver MRI in March 2018

23.2 Case 31 A 47-Year-Old Man with Advanced GIST Received Palliative Surgery and Third-Line Drugs Combined with PD-1 Therapy

Chun Zhuang and Haibo Qiu

23.2.1 Case Background

The patient, a 47-year-old man, visited the local hospital in August 2010 for investigation of a 2-month history of abdominal distention after eating. Gastroscopy revealed an ulcerative mass in the gastric body. The results of a biopsy of the mass showed that it was consistent with a spindle cell tumor, but only a small tissue sample was collected, so further diagnosis was recommended after operation. The patient visited the gastric surgery department of the cancer prevention and treatment center of Sun Yat-sen University. The outpatient doctor admitted the patient to the ward with the diagnosis of "Gastric mass, nature to be investigated."

23.2.1.1 Past History and Family History

The patient was previously healthy, and reported no history of drug allergies. The patient's parents were alive, and there was no similar medical history in the family.

23.2.1.2 Physical Examination

The patient's vital signs were stable, and the skin and mucous membranes were not yellowish or pale. The abdomen was flat, and no gastrointestinal or peristaltic waves were seen. The abdomen was soft, with no tenderness, rebound tenderness, or palpable mass in the abdomen. The bowel sounds were normal.

23.2.1.3 Auxiliary Examination

There were no obvious abnormalities in blood routine, blood biochemistry, or tumor markers.

Ultrasonic Gastroscopy An ulcer caused by a submucosal mass was revealed in the gastric body, which was considered as a possible mesenchymal malignant tumor.

Enhanced CT of Chest, Abdomen and Pelvis A mass (7.2 cm × 5.2 cm) was observed in the greater curvature of the gastric body, with deep ulcers extending to the lesion, and the possibility of GIST was considered (Fig. 23.10).

23.2.1.4 Preliminary Diagnosis

Space-occupying lesion of the gastric body: possible GIST.

23.2.2 Therapy

23.2.2.1 Case Analysis

The patient was a middle-aged man who presented to the doctor for investigation of abdominal distension after eating. The patient's current preliminary diagnosis was of a gastric body occupying lesion, considered to be possible GIST. The patient was generally in good condition, the primary tumor was assessed to be resectable, surgical treatment was recommended, and postoperative treatment should be based on the pathological test results.

23.2.2.2 Treatment

The patient underwent a gastric mass resection (partial gastrectomy) in September 2010, and the procedure went smoothly.

Postoperative Pathology Possible gastric GIST, 7 cm × 6 cm × 4.5 cm in size, mitotic count >50/50 HPF. The tumor was considered to be high risk based on the modified NIH recurrence risk classification.

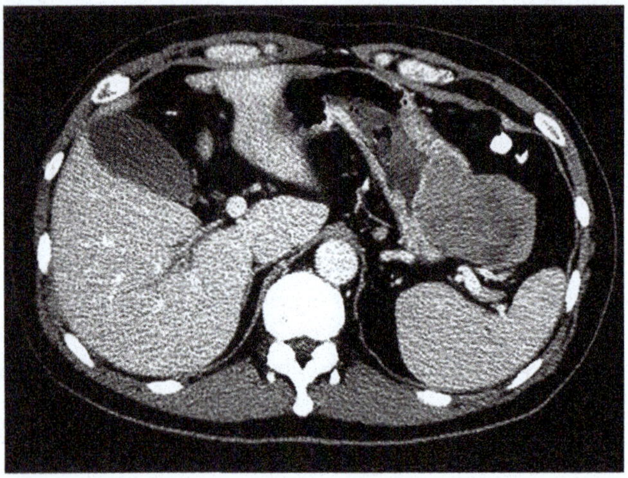

Fig. 23.10 CT showed a mass on the greater curvature of the stomach at the time of initial diagnosis

Immunohistochemistry CD117 (+), CD34 (+), DOG-1 (+), Ki-67 (Li: 30%).

The patient started taking imatinib 400 mg/d 1 month after the operation, and then stopped taking it arbitrarily 2 years later (drug course: October 10, 2010, to September 24, 2012). A chest, abdomen, and pelvic enhanced CT on November 6, 2013, showed a 5.6 cm × 4.3 cm mass below the gastric antrum and a 6.3 cm × 7.0 cm mass in the front of the rectum, which were considered to be GIST metastases (Fig. 23.11).

The patient resumed imatinib 400 mg/d in November 2013. At that time genetic testing revealed a *KIT* mutation in exon 11, W557-K558 deletion mutation, and *PDGFRA* was wild type. A CT scan in February 2014 showed that the mass below the gastric antrum (2.6 cm × 3.0 cm) and the mass in the front of the rectum (3.0 cm × 7.0 cm) were significantly smaller than before (Fig. 23.12).

The patient continued imatinib 400 mg/d. CT reexamination in June 2014 showed that the mass below the gastric antrum was slightly larger than the front the size of the mass in the front of the rectum did not change much, and the internal solid components were slightly more than before.

After MDT (multidisciplinary team) discussion, imatinib therapy was increased to 600 mg/d. A CT in October 2014 revealed that the anterior rectal mass was enlarged and fused (approximately 7.0 cm × 6.0 cm), and the mass below the gastric antrum was not obvious. The patient continued to maintain the original treatment regimen of imatinib 600 mg/d. A further CT in December 2014 showed that the size and number of ante-

Fig. 23.11 Enhanced CT of the chest, abdomen and pelvis in November 2013

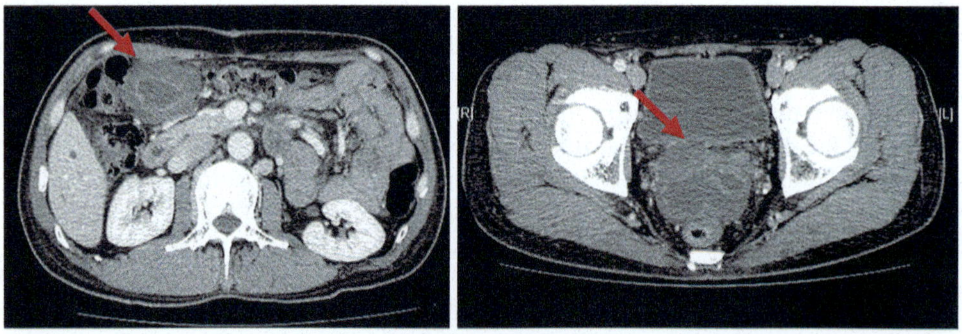

Fig. 23.12 CT reexamination in February 2014

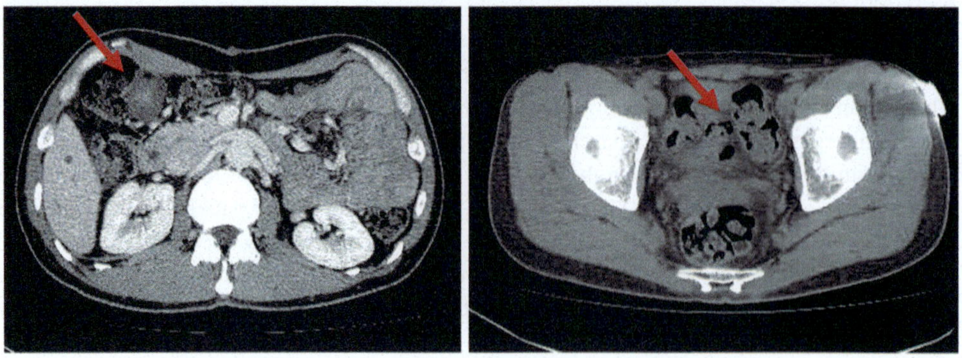

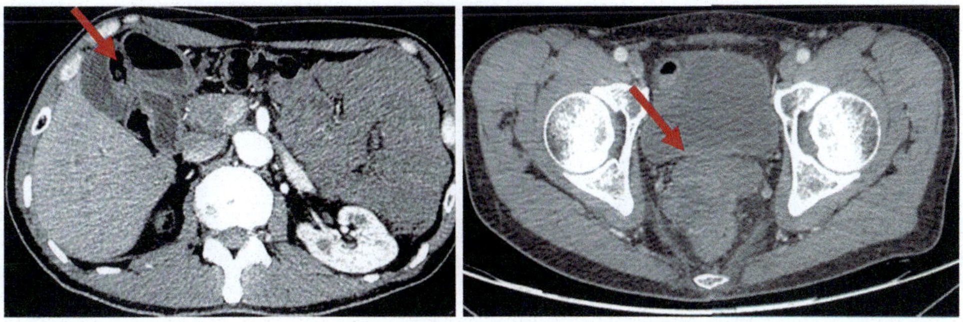

Fig. 23.13 CT reexamination in November 2015

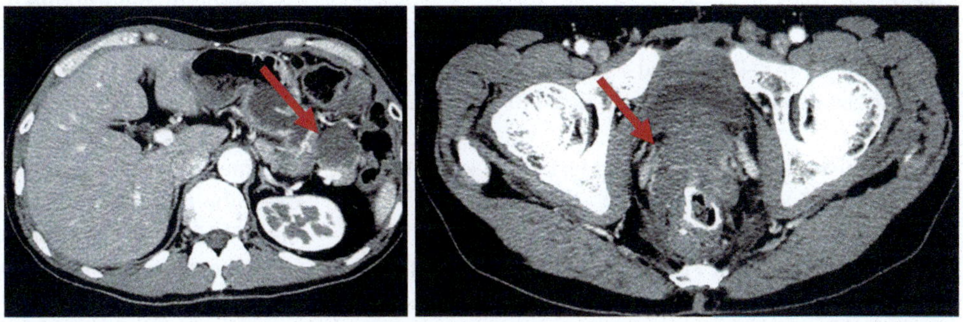

Fig. 23.14 CT reexamination in April 2016

rior rectal masses had increased (two lesions, 8.0 cm × 6.0 cm and 10.0 cm × 7.5 cm in size). After discussion, the patient's treatment was changed to sunitinib 37.5 mg/d. A CT scan in November 2015 showed that the anterior rectal masses were slightly smaller than before (approximately 6.0 cm × 5.0 cm and 7.0 cm × 3.6 cm) (Fig. 23.13).

After multidisciplinary consultation and discussion, surgery was recommended for the patient. The patient underwent rectal Dixon surgery and partial cystectomy in December 2015.

Postoperative Pathology The tumors were 6 cm × 6 cm × 4.5 cm and 7 cm × 4 cm × 3 cm in size, mitotic count 8/50 HPF, combined with immunohistochemistry, GIST was considered.

Immunohistochemistry CD117 (+), CD34 (+), Ki-67 (Li: 45%).

Genetic Testing There was a deletion mutation in *KIT* exon 11, W557-K558 was missing. Exons 9, 13, 17 of *KIT* and *PDGFRA* exons 12 and 18 were all wild type.

The patient started taking sunitinib 37.5 mg/d 3 weeks postoperatively. The patient had a CT scan on April 13, 2016, which revealed recurrence of tumors in the anterior rectum and gastro-pancreatic (Fig. 23.14).

Following this, the patient's medication was changed to pembrolizumab injection 100 mg once every 3 weeks and imatinib 400 mg/d. A CT scan of the chest, abdomen, and pelvis on June 18, 2016, revealed multiple masses in the space between the stomach and spleen, the space between the bladder and the rectum, and the back of the rectum. The size of the tumors had not changed much compared to the previous scan, but the degree of enhancement was significantly reduced. It was determined that the scans indicated SD. Following this scan, the patient's treatment was changed to pembrolizumab 100 mg once every 3 weeks and regorafenib 160 mg daily (3-weeks-on/1-week-off schedule). CT scans of the chest, abdomen, and pelvis on August 18, 2016 and December 28, 2017, showed the size of the mass in the gastrosplenic space was stable. The masses in the bladder-rectal space and multiple masses in the back of the rectum were slightly smaller than before. The masses were evaluated as SD statue (Fig. 23.15).

23.2.2.3 Postoperative Pathology and Genetic Testing

September 2010

Postoperative Pathology The tumor was 7.0 cm × 6.0 cm × 4.5 cm, mitotic count >50/50 HPF, the tumor was considered to be GIST.

Immunohistochemistry CD117 (+), CD34 (+), DOG1 (+), Ki-67 (Li: 30%).

November 2013

Genetic Testing Of a puncture biopsy sample revealed an exon 11 W557-K558 deletion mutation in *KIT*. *PDGFRA* was wild type.

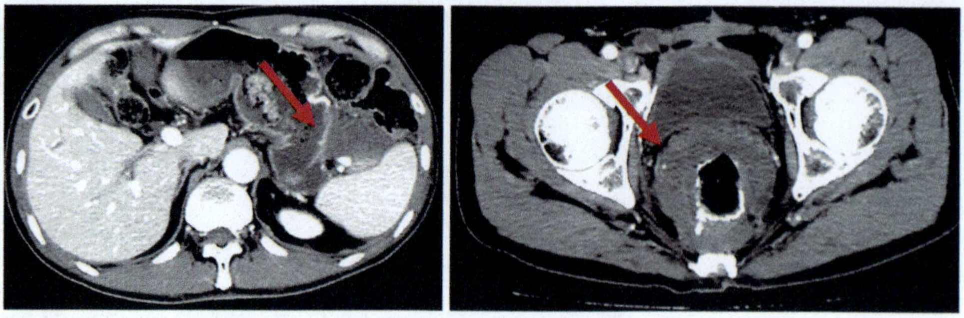

Fig. 23.15 CT reexamination in December 2017

December 2015

Postoperative Pathology The resected tumors were 6.0 cm × 6.0 cm × 4.5 cm and 7.0 cm × 4.0 cm × 3.0 cm in size, mitotic count 8/50 HPF, considered to be GIST.

Immunohistochemistry CD117 (+), CD34 (+), DOG1 (+), Ki-67 (Li: 45%).

Genetic Testing Exon 11 W557-K558 deletion mutation in *KIT*. Exons 9, 13, and 17 of *KIT*, and *PDGFRA* exons 12 and 18 were all wild type.

23.2.3 Prognosis

As of June 2018, the patient's condition was generally good, there were no obvious adverse drug reactions, and no signs of new tumor recurrence or metastases were found.

23.2.4 Experience of Diagnosis and Therapy

23.2.4.1 Targeted Therapy Is the Standard Treatment for Patients with Advanced GIST

In case 30, the primary tumor of the patient was a giant gastric malignant GIST. In 2004, TKI treatment was not yet universal, patients did not receive adjuvant therapy in time, and imaging follow-up was not performed regularly, which led to postoperative recurrence and metastasis, and the disease progressed to an advanced stage. The patient was diagnosed with recurrence and metastasis in 2011. After two kinds of TKI drugs used alone and in combination and one surgical intervention, the survival time was prolonged, and the quality of life was relatively good. From the perspective of the contribution of each treatment plan to the patient's disease control, imatinib provided disease control for nearly 4 years, sunitinib provided disease control for more than 6 months, and the disease progressed again within 6 months after surgical intervention. After progression, the combined application of imatinib and sunitinib achieved disease control for at least 2 months. The patient did not receive third-line drug regorafenib treatment for economic reasons. If there was a chance to receive this treatment, the survival period might have shown a certain benefit.

Although regorafenib was approved by the FDA in 2012, it was not available in China until 2017. At that time, domestic advanced GIST patients who were resistant to sunitinib were often treated with imatinib again for maintenance treatment, and a small number of patients obtained a short period of disease stabilization. In this case, the patient was resistant to second-line sunitinib in early 2016, and the treatment was changed back to imatinib, because regorafenib was not available at that time, and exploratory use of pembrolizumab was also administered. When regorafenib became available, the pembrolizumab treatment was maintained. The exploratory treatment of a PD-1 antagonist combined with TKI allows patients to obtain a longer survival time and improve their quality of life.

23.2.4.2 Tumor Heterogeneity Shown by Advanced GIST

In case 30, after the patient underwent palliative surgery, we conducted molecular pathological testing on each metastatic lesion, and found that the heterogeneity of each lesion was obvious, while some metastases were still the primary mutation type. Some metastatic foci had new secondary mutations of *KIT* exon 13 or *KIT* exon 17.

In case 31, the patient has a very interesting clinical phenomenon, that is, after treatment, drug resistance was demonstrated in the tumor below the gastric antrum and in front of the rectum. However, after the addition of imatinib, the rectal tumor was slightly larger than before, while the tumor below the gastric antrum disappeared, and there was no recurrence in the course of treatment. The authors conclude that the heterogeneity of tumors was responsible for the different drug responses in the two metastases.

Heterogeneity or polyclonal properties of tumors is a common phenomenon in advanced GIST and one of the main causes of treatment failure [1]. Studies published a few years ago in the *NEJM* on renal carcinoma and in *Science* on breast cancer showed that different metastases of tumors, even in the same metastasis at different locations, whose genetic tests showed different mutations, illustrated the heterogeneity of tumors [2, 3]. There are some complementarities in the effectiveness of sunitinib and regorafenib for different secondary mutations. Sunitinib and regorafenib showed certain complementarity in the effectiveness of different secondary mutations. The mutation in exon 13 of *KIT* was more sensitive to sunitinib and that in exon 17 of *KIT* was more sensitive to regorafenib [4]. In May 2020, the food and drug administration (FDA) approved ripretinib as a fourth-line therapeutic drug for GIST [5]. This new TKI showed a broad-spectrum inhibitory effect on *KIT* and *PDGFRA* genes in preclinical and clinical studies, bringing new possibilities for patients with advanced GIST with multiple drug resistance.

23.2.4.3 Whether Palliative Surgery Can Benefit Patients with Advanced Widespread Progression

The value of palliative surgery in advanced GIST has been recognized more in recent years. As early as 2006, Raut of Harvard Medical School found that among patients with advanced GIST, those who were responsive to TKI treatment could benefit from palliative surgery, while patients with extensive progress could not benefit from surgery [6]. In clinical work, surgeons need to consider the patient's condition, past surgical procedures, compliance, financial status, and their own experience and surgical ability (especially the ability to respond to intraoperative emergencies) in patients with advanced GIST, while carefully formulating a treatment plan. Surgeons should not rush to perform inappropriate surgeries which may increase medical risks and patient suffering, nor should they turn a blind eye and refuse surgery indefinitely to advanced patients whose drug control is ineffective [7].

The patient presented as case 30 underwent surgical intervention after extensive disease progression to relieve obstruction, and then re-advanced 6 months later. At that time fulminant growth of multiple lesions was evident in the liver, suggesting that surgical intervention in the extensive progression period had limited significance for disease control and prolonged survival, and only helped to manage complications caused by disease.

The patient presented as case 31 had a local lesion in the anterior rectum for a long period of time which was effectively controlled by the drugs, so palliative surgical resection could be considered. In fact, the patient missed an opportunity for palliative surgical resection during imatinib treatment, although after sunitinib treatment the tumor shrank again creating an opportunity for surgery and allowing for surgical resection. Unfortunately, however, the tumor recurred 5 months after resection.

23.3 Expert Comments

Ye Zhou

It is believed that most tumor progression after first-line treatment is due to a secondary mutation in *KIT*. Due to the heterogeneity of tumors, there are also heterogeneous manifestations of secondary mutations [8]. Different secondary gene mutations can be found not only in different lesions, but also within a single lesion. Many of the existing second-line and third-line drugs are multi-target TKI inhibitors [9]. Just as the first-line drug imatinib has a better effect on *KIT* exon 11, sunitinib and regorafenib have different effects on GIST at different mutation sites of *KIT*. The former has a better effect on site mutation in the activation ring region and the latter has a better effect on mutations in the ATP binding region. Ripretinib showed a certain tumor inhibitory effect for patients with advanced GIST with different secondary drug resistance mutations. In the INVICTUS study, compared to placebo, the risk of disease progression for patients treated with ripretinib was reduced by 85%, and the median PFS was 6.3 months, while the placebo group was only 1.0 months, which provided new opportunities for control of multiple drug resistant GIST [10]. Because puncture biopsies are invasive, tissue accessibility is low, and the tumor has spatial heterogeneity; therefore, a puncture biopsy cannot fully meet the sampling requirements for gene detection. Relatively speaking, the noninvasive operation of ctDNA technology is its biggest advantage, but it still has some disadvantages, such as a false negative rate, which is not completely consistent with the detection results of tissue samples [11].

For research on the position of surgical treatment in recurrent and metastatic GIST, due to the limitation of objective conditions, we cannot carry out strict prospective clinical research. However, in clinical practice, it can be found that patients can obtain a better tumor-free survival period with surgical resection under the conditions of well-controlled targeted therapy. For patients with localized progression, it may be necessary to strictly evaluate the complications of surgery and the possibility of complete resection to identify the possible beneficiaries.

References

1. Serrano C, George S. Gastrointestinal stromal tumor: challenges and opportunities for a new decade. Clin Cancer Res. 2020;26(19):5078–85. https://doi.org/10.1158/1078-0432.CCR-20-1706.
2. Ravaud A. A step ahead in metastatic renal cell carcinoma. N Engl J Med. 2021;384(14):1360–1. https://doi.org/10.1056/NEJMe2101777.
3. Kim M, Park J, Bouhaddou M, Kim K, Rojc A, Modak M, Soucheray M, McGregor MJ, O'Leary P, Wolf D, Stevenson E, Foo TK, Mitchell D, Herrington KA, Munoz DP, Tutuncuoglu B, Chen KH, Zheng F, Kreisberg JF, Diolaiti ME, Gordan JD, Coppe JP, Swaney DL, Xia B, van 't Veer L, Ashworth A, Ideker T, Krogan NJ. A protein interaction landscape of breast cancer. Science. 2021;374(6563):eabf3066. https://doi.org/10.1126/science.abf3066.
4. Klug LR, Khosroyani HM, Kent JD, Heinrich MC. New treatment strategies for advanced-stage gastrointestinal stromal tumours.

Nat Rev Clin Oncol. 2022;19(5):328–41. https://doi.org/10.1038/s41571-022-00606-4.

5. Kumar V, Doros L, Thompson M, Mushti SL, Charlab R, Spehalski EI, Zhao H, Thompson MD, Tang S, Pazdur R, Lemery SJ, Theoret MR, Fashoyin-Aje LA. FDA approval summary: ripretinib for advanced gastrointestinal stromal tumor. Clin Cancer Res. 2022;29:2020. https://doi.org/10.1158/1078-0432.CCR-22-2400.
6. Raut CP, Posner M, Desai J, Morgan JA, George S, Zahrieh D, Fletcher CD, Demetri GD, Bertagnolli MM. Surgical management of advanced gastrointestinal stromal tumors after treatment with targeted systemic therapy using kinase inhibitors. J Clin Oncol. 2006;24(15):2325–31. https://doi.org/10.1200/JCO.2005.05.3439.
7. Cao H, Wang M. Lancet in the era of targeted drug therapy: the role of surgery in the management of advanced gastrointestinal stromal tumor. Zhonghua Wei Chang Wai Ke Za Zhi. 2016;19(11):1211–6. Chinese. https://doi.org/10.3760/cma.j.issn.1671-0274.2016.11.003.
8. Serrano C, Marino-Enriquez A, Tao DL, Ketzer J, Eilers G, Zhu M, Yu C, Mannan AM, Rubin BP, Demetri GD, Raut CP, Presnell A, McKinley A, Heinrich MC, Czaplinski JT, Sicinska E, Bauer S, George S, Fletcher JA. Complementary activity of tyrosine kinase inhibitors against secondary kit mutations in imatinib-resistant gastrointestinal stromal tumours. Br J Cancer. 2019;120(6):612–20. https://doi.org/10.1038/s41416-019-0389-6.
9. Khosroyani HM, Klug LR, Heinrich MC. TKI treatment sequencing in advanced gastrointestinal stromal tumors. Drugs. 2023;83(1):55–73. https://doi.org/10.1007/s40265-022-01820-1.
10. Bauer S, Heinrich MC, George S, Zalcberg JR, Serrano C, Gelderblom H, Jones RL, Attia S, D'Amato G, Chi P, Reichardt P, Meade J, Su Y, Ruiz-Soto R, Blay JY, von Mehren M, Schoffski P. Clinical activity of ripretinib in patients with advanced gastrointestinal stromal tumor harboring heterogeneous KIT/PDGFRA mutations in the phase III INVICTUS study. Clin Cancer Res. 2021;27(23):6333–42. https://doi.org/10.1158/1078-0432.CCR-21-1864.
11. Falkenhorst J, Grunewald S, Krzeciesa D, Herold T, Ketzer J, Christoff M, Hamacher R, Kostbade K, Treckmann J, Koster J, Farzaliyev F, Fletcher BS, Dieckmann N, Kaths M, Muhlenberg T, Schildhaus HU, Bauer S. Plasma sequencing for patients with GIST-limitations and opportunities in an academic setting. Cancers (Basel). 2022;14(22):5496. https://doi.org/10.3390/cancers14225496.

Avapritinib Therapy in Advanced Gastrointestinal Stromal Tumor with *PDGFRA* Mutation

24

Xiaoqi Li, Xinli Ma, and Gang Zhao

Keywords

Gastrointestinal stromal tumor · D842V mutation · Metastatic tumor · Targeted therapy · Avapritinib

24.1 Case 32 A 54-Year-Old Man with a Recurrent Metastatic GIST with *PDGFRA* D842V Mutation

Xiaoqi Li and Xinli Ma

24.1.1 Introduction

As GIST with *PDGFRA* gene D842V mutation doesn't respond to targeted therapy, the previous primary treatment for patients with recurrent metastatic tumors with this mutation was active surgical treatment. The advent of avapritinib provided more treatment options for such patients. Targeted therapy can improve patient prognosis and create conditions for radical surgery. Therefore, in the future targeted therapy combined with surgery will play an extremely important role in the diagnosis and treatment of GIST with primary drug resistance, for example, D842V.

24.1.2 Case Background

The patient, a 54-year-old man, was treated for abdominal pain and abdominal distension for more than 1 week at another hospital on February 4, 2010. He was diagnosed with a space-occupying lesion in the great curvature of the stomach and admitted to another hospital for surgical treatment. The postoperative pathology showed a high-risk GIST in the stomach. The patient was not followed up and didn't receive targeted therapy after surgery. In April 2016, he underwent an abdominal tumor resection and small intestinal segment resection for treatment of tumor recurrence. The postoperative pathology showed high-risk GIST in the abdominal cavity and a D842V mutation in *PDGFRA* exon 18. After taking imatinib orally for 2 months, the doctor discontinued the medication based on the genetic test results. In October 2019, a CT scan revealed a huge metastasis in the right lobe of the liver, accompanied by intra-abdominal metastasis.

On October 5, 2019, the patient underwent transcatheter arterial chemoembolization (TACE) under digital subtraction angiography (DSA) and local anesthesia. After the operation, the patient visited hospital for medical consultation.

24.1.2.1 Past History and Family History

The patient was previously healthy and reported no history of drug allergies. The patient's parents were alive, and the family had no similar medical history.

24.1.2.2 Physical Examination

The patient's vital signs were stable, and the skin and mucous membranes were not yellowish or pale. The abdomen was flat, and no gastrointestinal or peristaltic waves were observed. The abdomen was soft, with no tenderness, or rebound tenderness. A large mass was palpable in the right abdomen. The bowel sounds were normal.

24.1.2.3 Preliminary Diagnosis

Postoperative liver and abdominal metastasis from gastric GIST.

X. Li · X. Ma (✉) · G. Zhao
Department of Gastrointestinal Surgery, Renji Hospital, Shanghai Jiaotong University School of Medicine, Shanghai, China

K. Tao, H. Cao (eds.), *Clinical Management of Gastrointestinal Stromal Tumor*, https://doi.org/10.1007/978-981-99-9392-5_24

24.1.3 Therapy

24.1.3.1 Auxiliary Examination

Abdominal CT A space-occupying lesion was found in the right lobe of the liver and abdominal cavity, 20 cm × 15 cm × 7 cm in size (Figs. 24.1 and 24.2).

24.1.3.2 Case Analysis

We conducted a MDT meeting to discuss the patient's condition. After the joint discussion and assessment with oncologists, liver surgeons, and gastrointestinal surgeons, it was considered that the patient had primary resistant GIST with *PDGFRA* exon 18 D842V mutation, for which the control of disease progression via targeted therapy was challenging. The hepatic metastasis was located in the right lobe of the liver while an isolated space-occupying lesion was seen in the abdominal cavity, and both metastases could be excised using surgery. After communication with the patient's family members, combined hepatic and gastrointestinal surgery, including right hemihepatectomy, partial enterectomy, resection of mesentery nodules of the small intestine, and cholecystectomy, was performed on November 12, 2019. During the surgery, a tumor in the right lobe of the liver, with a diameter of approximately 16 cm, without a capsule, and vascular invasion was found. The tumor bulged toward the thoracic cavity, with an old hemorrhagic focus, and without bile duct thrombi or portal vein thrombosis. Additionally, a tumor with a diameter of approximately 4 cm was seen in the abdominal cavity. This tumor involved part of the small intestine, and the involved portion of the intestine was excised. Scattered metastatic nodules were seen in the abdominal cavity and mesentery.

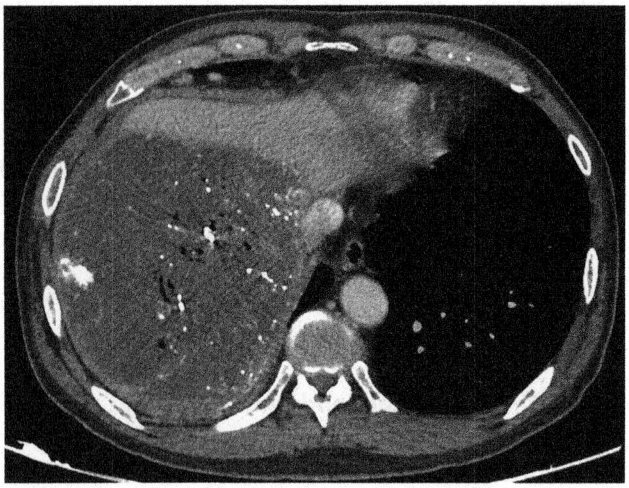

Fig. 24.1 Abdominal enhanced CT of the liver tumor

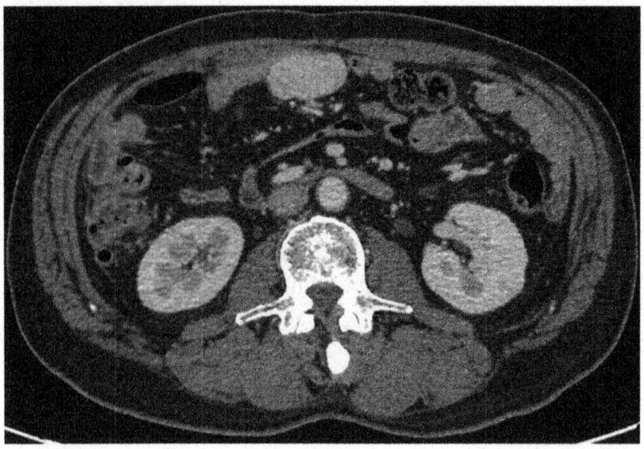

Fig. 24.2 Abdominal enhanced CT of the abdominal tumor

24.1.3.3 Postoperative Pathology, Genetic Testing, and Prognosis

Pathological Diagnosis The postoperative pathology indicated a partial liver tumor, 20 cm × 15 cm × 8 cm, with predominant necrosis and a small amount of degenerated GIST tumor tissue, which was consistent with post-treatment changes. The small intestinal tumor was a GIST, 3.5 cm × 3 cm × 3 cm in size, with a mitotic count > 10/50 HPF. The diagnosis was GIST in the mesentery nodule of the small intestine.

Immunohistochemistry CD117 (+), CD34 (−), DOG-1 (+), SMA (−), and Ki-67 (Li: >70%).

Genetic Testing The results indicated a D842V mutation in *PDGFRA* exon 18.

24.1.4 Prognosis

After the third surgery, a new tumor, 4.0 cm in size, was found in the patient's abdominal cavity upon reexamination in another hospital on December 25th, 2019, and extensive millet-like nodules were seen in the mesentery of the small intestine. In January 2020, the patient underwent avapritinib therapy for a month. Following initial treatment, a repeat contrast-enhanced CT of thoracic, abdominal, and pelvic cavities suggested a decrease in the size of the abdominal metastasis from 4.0 to 0.9 cm. After 3 months of avapritinib treatment, a contrast-enhanced CT of the thoracic, abdominal, and pelvic cavities revealed no obvious tumors.

24.1.5 Experience in Diagnosis and Therapy

24.1.5.1 Therapy for Metastatic GIST Patients with D842V Mutation

Previous literature has shown that imatinib targeted therapy was the main therapeutic option for recurrent metastatic

GIST, but the 5-year PFS was only 20%, and half of the patients exhibited a secondary drug-resistant mutation after 2 years of treatment [1]. Therefore, most patients still needed complete tumor resection or cytoreductive surgery. Many small-sample single-center retrospective studies [2–5] showed that patients with stable disease (SD) or partial response (PR) after imatinib (IM) treatment might benefit from R0/R1 surgery. Nevertheless, patients with poor efficacy in targeted therapy and widespread disease progression can still exhibit tumor recurrence within a short term even after R0/R1 treatment. The D842V mutation is a type of primary drug-resistant mutation, and IM treatment was ineffective, so it was difficult to achieve SD or PR through targeted therapy in this case. Even if the efficacy of surgery alone was poor, if patients had no prominent surgical contraindication, surgery was the only therapeutic means that could improve the prognosis of such patients. For this reason, whether there was targeted therapy for GIST patients with the D842V mutation became a key factor to improve patients' prognosis.

24.1.5.2 The Noble Medicine Avapritinib for GIST Patients with D842V Mutation

Avapritinib (sold under the brand name AYVAKIT™), i.e., BLU-285, was developed by Blueprint Medicines. In the Phase, I clinical study NAVIGATOR (NCT02508532) [6], the overall response rate (ORR) of 56 GIST patients with *PDGFRA* exon 18 D842V mutation was assessed. The ORR was 91% (51/56 patients). The clinical benefit rate (CBR) was 98% (55/56 patients). The median disease control rate (DOR) was 27.6 months. Therefore, this drug was approved [7] by the U.S. Food and Drug Administration on January 9, 2020, for patients with advanced GIST patients with unresectable and metastatic tumors with *PDGFRA* exon 18 mutations (including D842V mutation). Meanwhile, the NCCN Guidelines published in February 2020 [8] recommended avapritinib for patients with *PDGFRA* exon 18 mutation (including D842V mutation) for the first time. The recommended dose was 300 mg (or the maximum dose was 400 mg) once a day, which should be taken on an empty stomach. During avapritinib treatment, the major reported adverse reactions included edema, the adverse reaction in the digestive tract, hair discoloration, hyperdacryosis, and fatigue. In addition, there were some reports of intracranial hemorrhage and toxic side effects in the central nervous system.

Surgical resection has previously been the predominant treatment for patients with recurrent metastatic GIST with D842V mutation since this gene mutation does not respond to traditional targeted therapy. However, the emergence of avapritinib provides more options for treating such patients, improves the patients' prognosis through targeted therapy, and creates a favorable condition for radical surgery. It can be seen from this case report, that the combination of targeted therapy and surgery may play a crucial role in the treatment of imatinib-resistant GIST with primary D842V resistance mutation.

24.2 Case Review

Gang Zhao

This patient has a total course of disease of more than 10 years, during which he underwent three laparotomies and one TACE procedure. Now, he is receiving avapritinib targeted therapy and has met the diagnostic criteria for PR. During the treatment of this patient, 3 R0/R1 surgeries with complete tumor resection played a vital role in prolonging survival. Although there was no consensus on adjuvant therapy on GIST among Chinese experts in 2010, and no effective drug for targeted therapy of D842V mutation, after the first resection, the PFS of this patient still reached a considerable 74 months. After the second resection, the PFS of this patient was 42 months. Therefore, the active R0/R1 radical resection on recurrent metastatic GIST patients with local progression can significantly prolong the PFS and OS. After the third R2 resection for liver metastasis and extensive abdominal metastasis, the patient suffered from a recurrence of the abdominal tumor in a short period (PFS = 1 month), indicating that this patient had entered a period of rapid progression. If we were confined to the previous therapeutic options for patients with D842V mutations, the prognosis of this patient would have been poor. In this case, avapritinib, a targeted drug for patients with D842V mutation entered the clinical stage in China, and this patient was fortunate enough to pass screening and receive treatment with 300 mg/d avapritinib. The results indicated that after 4 months of targeted therapy, the patient achieved PR again, improved prognosis, and prolonged his life. For this reason, the comprehensive diagnosis and treatment mode of surgery combined with targeted therapy has good efficacy for GIST patients with recurrent metastatic D842V mutation.

References

1. Blanke CD, Demetri GD, von MM HMC, Eisenberg B, Fletcher JA, Corless CL, Fletcher CD, Roberts PJ, Heinz D, Where E, Nikolova Z, Joensuu H. Long-term results from a randomized phase II trial of standard- versus higher-dose imatinib mesylate for patients with unresectable or metastatic gastrointestinal stromal tumors expressing KIT. J Clin Oncol. 2008;26(4):620–5. https://doi.org/10.1200/JCO.2007.13.4403.
2. Raut CP, Posner M, Desai J, Morgan JA, George S, Zahrieh D, Fletcher CD, Demetri GD, Bertagnolli MM. Surgical management of advanced gastrointestinal stromal tumors after treatment with targeted systemic therapy using kinase inhibitors. J Clin Oncol. 2006;24(15):2325–31. https://doi.org/10.1200/JCO.2005.05.3439.

3. Dematteo RP, Maki RG, Singer S, Gonen M, Brennan MF, Antonescu CR. Results of tyrosine kinase inhibitor therapy followed by surgical resection for metastatic gastrointestinal stromal tumor. Ann Surg. 2007;245(3):347–52. https://doi.org/10.1097/01.sla.0000236630.93587.59.
4. Gronchi A, Fiore M, Miselli F, Lagonigro MS, Coco P, Messina A, Pilotti S, Casali PG. Surgery of residual disease following molecular-targeted therapy with imatinib mesylate in advanced/metastatic GIST. Ann Surg. 2007;245(3):341–6. https://doi.org/10.1097/01.sla.0000242710.36384.1b.
5. Bauer S, Rutkowski P, Hohenberger P, Miceli R, Fumagalli E, Siedlecki JA, Nguyen BP, Kerst M, Fiore M, Nyckowski P, Hoiczyk M, Cats A, Casali PG, Treckmann J, van CF, Gronchi A. Long-term follow-up of patients with GIST undergoing metastasectomy in the era of imatinib – analysis of prognostic factors (EORTC-STBSG collaborative study). Eur J Surg Oncol. 2014;40(4):412–9. https://doi.org/10.1016/j.ejso.2013.12.020.
6. Jones RL, Serrano C, Von Mehren M, George S, Heinrich MC, Kang YK, Schöffski P, Cassier PA, Mir O, Chawla SP, Eskens F, Rutkowski P, William D, Teresa Z, Roche M, Bauer S. Avapritinib in unresectable or metastatic PDGFRA D842V-mutant gastrointestinal stromal tumors: long-term efficacy and safety data from the NAVIGATOR phase I trial. Eur J Cancer. 2021;145(1):132–42. https://doi.org/10.1016/j.ejca.2020.12.008.
7. Dhillon S. Avapritinib: first approval. Drugs. 2020;80(4):433–9. https://doi.org/10.1007/s40265-020-01275-2.
8. NCCN. NCCN clinical practice guidelines in oncology, soft tissue sarcoma (version 6. 2019). https://www.nccn.org/

Therapy for Advanced Gastrointestinal Stromal Tumors

25

Xinli Ma, Ming Wang, Kuntang Shen, Xinhua Zhang, Bo Ni, Linxi Yang, and Hui Cao

Keywords

Gastrointestinal stromal tumor · Radiofrequency ablation · Combination therapy · Imatinib · Ripretinib ctDNA · Surgery

25.1 Case 33 A 50-Year-Old Man with Advanced GIST Underwent RFA and TKI Therapy

Xinli Ma and Ming Wang

25.1.1 Introduction

The emergence of molecularly targeted drugs, initially represented by imatinib, changed the traditional treatment regimen of GIST and formed a concept of surgery combined with molecular-targeted drugs. Although most GISTs are sensitive to imatinib at the beginning of treatment, more than 50% will eventually develop imatinib resistance. Thus, managing advanced GIST has become a key issue. Patients with advanced GIST who do not respond to standard-dose imatinib treatment can proceed with individualized therapies including high-dose imatinib, second-line or third-line medications, TKI combined with radiofrequency ablation (RFA), or first-line plus second-line combination medication. Systemic therapy is often needed for patients with advanced GIST and combined surgical intervention can reduce tumor burden and prolong survival. However, determining how to apply these treatments rationally is a clinical problem that needs to be solved urgently. Therefore, it is necessary to make full use of the multidisciplinary treatment model to weigh the risks and benefits and obtain the best clinical effect.

25.1.2 Case Background

The patient, a 50-year-old man, was admitted to the emergency room on November 12, 2012, with a 9-hour history of abdominal pain. A CT examination revealed that the small intestinal lumen was entangled in clusters in the left lower abdomen, with possible intestinal torsion and a slightly hypointense shadow in the left lateral lobe of the liver, the nature of which was to be determined (Fig. 25.1).

An emergency exploratory laparotomy was performed. An exophytic mass, 10 cm × 8 cm × 6 cm in size, was found in the sigmoid colon, and the mass invaded a local segment of the small intestine, located 1.5 m from the ileocecal region (Fig. 25.2).

Postoperative pathology showed a sigmoid GIST (12 cm × 5 cm × 5 cm) with necrosis and mitotic count 5/50 HPF, graded as high risk by the modified NIH risk classification. Tumor involvement was seen in the intestinal wall of the small intestinal segment. Tumor cells were CD117(+), CD34(−), DOG-1(+), SMA (−), Actin (−), S-100(−), FN (−), Ki-67 (Li: 10%). Genetic testing suggested a heterozygous deletion mutation in *KIT*, with the deletion starting at the first 3 bases of exon 11 and ending at base 1761 (CAG AAA CCC ATG TAT GAA GTA CAG TGG AAG). *KIT* exons 9, 13, and 17, as well as *PDGFRA* exons 12 and 18, were wild types. The patient was discharged after a good postoperative recovery. Imatinib 400 mg/d was initiated 1 month after surgery and regular reexamination was conducted. On May 8, 2013, enhanced CT showed postoperative changes in the colon, and abnormal density shadow in the

X. Ma · M. Wang (✉) · B. Ni · L. Yang (✉) · H. Cao
Department of Gastrointestinal Surgery, Renji Hospital, Shanghai Jiaotong University School of Medicine, Shanghai, China

K. Shen
Department of Gastrointestinal Surgery, Zhongshan Hospital, Fudan University, Shanghai, China
e-mail: shen.kuntang@zs-hospital.sh.cn

X. Zhang (✉)
Department of Gastrointestinal Surgery, The First Affiliated Hospital of Sun Yat-sen University, Guangzhou, China

K. Tao, H. Cao (eds.), *Clinical Management of Gastrointestinal Stromal Tumor*, https://doi.org/10.1007/978-981-99-9392-5_25

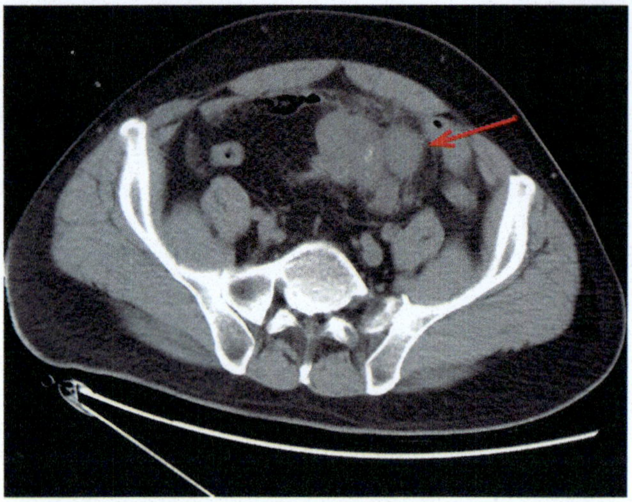

Fig. 25.1 CT showed that a soft tissue mass in the lower abdomen and the peripheral intestines were tangled together

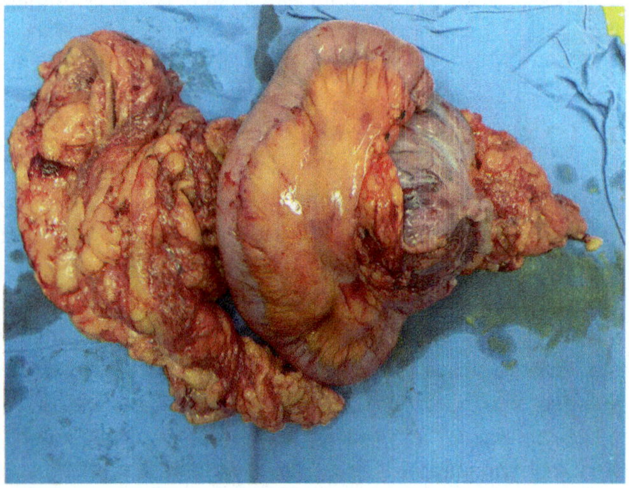

Fig. 25.2 The gross specimen

left lobe of the liver, with a high probability of metastatic tumor. Imatinib 400 mg/d was continued with regular reexamination. A CT in October 2013 showed a nodule in the left lobe of the liver, consistent with a metastatic tumor. The patient was admitted to the hospital for further treatment.

25.1.2.1 Past History and Family History

The patient was previously healthy and reported no history of drug allergies. The patient's parents were alive and there was no similar medical history in the family.

25.1.2.2 Physical Examination

The patient's vital signs were stable, and the skin and mucosa were not yellowish or pale. The abdomen was flat, with no gastrointestinal or peristaltic waves. A surgical scar was seen in the mid-abdomen. The abdomen was soft, with no rebound tenderness. The bowel sounds were normal.

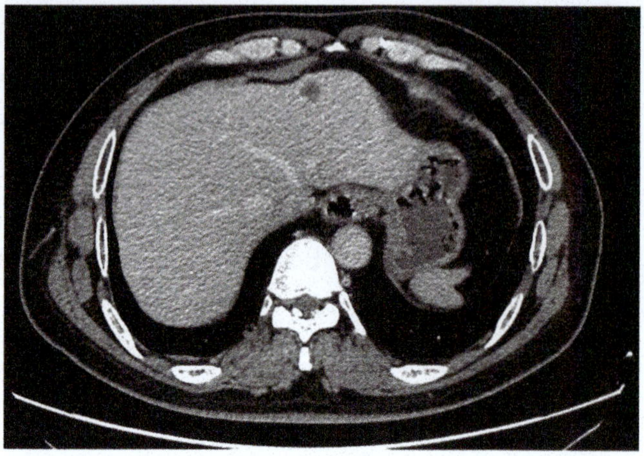

Fig. 25.3 MRI of the liver before radiofrequency ablation

25.1.2.3 Auxiliary Examination

PET-CT Low-density lesions were observed in the left lobe of the liver, with no obvious FDG uptake; the findings were consistent with possible benign lesions.

Abdominal MRI The nodular lesions in the left lobe of the liver were slightly larger than those in the anterior film, and the size was about 17 mm. The lesions were considered to be inflammatory granulomatous lesions, possibly due to GIST metastasis (based on patient history), and there were annular active components at the edge (Fig. 25.3).

25.1.2.4 Preliminary Diagnosis

Postoperative liver metastasis from colon GIST.

25.1.3 Therapy

25.1.3.1 Case Analysis

The patient was a middle-aged man, with a prior history of high-risk GIST in the colon who was receiving imatinib therapy. There was a progressive increase in the size of the suspected metastasis in the liver. The location and diameter of the tumor should be evaluated, and radiofrequency ablation should be performed after a puncture biopsy to clarify the nature of the lesion.

25.1.3.2 Treatment

The patient underwent RFA of a liver tumor on June 10, 2014. Intraoperative ultrasound showed that the tumor was located in the left lateral lobe of the liver, with a diameter of approximately 1.8 cm. The tumor was first biopsied, and the sample was sent for pathological analysis. The needle was inserted into the center of the tumor under ultrasound guidance, and the power was set at 100 W. Radiofrequency ablation was performed on the tumor until it was completely covered by a strong echo. The operation was performed smoothly.

25.1.3.3 Postoperative Pathology and Genetic Testing

Pathological Diagnosis Liver tumor biopsy showed a small amount of GIST in the liver tissue.

Immunohistochemistry CD117(+), DOG-1(+), CD34(−), Vim (+), S-100(−), SMA (−), Ki-67 (Li: 3%).

Genetic Testing The amount of tissue collected was insufficient and genetic testing could not be performed.

25.1.4 Prognosis

The patient continued to take oral imatinib 400 mg/d after RFA and was regularly followed up with liver-enhanced MRI in the outpatient clinic. By July 2020, the liver metastases were assessed as SD (Fig. 25.4). In November 2020, an enhanced MRI of the upper abdomen suggested partial progression of the patient's liver metastases, and RFA was performed again. After that, the drug treatment was changed to sunitinib 37.5 mg/d. Upon review 4 months later, the liver metastasis was still progressing, and both RFA and TACE were performed. The MRI was still suggestive of progression on review after 2 months, after which the patient switched to regorafenib 120 mg/d and a review after 40 days suggested continued progression (Fig. 25.5). The patient declined fourth-line ripretinib treatment due to financial factors, and a hepatic segment resection with cholecystectomy and intraoperative RFA was subsequently performed on September 15, 2021. Intraoperatively, dense adhesions in the upper abdomen were seen, and the liver was soft after the decomposition of the adhesions. There was no visible cirrhosis or ascites, and the spleen was normal. The tumor was located in the right anterior S5 segmental septum, exhibited dense adhesion with the right abdominal wall, was approximately 8 × 6 cm in size, and exhibited no envelope, invasion of blood vessels, cancerous thrombus in the bile duct, or portal thrombus. Multiple sub-foci in the right and left liver were treated with intraoperative RFA. At the site of the original RFA treatment in the right lobe of the liver, a huge purulent lesion, approximately 5 cm in size, was found attached to the abdominal wall. Approximately 200 mL of pus was visible after the incision of this lesion. Postoperative pathology showed that the first specimen from the liver with hemorrhagic degeneration necrosis and cystic degeneration was consistent with recurrent GIST. Several nodules were identified, with a maximal diameter of approximately 1–1.5 cm, likely representing the effects of therapy. The second specimen from the liver showed fibrous tissue with hemorrhage, extensive degeneration, and inflammatory cell infiltration, consistent with recurrent GIST. Immunohistochemistry showed CD117(+), CD34(−), DOG-1(+), S-100(−), Ki-67 (Li: 10%). Genetic testing revealed an exon 11 deletion mutation in *KIT* without secondary mutations. The patient completed baseline upper abdominal enhancement MRI and resumed imatinib 400 mg/d therapy after 2 months with no new metastatic lesions in the liver at follow-up until March 2022 (Fig. 25.6).

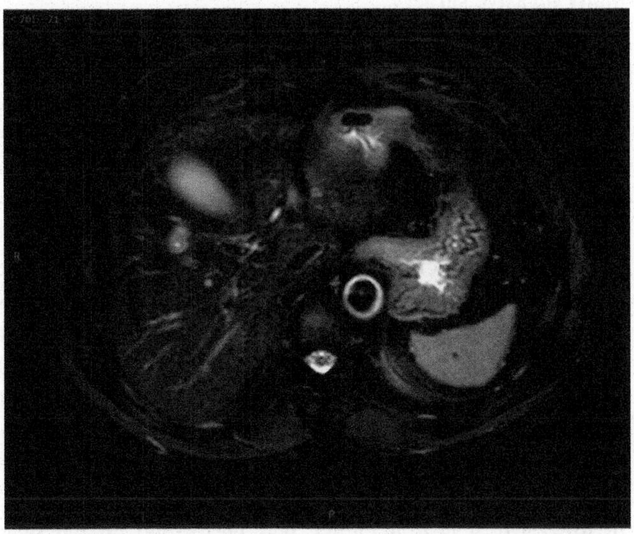

Fig. 25.4 Enhanced MRI of the upper abdomen demonstrated SD 6 years after RFA

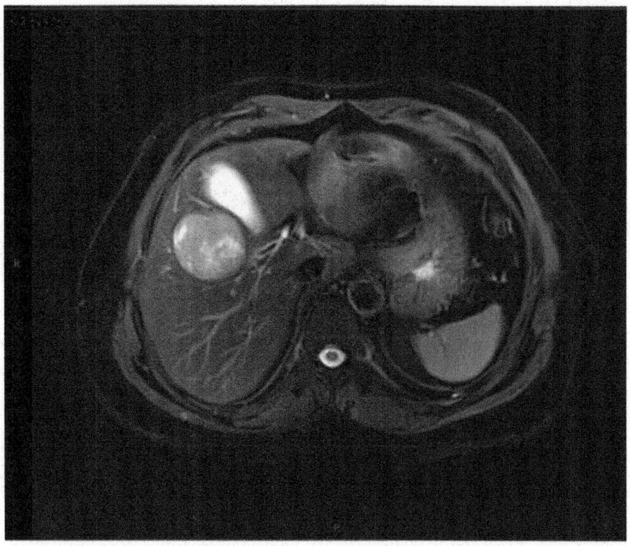

Fig. 25.5 Enhanced MRI of the upper abdomen in November 2020

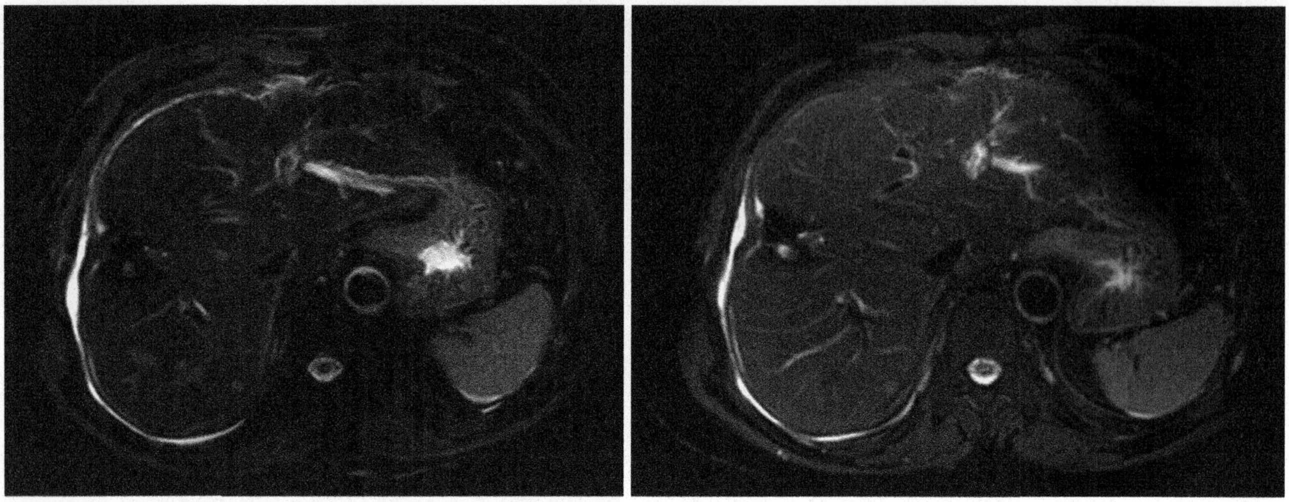

Fig. 25.6 Postoperative baseline in October 2021 and 6-month postoperative enhanced MRI of the upper abdomen

25.1.5 Experience in Diagnosis and Therapy

25.1.5.1 The Role of Imaging in Diagnosing GIST Liver Metastasis

Common imaging modalities for GIST include conventional methods (CT) and alternative methods (MRI, PET-CT). CT is commonly used and widely available, and plays a key role in the localization of the tumor, estimation of tumor burden and metastasis, evaluation of invasive lesions, and responses to medical management. MRI and PET-CT are used as alternatives when CT-enhanced scanning is contraindicated or when previous diagnostic studies are inconclusive. For suspected liver metastases, MRI has certain advantages over CT. Diffusion-weighted MRI (DWI) can help detect small metastatic lesions and evaluate the efficacy of targeted therapy. It can also be used to evaluate the efficacy of targeted therapy early in the treatment course. It is difficult to assess whether liver nodules, especially those in the left lateral hepatic lobe, are benign or malignant using CT scans during routine follow-ups. Based on the lesions found in enhanced MRI combined with the slow progression and history of GIST, the diagnosis of GIST with liver metastasis was made for this patient. Interestingly, the patient did undergo PET-CT imaging previously, but no increased FDG uptake of the lesion was noted. This may be related to the inhibition of tumor activity during targeted drug treatment.

25.1.5.2 Choosing the Proper Treatment Strategy for GIST with Liver Metastases

The current domestic [1, 2] and international guidelines [3] have pointed out that for some patients with liver metastases from GIST who cannot undergo surgery, arterial embolization and RFA can also be considered palliative treatments. Patients with locally progressive lesions who are not candidates for localized treatment are advised to use sunitinib or high-dose imatinib. In this case, there was the progression of a liver lesion during targeted therapy, which indicated that drug resistance may have occurred. If the original targeted therapy is maintained, the disease is expected to progress further. However, unlike extensive progression, the patient did not have metastases in the abdominal or pelvic cavities. If isolated drug-resistant lesions can be appropriately treated, second-line targeted drugs may not be needed. Treatment of isolated liver metastasis includes surgical resection and RFA [4]. Considering the size and location of the metastases, the patient in this case finally received RFA treatment, and they recovered after surgery, reflecting the advantages of minimally invasive surgery.

The patient had been diagnosed with high-risk colonic GIST and had surgery 10 years ago, followed by radiofrequency ablation 6 years ago. No doubt targeted drugs greatly contributed to prolonging the survival of this patient, although the RFA treatment of liver metastases also played an important role in avoiding the possible complications of open surgery. The treatment with RFA also avoids prematurely switching to second-line drugs, which are costly and associated with side effects. When both TKI-targeted therapy and interventional therapy fail to benefit patients, accurate assessment of status and timely and effective surgical intervention can provide longer survival benefits.

25.1.5.3 Proper Use of Needle Biopsy

In this case, a needle biopsy was performed on the liver metastases, although molecular pathological examinations could not be completed because an insufficient volume of tissue was collected. Molecular pathology detection of drug-resistant lesions is very important, and the detection of new drug-resistant mutations can guide the selection of targeted molecular therapy. The GIST pathology community tends to collect the smallest volume of specimens to complete the tests that are sufficient to diagnose GIST (for example, immunohistochemistry tests may only be performed for CD117 and DOG-1) so that only enough specimens are collected for specific molecular testing.

25.1.5.4 The Therapeutic Value of RFA During GIST Drug Therapy for Advanced Liver Metastases

The value of local therapy for patients with advanced GIST was proven as early as 2006 by Raut et al. [5] from Harvard Medical School. A study published in the *Journal of Clinical Oncology* showed that patients with advanced GIST who can achieve stable or local progression under drug treatment may benefit from surgical resection, whereas patients with extensive progression are more suitable for local treatment using RFA. Under the overall control of drug therapy for advanced GIST where certain liver lesions are poorly controlled, local treatments can be actively applied, including treatments, such as RFA [6], interventional embolization, and absolute alcohol injection. In this case, even when the patient showed partial progression of liver tumor and poor efficacy of TKI drugs, the growth of liver metastases was slowed by RFA and TACE, which helped delay progressive metastasis of the disease.

25.2 Expert Comments

Kuntang Shen

A 2006 *JCO* study [5] showed that patients with stable or locally progressive advanced GIST can benefit from surgical resection, while the survival of patients with extensive progression cannot be prolonged with surgical management. However, the current domestic and international guidelines have pointed out that for some patients with liver metastases from GIST for whom surgery is not appropriate, arterial embolization and RFA can also be considered for palliative treatment. Patients with local progression where local treatment is not appropriate should switch to Sunitinib or high-dose imatinib.

In conclusion, surgeons need to consider the patient's condition, compliance, economic status, previous surgical procedures, and their own experience and surgical capabilities (especially the ability to respond to intraoperative emergencies), and carefully plan treatment for patients with advanced GIST. We should not rashly perform improper surgery which increases medical risks and patient suffering, nor should we ignore patients' needs.

25.3 Case 34 A 47-Year-Old Woman with Advanced GIST Treated with Ripretinib as Second-Line After Progression with First-Line Imatinib Therapy

Xinli Ma and Xinhua Zhang

25.3.1 Introduction

Although imatinib is effective for many patients with GISTs, tumor resistance to imatinib is common. Ripretinib is a type II switch-controlled TKI, which aims to control broad-spectrum mutations in KIT and PDGFRA. It has a favorable response in patients with refractory advanced GIST and has become an innovative treatment for heterogeneity of drug resistance mechanisms.

25.3.2 Case Background

A 47-year-old woman was diagnosed with GIST with liver metastases in June 2015 following a 1-year history of repeated abdominal pain and distension. At the time of diagnosis, CT revealed a tumor, approximately 12.4 cm × 12.9 cm in size, located between the greater curvature of the gastric fundus and spleen with metastases in liver S5/6, and a core-needle biopsy confirmed a diagnosis of GIST. Immunohistochemistry suggested tumor cells were positive for CD117, CD34, PDGFRA, and Ki-67. Based on the management guideline for GIST, the patient began to take imatinib 400 mg/d as first-line therapy. Regular reviews over 8 months of imatinib therapy showed the tumor had significantly reduced in size. The imatinib therapy was considered to have proved a PR. Subsequently, the patient underwent resection of the gastric fundus tumor and wedge gastrectomy in February 2016 in a tertiary teaching hospital, but liver metastases were not resected (R2 resection). Following this, she received postoperative imatinib maintenance treatment and regular surveillance showed disease control for 2.5 years. However, ceased imatinib treatment in July 2018 because she experienced side effects of alopecia, nausea, and fatigue.

In May 2019, 10 months after discontinuation of imatinib treatment, a CT scan indicated enlargement and new liver metastases and abdominal metastases. From that time on, imatinib 300 mg/d was resumed regularly, with acceptable plasma imatinib concentration. The patient regained PR from the therapy. However, CT and PET-CT scans on May 18, 2021, indicated a new metastasis, approximately 4.3 cm × 4.4 cm in size, in the hepatorenal recess, and multiple small lesions in the abdominal cavity. The size of the initial liver metastases was still stable. A biopsy of the lesion in the hepatorenal recess confirmed GIST, with Ki-67 50% positive. Mutational analysis demonstrated that the mutation abundance of *KIT* exon 11 K558_E562del and exon 17 D816del were 4.0% and 2.6%, respectively, in peripheral blood (ctDNA), while those in tissues sample were 49.7% and 26.1%, respectively. In addition, a nonsense mutation in *PDGFRA* exon 3 tested positive on ctDNA testing.

25.3.2.1 Past History and Family History

The patient had a more than 20-year history of hypertension, which was well controlled by drugs. The patient reported no drug allergies. The patient's parents were deceased and there was no similar medical history in the family.

25.3.2.2 Physical Examination

The patient's vital signs were stable, the patient showed no signs of anemia, and the skin and mucous membranes were free of yellow staining. The abdomen was flat and soft, with no rebound tenderness, abdominal masses or muscle guarding. The bowel sounds were normal.

25.3.2.3 Preliminary Diagnosis

Gastric GIST with liver metastasis.

25.3.3 Therapy

25.3.3.1 Case Analysis

This was a patient who had extensive progression of gastric GIST with liver metastases after first-line imatinib treatment. The preferred treatment would be second-line systematic targeted therapy. However, there were few progressive lesions and a relatively low tumor burden, including the original lesions and new lesions which were potentially resectable. If there was an opportunity for effective systemic treatment, another satisfactory cytoreductive surgery (CRS) might increase the patient's benefit and prolong survival. However, tumors with *KIT* exon 17 mutation are not sensitive to sunitinib, which is the standard second-line therapy for GISTs. Limited evidence suggested that the usual third- and fourth-line therapies regorafenib and ripretinib, respectively, may both be effective for GISTs with this mutation, and that the ORR for ripretinib may be better and that the safety was certainly superior to that of regorafenib. The MDT discussion recommended ripretinib or regorafenib for treatment choice, with ripretinib more favorably recommended.

25.3.3.2 Treatment

After MDT discussion and sufficient explanation, the patient gave informed consent and commenced ripretinib 150 mg/d from June 1, 2021. In order to obtain an earlier assessment of ripretinib therapy, a plasma ctDNA test was conducted after 2 weeks of treatment, and this showed that the mutation abundance of *KIT* exons 11 and 17 had decreased to zero. MRI indicated SD after 4 weeks of treatment. A repeat MRI and CT scan after 80 days of ripretinib treatment showed that the lesion in the hepatorenal recess had shrunk about 17% in diameter, which met treatment expectations (Fig. 25.7). After a subsequent MDT discussion, the patient underwent laparotomy in our hospital.

The main imatinib-resistant lesion was located in the hepatorenal recess, which showed effective changes after treatment. The texture was soft, and it was surrounded by a thickened peritoneal capsule and fascia. Most of the other

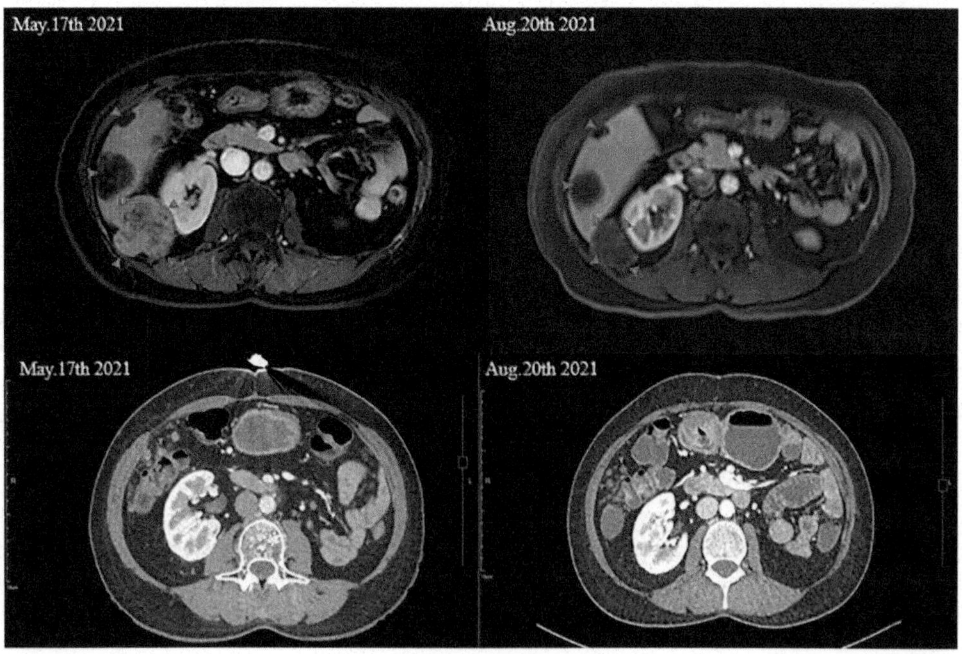

Fig. 25.7 MRI and CT results after ripretinib treatment for 80+ days on August 20, 2021, compared with the baseline on May 17, 2021

scattered peritoneal implant metastases were located in the right-sided greater omentum, and a few were located in the right diaphragmatic peritoneum. Liver metastases in S1, S5, and S6 appeared to demonstrate effective changes under targeted therapy. All visible lesions were removed, and a R0/1 resection was accomplished (Fig. 25.8).

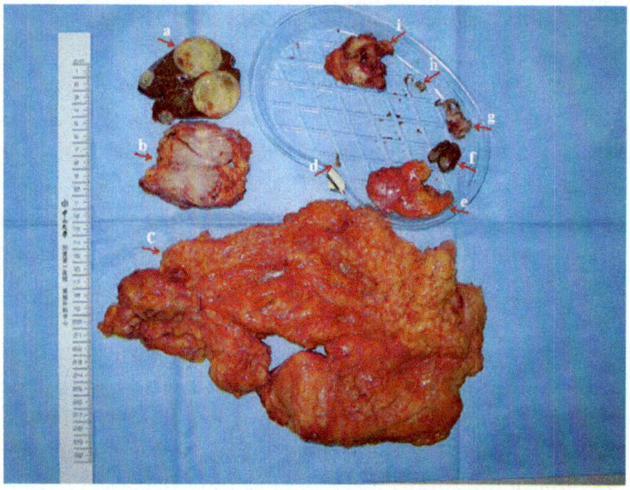

Fig. 25.8 **a** Metastatic tumors of liver S5 and S6; **b** Hepatorenal recess metastasis; **c** Omentum and small metastatic lesions; **d** Diaphragmatic tubercle (1); **e** Ligamentum teres hepatis; **f** Metastatic tumor of liver S1; **g** Diaphragmatic peritoneal tubercle; **h** Diaphragmatic tubercle (2); **i** Adrenal tumor (myelolipoma)

25.3.3.3 Postoperative Pathology and Genetic Testing

Postoperative pathology confirmed GIST. Plasma ctDNA before surgery indicated that the mutation abundance of both *KIT* exon 11 and 17 deletion remained at zero, while *PDGFRA* exon 3 increased slightly from 0.9% to 1.0% (Fig. 25.9). Analysis of all resected tissues did not find any new mutation in *KIT* (Fig. 25.10).

Tumor specific mutation(%)	May.19th 2021	Jun. 14th 2021	Aug. 28th 2021
KIT p.K558_E562del	4.00	0	0
KIT p.D816del	2.60	0	0
PDGFRB p.S55*	0.70	0.90	1.00

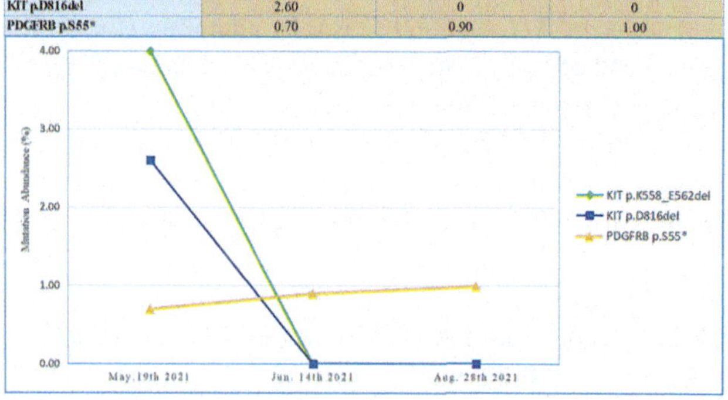

Fig. 25.9 ctDNA level before taking ripretinib (May 19, 2021), 2 weeks after ripretinib therapy (June 14, 2021) and 80 days after ripretinib therapy (August 28, 2021)

25.3.4 Prognosis

Considering that there was a secondary *KIT* exon 17 mutation in multiple peritoneal metastases, suggesting that drug-resistant lesions were widely distributed, it was recommended that ripretinib treatment be resumed. The patient recovered well and was discharged on the 8th POD. During ripretinib treatment, mild adverse reactions, such as alopecia, palmar-plantar erythrodysesthesia syndrome, and mild anemia (Hb: 106–113 g/L), were present. The patient tolerated the therapy well and there were no interruptions in treatment. The patient stopped ripretinib for 5 days before operation, and resumed ripretinib at 150 mg/d on the 7th day postoperatively.

Gene	AAChange	Diaphragmatic tubercle(1)	Diaphragmatic peritoneal tubercle	Diaphragmatic tubercle(2)	Metastatic tumor of liver S1	Metastatic tumor of liver S5	Metastatic tumor of liver S6	Omentum and metastasis	Hepatorenal recess tubercle	
KIT	c.1673_1687del (p.K558_E562del)	34.5%	19.2%	41.4%	14.0%	27.0%	38.1%	44.3%	46.9%	
KIT	c.2446_2448del (p.D816del)	19.2%	9.7%	21.8%	-	-	-	24.2%	25.8%	
PDGFRB	c.164C>A(p.S55*)	-	-	-	-	-	-	-	-	
NOTCH1	c.4423G>A (p.D1475N)	4.3%	-	-	-	-	-	-	-	
PIK3CA	c.323G>A (p.R108H)	-	5.0%	-	-	-	-	-	-	
BMPR1A	-	-	-	CN：0.9	-	-	-	CN：0.8	CN：0.8	
PTEN	-	CN：1.1	-	CN：0.9	-	-	-	CN：0.9	CN：0.9	

Fig. 25.10 Mutation types and their abundance in all resected tissues

25.3.5 Experience of Diagnosis and Therapy

Activating genomic alterations in *KIT* or *PDGFRA* drive cellular growth in most GISTs. Targeted therapy with TKIs has revolutionized the treatment of GIST. Initially, imatinib was approved for patients with *KIT* positive unresectable and/or metastatic malignant GISTs. Although more than 80% of patients with GIST receive clinical benefit from imatinib monotherapy, development of imatinib resistance is common, with more than half of patients developing progressive disease in approximately 2 years, mostly attributed to acquisition of secondary *KIT* mutations. These resistance mutations could be heterogeneous, with multiple secondary mutations from different lesions, or different mutations in a single lesion from one patient. Given this heterogeneity, an unmet need existed for a drug that inhibited a broad spectrum of *KIT* and *PDGFRA* mutants, thus, blocking the various resistance mutations and limiting the impact of further resistance mutations. In May 2020, oral ripretinib first received FDA approval for patients with advanced GIST who had received prior treatment with ≥3 TKIs. Ripretinib is the first switch-controlled TKI which can control broad-spectrum mutations in *KIT* and *PDGFRA* by inhibiting the switch pocket and activation ring switch, as proven theoretically and using preclinical cellular proliferation tests [7, 8].

For advanced GISTs which are resistant or intolerant to imatinib, sunitinib is the standard second-line treatment for progressive GISTs [9]. However, sunitinib is likely to be ineffective for this patient due to secondary mutations in *KIT* exon 17. After the failure of sunitinib treatment, the median PFS for regorafenib has been shown as 4.8 months, with an ORR of 4.5% [10]. Studies have shown that some GISTs with *KIT* exon 17 mutations are also resistant to regorafenib, and the drug-related adverse reactions (including hand and foot skin reactions, hypertension, and diarrhea) are experienced relatively more frequently in Asian patients [11]. Based on the phase I study of ripretinib, the median PFS of and ORR second-line treatment with ripretinib in patients with advanced GIST after imatinib resistance are 10.7 months and 19.4%, respectively [8]. This shows potential applied value in terms of efficacy and safety of the drug. As can be seen from the whole process of treatment, this patient was successfully treated with ripretinib. The administration of ripretinib for systematic control and tumor shrinkage gave the patient an opportunity to obtain a non-evidence disease (NED) cytoreductive surgery. Although ripretinib was not superior to sunitinib in terms of PFS in the phase III trial (INTRIGUE, NCT03673501) [12], meaningful clinical activity, fewer grade 3/4 treatment-emergent adverse events, and improved tolerability were observed with ripretinib.

Before the second operation, the patient had a good response to ripretinib, and the ctDNA tests became negative. Imaging showed that the tumor focus was smaller than before treatment, and most of the adverse reactions related to the treatment of ripretinib were grade 1 and tolerable, suggesting that the treatment was effective and safe. As a minimally invasive detection technique, peripheral blood ctDNA detection has the advantages of being non-invasive, safe, flexible and convenient, overcomes tumor heterogeneity, and allows a series of evaluations over time [13]. It is widely used in the diagnosis of lung cancer and breast cancer, the exploration of drug resistance mechanisms, postoperative minimal residual disease (MRD) monitoring, prognosis, and so on. With regard to this patient, ctDNA tests were negative in the early stage of ripretinib treatment, which showed an effective treatment response earlier than imaging re-examination, and for a drug whose mechanism of drug resistance is not clear, early efficacy evaluation is crucial to doctors' decision-making. The therapeutic effect with dynamic monitoring of ctDNA in this patient was highly consistent with that of imaging and demonstrated the effective therapeutic response earlier than imaging could. Although there are fewer ctDNA exfoliated in GIST than in other tumors, continuous monitoring can reflect the dynamic changes of the tumor when ctDNA is positive [14]. It is a feasible and promising method to guide the treatment and predict the prognosis of patients with advanced GIST. It is expected to become a biomarker for non-invasive dynamic detection of GIST.

The target treatment effect of ripretinib was met before the operation. The genotyping of the resected specimens demonstrated that lesions which appeared after the patient developed resistance to first-line treatment (diaphragm, peritoneum, hepatorenal recess nodule) all carried a mutation in *KIT* exon 17, which indicated that secondary drug-resistant tissues might be widely distributed. If imatinib was resumed after operation, it was likely to lead to further tumor recurrence or metastasis in a short period of time, so continuation of ripretinib was recommended after comprehensive consideration. It should be pointed out that there was also a certain risk in the decision to continue postoperative ripretinib maintenance treatment as the mechanism of ripretinib resistance is not yet clear. If the patient develops ripretinib resistance in the future, the choice of the subsequent treatments is still uncertain.

25.4 Case 35 A 39-Year-Old Woman with Advanced GIST Who Underwent Cytoreductive Surgery After Fourth-Line Ripretinib Therapy

Bo Ni and Linxi Yang

25.4.1 Case Background

The patient, a 39-year-old woman, underwent partial small bowel resection of a pelvic mass at her local hospital in September 2016. Intraoperative exploration revealed that the tumor had ruptured. The postoperative pathology showed small intestinal GIST, with a maximal diameter of

12 cm, and no clear mitoses were found. Genetic testing revealed a heterozygous deletion mutation in *KIT* exon 11, and codons 559–565 were deleted. The patient did not receive adjuvant therapy after surgery and was followed up regularly. On February 12, 2018, a CT scan in our hospital revealed multiple pelvic masses, and the recurrence was considered (Fig. 25.11). The patient then started imatinib 400 mg standard treatment, and the whole abdomen enhanced CT was reviewed every 3 months. On September 20, 2019, the abdominal enhanced CT showed that the multiple nodules in the pelvis were smaller than before, and the enhancement degree was weakened (Fig. 25.12). After 23 months of imatinib treatment, the abdominal CT scan showed disease progression (Fig. 25.13), and the patient was switched to sunitinib 37.5 mg/d. After 80 days, the disease was assessed as PD on the abdominal CT scan (Fig. 25.14). After 83 days of 120 mg/d regorafenib treatment, an abdominal CT scan showed further progression of the disease (Fig. 25.15). The patient started daily treatment with ripretinib 150 mg in August 2020, with regular review. Thirteen months later, the abdominal CT scan again showed tumor progression.

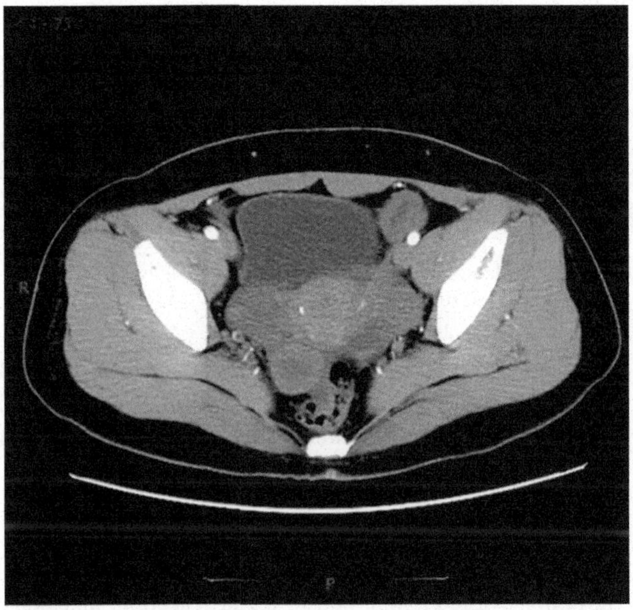

Fig. 25.11 The CT found tumor recurrence

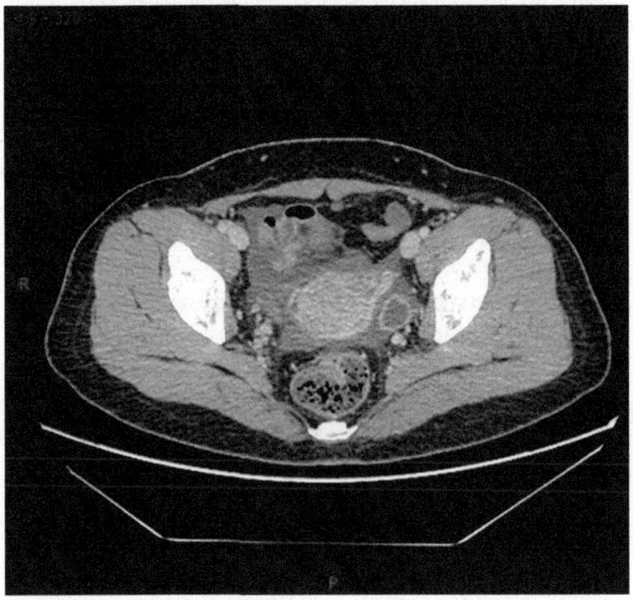

Fig. 25.12 CT after 20 months of imatinib treatment

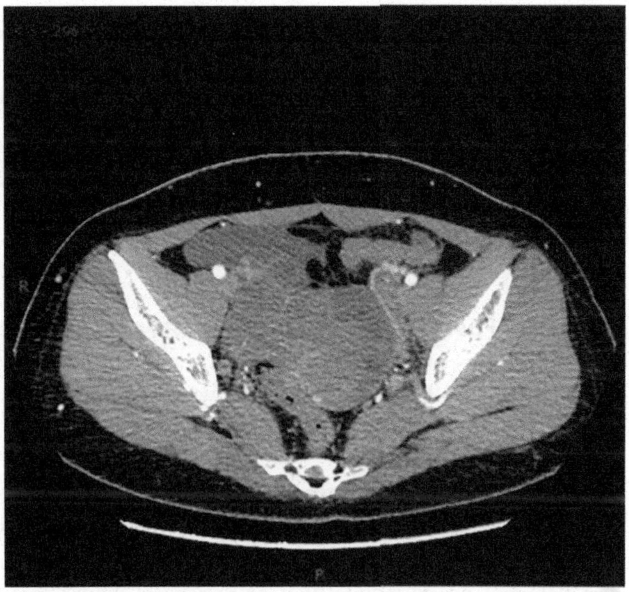

Fig. 25.13 CT after 23 months of imatinib treatment (tumor progression)

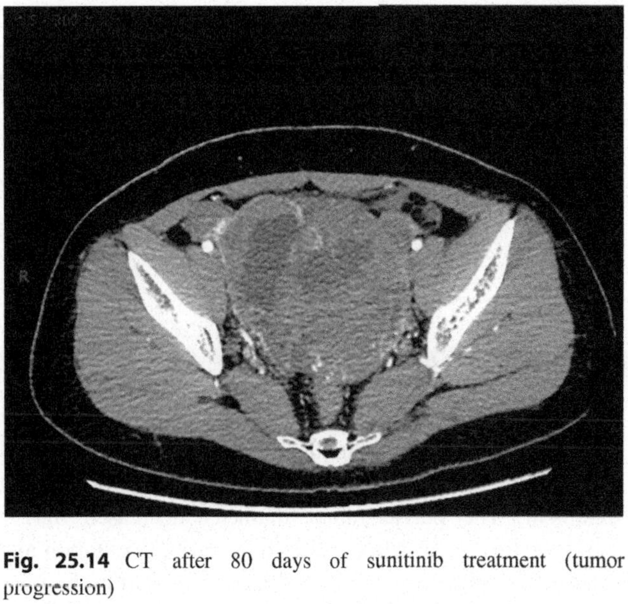

Fig. 25.14 CT after 80 days of sunitinib treatment (tumor progression)

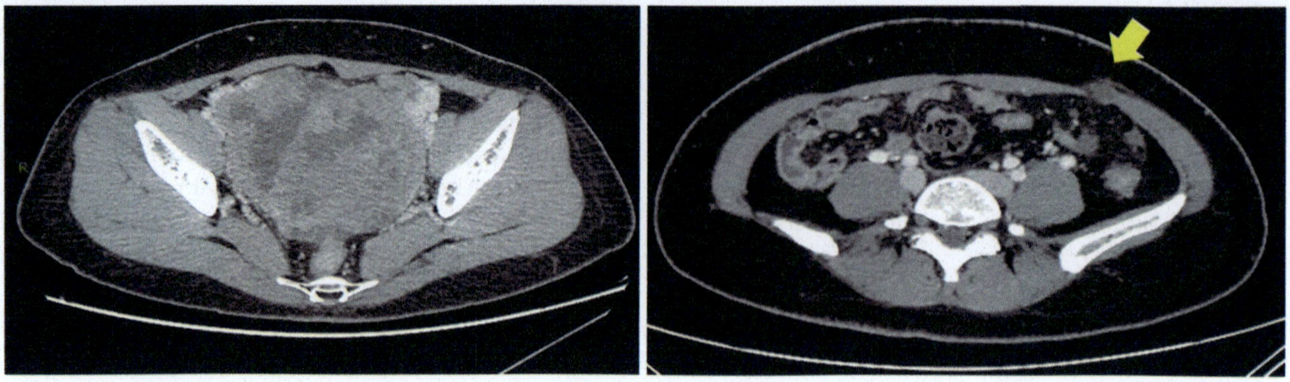

Fig. 25.15 CT after 83 days of regorafenib treatment (tumor progression)

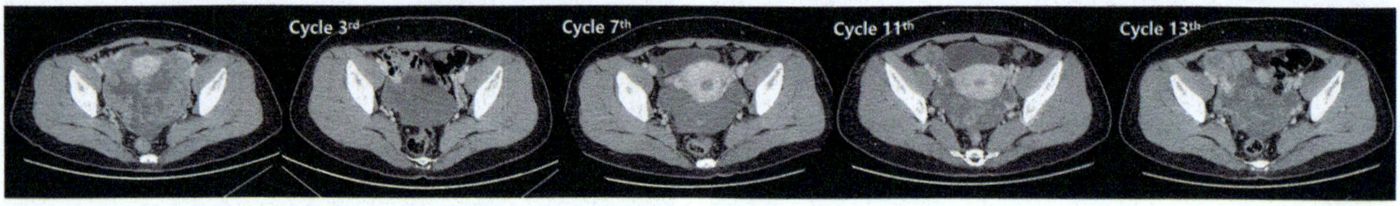

Fig. 25.16 Repeated CT after ripretinib treatment, tumor progression after the 13th cycle

25.4.1.1 Past History and Family History

The patient was previously healthy and reported no history of drug allergies. The patient's parents were alive, and there was no similar medical history in the family.

25.4.1.2 Physical Examination

The patient's vital signs were stable, and the skin and mucous membranes were neither yellowish nor pale. The abdomen was flat, and no gastrointestinal or peristaltic waves were seen. An old surgical scar was seen in the mid-abdomen. The abdomen was soft, with no rebound tenderness or palpable mass in the abdomen. The bowel sounds were normal.

25.4.1.3 Auxiliary Examination

Abdominal CT Multiple patchy nodular foci were observed in the left lower abdominal wall and pelvic cavity, considered to represent GIST tumor spread and implantation. The number of nodules in the pelvis had increased and some were enlarged compared to the previous images (June 17, 2021) (Fig. 25.16).

25.4.2 Therapy

25.4.2.1 Case Analysis

The patient is a young to middle-aged woman with advanced GIST of focal disease progression under fourth-line drug treatment. The pelvic tumor diameter decreased during ripretinib treatment. After multidisciplinary consultation and discussion, despite the tumor was closely related to the uterine appendages and the rectosigmoid colon, it was deemed that the pelvic progressive lesions were still resectable, and surgical treatment was recommended for tumor cytoreduction and resistance mutations.

25.4.2.2 Treatment

The patient underwent laparotomy with abdominal and pelvic tumor cytoreduction, partial rectal resection, and bilateral adnexectomy in our hospital on August 26, 2021. The tumors were mostly located in the pelvis: scattered in the uterine bladder depression, rectum uterine depression, pelvic floor peritoneum, and invading the rectosigmoid junction and bilateral appendages, with a maximum diameter of about 12 cm. The tumor near the right appendix was approximately 7 cm, and a mass of approximately 1 cm in diameter was found in the abdominal wall next to the original surgical incision on the left (Fig. 25.17). No obvious metastasis was found in the liver, and the ascites was about 100 mL.

25.4.2.3 Postoperative Pathology and Genetic Testing

Pathological Diagnosis The pelvic mass, uterus-vesical indentation nodule, abdominal wall nodule, pelvic floor nodule, left paraovarian nodule, sigmoid mesenteric nodule, and right para-adnexal mass were all GIST metastases (after targeted drug therapy). Among them, the uterus-vesical nodule, abdominal wall nodule, pelvic floor nodule, left paraovarian nodule, and sigmoid mesenteric nodule had sparse tumor cell density, interstitial fibrosis, and obvious changes after treatment. The tumor cells of the pelvic tumor and right adnexal

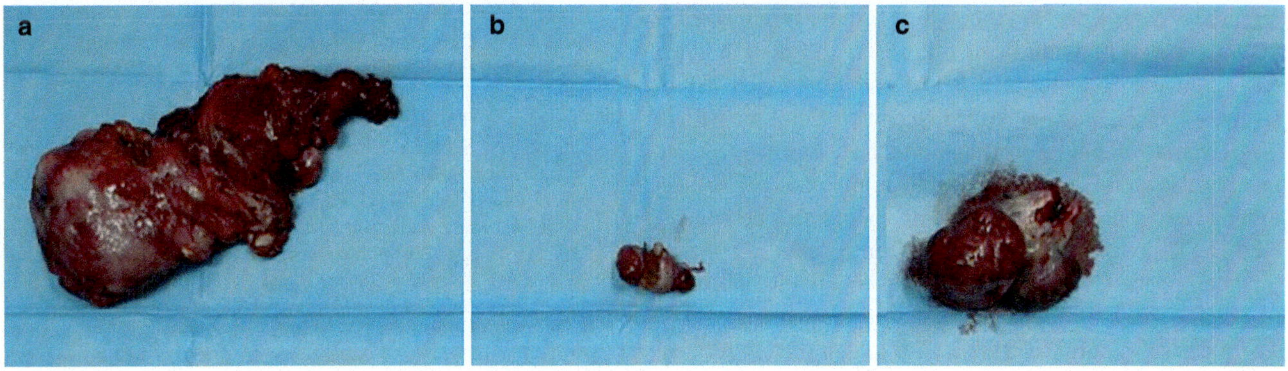

Fig. 25.17 The gross specimen. **a** Pelvic tumor; **b** Next to the left adnexa; **c** Next to the right adnexa

tumor had partially retreated, with interstitial fibrosis and focal necrosis. High tumor cell density areas were still visible (20% of all tissues in the pelvic mass and 80% of all tissues in the right para-adnexal tumor). In the active area of tumor cell proliferation, tumor cells were distributed in clusters around blood vessels, with a mitotic count >10/50 HPF, which was in line with partial response to treatment.

Immunohistochemistry Ki-67 (Li: 40%), VIM (+), CD117 (+), CD34 (+), DOG-1 (+), SMA (−), S-100 (−), SDHB (+), ALK-D5F3 (−), BRAF (−), Pan-TRK (−), C-MYC (−), P53 (+).

Genetic Testing Right adnexal tumor and pelvic tumor: Heterozygous mutation in exon 11 of *KIT*, 558–565 loss, heterozygous mutation in exon 13 of *KIT*, 654GTG > GCG, and a heterozygous mutation in exon 17 of *KIT*, 823TAT > GAT.

Uterus-vesical nodule, abdominal wall nodule, pelvic floor nodule, left paraovarian nodule, and sigmoid mesenteric nodule: Heterozygous mutation in exon 11 of *KIT*, 558–565 loss. Exons 9, 13 and 17 of *KIT*, as well as exons 12 and 18 of *PDGFRA*, were all wild type.

25.4.3 Prognosis

The patient completed a baseline CT postoperatively and was discharged 8 days after surgery. Due to economic factors, the patient chose to continue regorafenib maintenance therapy after surgery, and the CT scan showed no obvious progression of the remaining multiple small nodules in the pelvis 6 months after surgery.

25.4.4 Experience of Diagnosis and Therapy

25.4.4.1 A New Treatment Option for Patients with Advanced GIST-Ripretinib

The patient was initially diagnosed with small intestine GIST, and the intraoperative exploration revealed that the tumor had ruptured. For economic reasons, she did not receive adjuvant imatinib therapy at that time, resulting in multiple abdominal and pelvic metastases. After 23 months of standard first-line treatment with imatinib, her disease showed signs of progression neither sunitinib nor regorafenib provided significant treatment benefit, which may be related to secondary multidrug resistance mutations. Fortunately, the patient was treated with the newer TKI drug, ripretinib. Ripretinib, as a broad-spectrum *KIT/PDGFRA* inhibitor designed with a switch pocket, has efficient inhibitory effects on GIST of different gene mutation types. This treatment provided the patient with a PFS of 13 months, which was already much higher than the median PFS reported as a result of the INVICTUS study (6.3 months), and the reliable efficacy of subsequent line therapy had been proven. Ripretinib is a new treatment option for patients with advanced GIST, especially those with confirmed multidrug-resistant mutations after progression [7, 8].

25.4.4.2 Selection and Grasp of Timing for Surgical Intervention in Advanced GIST

In the course of targeted drug therapy, the patient actually had more than one opportunity for surgical intervention: when recurrence and metastasis were found, when imatinib resistance was identified after 23 months of treatment, and when ripretinib resistance was identified after 13 months of treatment. At all three time points, the tumor had not progressed extensively, and multi-organ resection was not required for surgery. However, when tumors became resistant to second and third-line drugs and the disseminated lesions in the abdomen and pelvis had progressed extensively, surgery should not be the first choice. Since the patient was a woman of childbearing age, and the tumor happened to involve the uterus and double adnexa, the changes in hormone levels caused by adnexectomy should also be considered in the preoperative evaluation. The success of surgical treatment depends on the ability to effectively intervene before the disease progresses widely in the patient's body. The purpose of surgical treatment is to completely remove drug-resistant lesions, and to remove as many lesions that respond to treatment as possible without increasing the risk, so as to prolong and slow down the re-progression time of tumor lesions as much as possible.

25.5 Expert Comments

Hui Cao

Gastrointestinal stromal tumors are the most common mesenchymal tumors of the alimentary tract, which are more common in the stomach (50–60%). The most common metastatic sites after radical resection are the liver and peritoneum, and 70–80% of activating mutations in *KIT* and *PDGFRA* are considered the main oncogenic drivers of GIST. Imatinib is the first-line standard treatment for GIST. Although imatinib is effective for many patients with GISTs, tumor resistance to imatinib is common. Ripretinib is a type II switch-controlled TKI, which aims to control broad-spectrum mutations in *KIT* and *PDGFRA*. It has favorable responses for patients with refractory advanced GIST and has become an innovative treatment for heterogeneity of drug resistance mechanisms.

Case 34 shows us the successful application of molecular detection prediction, individualized second-line treatment with ripretinib after first-line imatinib progression, dynamic monitoring of efficacy with ctDNA and, once again, cytoreductive surgery, which may provide reference for the selective application of ripretinib combined with surgery in later line treatment for metastatic GISTs.

References

1. Expert Committee of Gastrointestinal Stromal Tumor of Chinese Society of Clinical Oncology. Chinese consensus on diagnosis and treatment of gastrointestinal stromal tumor (2017 edition). Chin J Cancer Res. 2017;29(4):281–93. https://doi.org/10.21147/j.issn.1000-9604.2017.04.01.
2. Professional Committee for Gastrointestinal Stromal Tumor Diagnosis and Treatment of the Chinese Medical Doctor Association, Surgery Branch of the Chinese Medical Association. Chinese expert consensus on standardized surgical treatment of gastrointestinal stromal tumor (2018 edition). Chin J Pract Surg. 2018;38(9):965–73. https://doi.org/10.19538/j.cjps.issn1005-2208.2018.09.01.
3. von Mehren M, Randall RL, Benjamin RS, Boles S, Bui MM, Ganjoo KN, George S, Gonzalez RJ, Heslin MJ, Kane JM, Keedy V, Kim E, Koon H, Mayerson J, McCarter M, McGarry SV, Meyer C, Morris ZS, O'Donnell RJ, Pappo AS, Paz IB, Petersen IA, Pfeifer JD, Riedel RF, Ruo B, Schuetze S, Tap WD, Wayne JD, Bergman MA, Scavone JL. Soft tissue sarcoma, version 2.2018, NCCN clinical practice guidelines in oncology. J Natl Compr Cancer Netw. 2018;16(5):536–63. https://doi.org/10.6004/jnccn.2018.0025.
4. Jones RL, McCall J, Adam A, O'Donnell D, Ashley S, Muderis O, Thway K, Fisher C, Judson IR. Radiofrequency ablation is a feasible therapeutic option in the multimodality management of sarcoma. Eur J Surg Oncol. 2010;36(5):477–82. https://doi.org/10.1016/j.ejso.2009.12.005.
5. Raut CP, Posner M, Desai J, Morgan JA, George S, Zahrieh D, Fletcher CD, Demetri GD, Bertagnolli MM. Surgical management of advanced gastrointestinal stromal tumors after treatment with targeted systemic therapy using kinase inhibitors. J Clin Oncol. 2006;24(15):2325–31. https://doi.org/10.1200/jco.2005.05.3439.
6. Patterson T, Li H, Chai J, Debruyns A, Simmons C, Hart J. Locoregional treatments for metastatic gastrointestinal stromal tumor in British Columbia: a retrospective cohort study from January 2008 to December 2017. Cancers. 2022;14(6):1477–92. https://doi.org/10.3390/cancers14061477.
7. Dhillon S. Ripretinib: first approval. Drugs. 2020;80(11):1133–8. https://doi.org/10.1007/s40265-020-01348-2.
8. Janku F, Abdul Razak AR, Chi P, Heinrich MC, von Mehren M, Jones RL, Ganjoo K, Trent J, Gelderblom H, Somaiah N, Hu S, Rosen O, Su Y, Ruiz-Soto R, Gordon M, George S. Switch control inhibition of KIT and PDGFRA in patients with advanced gastrointestinal stromal tumor: a phase I study of ripretinib. J Clin Oncol. 2020;38(28):3294–303. https://doi.org/10.1200/JCO.20.00522.
9. Heinrich MC, Maki RG, Corless CL, Antonescu CR, Harlow A, Griffith D, Town A, McKinley A, Ou WB, Fletcher JA, Fletcher CD, Huang X, Cohen DP, Baum CM, Demetri GD. Primary and secondary kinase genotypes correlate with the biological and clinical activity of sunitinib in imatinib-resistant gastrointestinal stromal tumor. J Clin Oncol. 2008;26(33):5352–9. https://doi.org/10.1200/JCO.2007.15.7461.
10. Demetri GD, Reichardt P, Kang YK, Blay JY, Rutkowski P, Gelderblom H, Hohenberger P, Leahy M, von Mehren M, Joensuu H, Badalamenti G, Blackstein M, Le Cesne A, Schöffski P, Maki RG, Bauer S, Nguyen BB, Xu J, Nishida T, Chung J, Kappeler C, Kuss I, Laurent D, Casali PG, GRID study investigators. Efficacy and safety of regorafenib for advanced gastrointestinal stromal tumours after failure of imatinib and sunitinib (GRID): an international, multicentre, randomised, placebo-controlled, phase 3 trial. Lancet. 2013;381(9863):295–302. https://doi.org/10.1016/S0140-6736(12)61857-1.
11. Xie G, Gong Y, Wu S, Li C, Yu S, Wang Z, Chen J, Zhao Q, Li J, Liang H. Meta-analysis of regorafenib-associated adverse events and their management in colorectal and gastrointestinal stromal cancers. Adv Ther. 2019;36(8):1986–98. https://doi.org/10.1007/s12325-019-01013-5.
12. Bauer S, Jones RL, Blay JY, Gelderblom H, George S, Schöffski P, von Mehren M, Zalcberg JR, Kang YK, Razak AA, Trent J, Attia S, Le Cesne A, Su Y, Meade J, Wang T, Sherman ML, Ruiz-Soto R, Heinrich MC. Ripretinib versus sunitinib in patients with advanced gastrointestinal stromal tumor after treatment with imatinib (INTRIGUE): a randomized, open-label, phase III trial. J Clin Oncol. 2022;40(34):3918–28. https://doi.org/10.1200/JCO.22.00294.

13. Xu H, Chen L, Shao Y, Zhu D, Zhi X, Zhang Q, Li F, Xu J, Liu X, Xu Z. Clinical application of circulating tumor DNA in the genetic analysis of patients with advanced GIST. Mol Cancer Ther. 2018;17(1):290–6. https://doi.org/10.1158/1535-7163.MCT-17-0436.
14. Liu MC, Oxnard GR, Klein EA, Swanton C, Seiden MV, CCGA Consortium. Sensitive and specific multi-cancer detection and localization using methylation signatures in cell-free DNA. Ann Oncol. 2020;31(6):745–59. https://doi.org/10.1016/j.annonc.2020.02.011.

Management of Targeted Drug Adverse Reaction

26

Bo Ni, Jian Li, and Lin Shen

Keywords

Gastrointestinal stromal tumor · Targeted therapy
Adverse reaction

26.1 Case 36 A 63-Year-Old Woman with GIST Who Suffered from Interstitial Lung Disease During Imatinib-Targeted Therapy

Bo Ni and Jian Li

26.1.1 Introduction

Imatinib is an effective treatment for GIST. The majority of patients with GIST benefit from imatinib treatment, but adverse reaction is inevitable during the course of medication. A small number of patients cannot tolerate imatinib due to serious adverse reaction, so they require second-line therapies. Targeted drugs can cause interstitial lung disease, mainly by affecting the EGFR signal pathway, but the mechanism is not completely clear. Similar findings have been found in the pulmonary toxicity of other chemotherapeutic drugs, such as gemcitabine and paclitaxel.

26.1.2 Case Background

The patient, a 63-year-old woman, presented with right abdominal pain and diagnosed as a hysteromyoma at the local hospital in June 2006. Gynecological exploratory surgery found small intestinal tumor. There was no tumor rupture or peritoneal or liver metastasis. A complete tumor resection was performed. Postoperative pathology testing revealed a small intestinal GIST, 4 cm × 3 cm in size, with a mitotic count >5/50 HPF. Immunohistochemistry showed CD117 (+), DOG1 (+), desmin (−), SMA (−), S-100 (−). Genetic detection showed a point mutation in *KIT* exon 11. Imatinib 600 mg/d was taken orally after surgery, and mild chest tightness occurred after 45 days of treatment. Chest CT showed mild interstitial affecting both pulmonary lobes (Fig. 26.1).

Imatinib was reduced to 400 mg/d, but the symptoms of chest tightness were aggravated, and fever occurred. Re-evaluation of the chest CT scan revealed extensive ground-glass opacities affecting both pulmonary lobes (Fig. 26.2).

Upon discontinuation of imatinib and initiation of symptomatic management, there was a subsequent resolution of the interstitial lesions in both pulmonary lobes (Fig. 26.3).

Approximately 1 year after imatinib withdraw, a CT revealed multiple pelvic metastases. And she was admitted to the Department of Gastroenterology and Oncology, Peking University Cancer Hospital.

B. Ni
Department of Gastrointestinal Surgery, Renji Hospital, Shanghai Jiaotong University School of Medicine, Shanghai, China

J. Li (✉) · L. Shen
Department of Gastrointestinal Oncology, Peking University Cancer Hospital & Institute, Beijing, China
e-mail: lin100@medmail.com.cn

K. Tao, H. Cao (eds.), *Clinical Management of Gastrointestinal Stromal Tumor*, https://doi.org/10.1007/978-981-99-9392-5_26

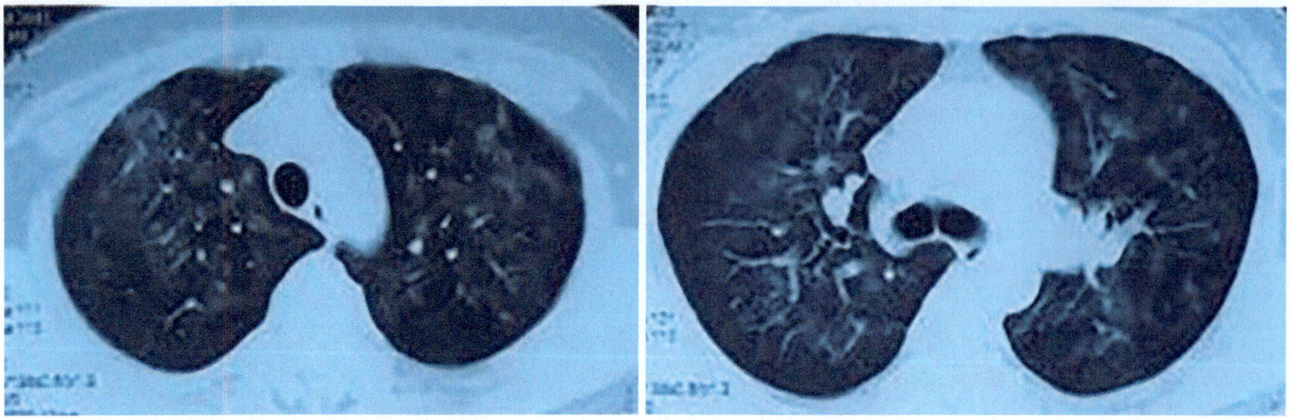

Fig. 26.1 Chest CT showed mild interstitial changes affecting both pulmonary lobes with pleural effusion

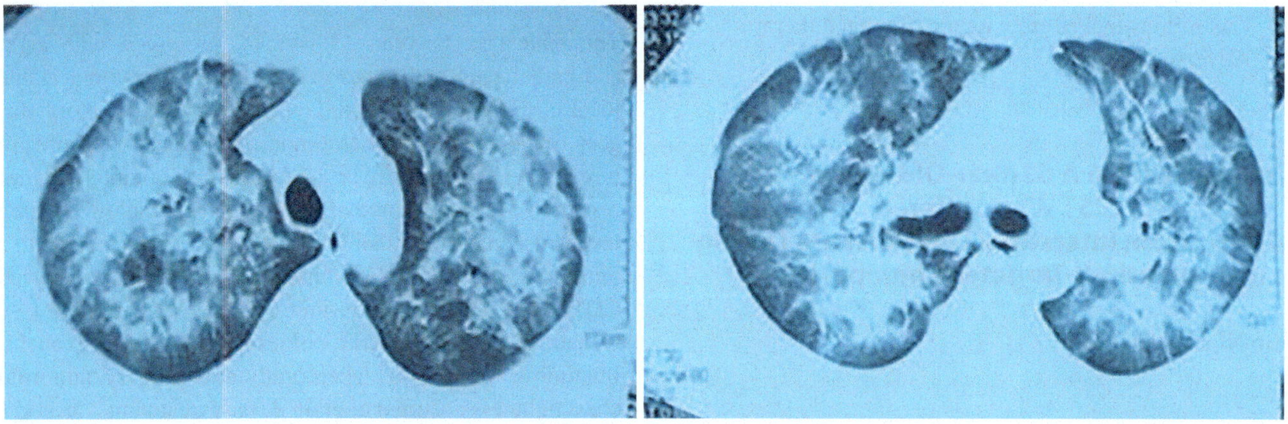

Fig. 26.2 Chest CT showed extensive ground-glass opacities affecting both pulmonary lobes

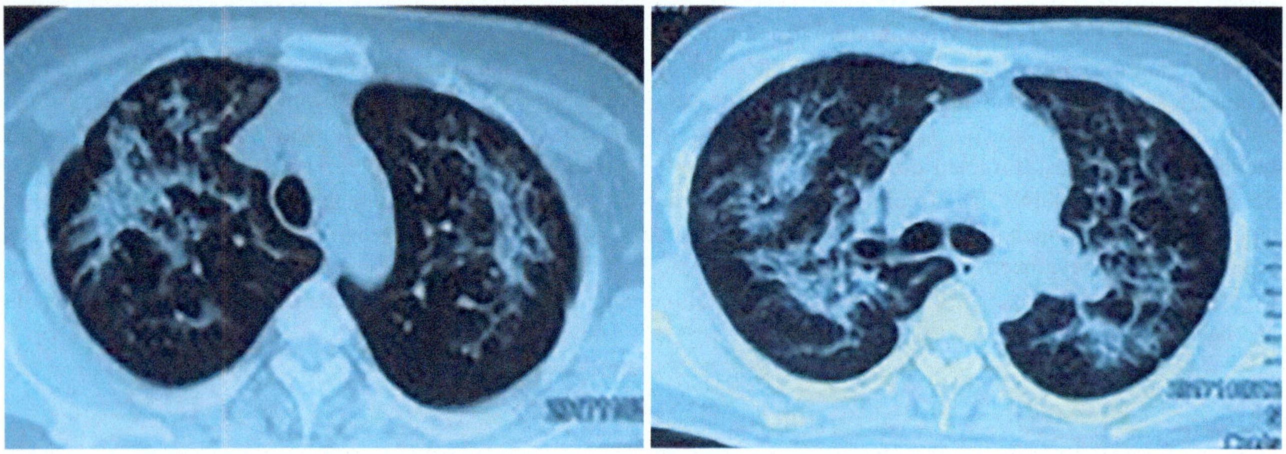

Fig. 26.3 Resolution of bilateral pulmonary interstitial lesions

26.1.2.1 Past History and Family History

The patient reported no previous history of hypertension, infectious diseases, such as hepatitis and tuberculosis, heart disease, diabetes, trauma, food and drug allergies, blood transfusions, and genetic history.

26.1.2.2 Physical Examination

The patient had mild anemia, no jaundice on the skin or mucous membrane of the whole body, and a flat abdomen. An abdominal surgical incision is visible. There were no varicose veins on the abdominal wall, no intestinal type, soft abdomen, rebound tenderness, and the liver and spleen were not palpable below the costal margin. Murphy's sign was negative, no mobile voiced sound, no palpable mass, normal bowel sounds, and no sounds of air or water.

26.1.2.3 Auxiliary Examination

Blood Routine WBC 6.45 × 10^9 /L, RBC 3.6 × 10^{12}/L ↓, Hb 106 g/L ↓, PLT 148 × 10^9/L, NEUT% 66.5%, LY% 31.5%.

26.1.2.4 Preliminary Diagnosis

1. Postoperative GIST
2. Multiple pelvic metastases
3. Interstitial lung disease
4. Hysteromyoma

26.1.3 Therapy

26.1.3.1 Case Analysis

According to the medical history, the previous pulmonary interstitial fibrosis was caused by imatinib therapy. The pelvic multiple metastases of GIST were not candidates for surgical treatment. Imatinib treatment was expected to be effective, but it was also likely to lead to repeat interstitial lung disease (ILD). Considering his families' willings, it was recommended that sunitinib 37.5 mg/d be administered as second-line treatment. While the patient decided the rechallenge of imatinib treatment, a reduced dose of 300 mg/d was administrated, and close observation of adverse reaction was performed.

26.1.3.2 Treatment

After more than 2-week treatment of 300 mg/d imatinib, the patient felt mild respiratory distress. A CT scan showed a small amount of ground-glass opacity affecting the left pulmonary lobe. Considering the recurrence of drug-related ILD, the targeted therapy with imatinib was replaced with 37.5 mg/d sunitinib.

26.1.4 Prognosis

Upon re-examination, the metastatic burden was slightly smaller than before and there was no obvious pulmonary interstitial change on chest CT, but the adverse reaction of hand-foot erythrodysesthesia was obvious, resulting in the reduction of sunitinib to 25 and 37.5 mg/d alternately. The patient has been taking medicine intermittently until now. The CT scan obtained at the most recent follow-up revealed stable pelvic metastases, with no evidence of interstitial pulmonary changes.

26.1.5 Experience of Diagnosis and Therapy

The adverse reaction of imatinib are important factors which determine medication compliance. Many patients reduce their imatinib compliance due to improper treatment of drug adverse reaction, which affects the treatment effect [1]. Interstitial lung disease is a relatively rare adverse reaction during the TKI treatment of patients with GIST. However, once diagnosed as interstitial lung disease caused by TKI, the patients need close attention and appropriate treatment. Limited literature suggests that interstitial lung disease may affect individuals of Asian descent more than other races and males more than females [2]. It is proved that the existence of interstitial lung disease before treatment is the risk factor of this disease resulted from TKI therapy [3]. The mechanisms of interstitial lung disease caused by TKI remain debatable. The main hypotheses are hypersensitivity reaction, the pharmacological action of TKI, the inhibition of PDGFRA inducing pulmonary fibrosis, and inflammatory cell infiltration [4, 5]. The symptoms are usually fever of unknown origin, cough, dyspnea, and hypereosinophilia. Chest X-ray, CT, and high-resolution CT may help diagnose interstitial lung disease. Typical CT characteristics include ground-glass attenuation, irregular liner or reticular areas of attenuation with bronchiectasis and bronchiectasis. Among the thousands of GISTs treated in our center, only four cases of pulmonary interstitial fibrosis secondary to imatinib therapy have been encountered, which is consistent with the overall incidence reported in the literature [6]. The patient experienced severe pulmonary interstitial fibrosis, and the timing of occurrence was consistent with a previous literature report. Regardless of the improper selection of the initial treatment dose, the time and course of pulmonary interstitial fibrosis showed a significant correlation with imatinib treatment. At the same time, mild interstitial changes in both lungs were seen in the first CT. From the perspective of treatment, the possibility of adverse reactions related to imatinib treatment should be considered at that time, and imatinib treatment should be terminated immediately, which may avoid the aggravation of subsequent lung injury. In this case, the patient's condition was relieved after drug withdrawal, so it could be determined that imatinib treatment caused the interstitial pneumonia. For such patients with serious side effects, they should resolutely choose to stop the drug before further treatment. For example, the continued application of imatinib can lead to repeated attacks of interstitial pneumonia, severe pulmonary fibrosis, and respiratory failure. Since the blood concentration of imatinib had not been measured prior to ceasing therapy, only sunitinib (second-line drug) could be selected.

The measurement of blood drug concentration is an important index to evaluate the bioavailability of drugs. At the same time, we have also found that a higher blood drug concentration is associated with more serious side effects. Given our understanding of imatinib's bioavailability, for patients experiencing severe adverse reaction, we can adjust the dosage based on blood concentration levels. This allows us to reduce the severity of adverse reaction, enabling patients to use the medication more safely and rationally.

26.2 Expert Comments

Lin Shen

The reported incidence of interstitial lung disease, also known as interstitial pneumonia, caused by imatinib is about 0.5% [6]. In addition, interstitial lung disease has also been reported in the course of treatment with many small molecule TKIs, such as gefitinib and afatinib [7]. Interstitial lung disease caused by imatinib is mostly reversed after termination of imatinib treatment, without serious complications [8]. Therefore, there is no need to be too concerned about similar adverse reactions. The key to treatment lies in early evaluation and accurate diagnosis. Once it is diagnosed as lung injury caused by a TKI, the offending medication should be ceased immediately [9].

At present, the clinical problem is whether imatinib can continue to be used for follow-up treatment once it is determined that imatinib causes interstitial lung disease and the patient's lung injury recovers.

Among the four patients with interstitial lung disease encountered in our center, one patient with mild pulmonary interstitial fibrosis was treated with imatinib again without lung injury, and the other three patients, who experienced relatively severe pulmonary interstitial fibrosis, had their therapy replaced with second-line drugs. Therefore, the follow-up treatment after the incidence of interstitial lung disease should be comprehensively considered in combination with various factors, such as the patient's condition, GIST status, status of basic lung diseases, severity of pulmonary interstitial fibrosis, patient's willingness to continue treatment, and replacement second-line drug treatment. The changes of chest CT should also be closely monitored during follow-up treatment.

References

1. Blay JY, Rutkowski P. Adherence to imatinib therapy in patients with gastrointestinal stromal tumors. Cancer Treat Rev. 2014;40(2):242–7. https://doi.org/10.1016/j.ctrv.2013.07.005.
2. Loong HH, Yeo W. Imatinib-induced interstitial lung disease and sunitinib-associated intra-tumour haemorrhage. Hong Kong Med J. 2008;14(6):495–8.
3. Bergeron A, Bergot E, Vilela G, Ades L, Devergie A, Espérou H, Socié G, Calvo F, Gluckman E, Ribaud P, Rousselot P, Tazi A. Hypersensitivity pneumonitis related to imatinib mesylate. J Clin Oncol. 2002;20(20):4271–2. https://doi.org/10.1200/JCO.2002.99.179.
4. Yamasawa H, Sugiyama Y, Bando M, Ohno S. Drug-induced pneumonitis associated with imatinib mesylate in a patient with idiopathic pulmonary fibrosis. Respiration. 2008;75(3):350–4. https://doi.org/10.1159/000091272.
5. Min JH, Lee HY, Lim H, Ahn MJ, Park K, Chung MP, Lee KS. Drug-induced interstitial lung disease in tyrosine kinase inhibitor therapy for non-small cell lung cancer: a review on current insight. Cancer Chemother Pharmacol. 2011;68(5):1099–109. https://doi.org/10.1007/s00280-011-1737-2.
6. Ohnishi K, Sakai F, Kudoh S, Ohno R. Twenty-seven cases of drug-induced interstitial lung disease associated with imatinib mesylate. Leukemia. 2006;20(6):1162–4. https://doi.org/10.1038/sj.leu.2404207.
7. Ohmori T, Yamaoka T, Ando K, Kusumoto S, Kishino Y, Manabe R, Sagara H. Molecular and clinical features of EGFR-TKI-associated lung injury. Int J Mol Sci. 2021;22(2):792. https://doi.org/10.3390/ijms22020792.
8. Go SW, Kim BK, Lee SH, Kim TJ, Huh JY, Lee JM, Hah JH, Kim DW, Cho MJ, Kim TW, Kang JY. Successful rechallenge with imatinib in a patient with chronic myeloid leukemia who previously experienced imatinib mesylate induced pneumonitis. Successful rechallenge with imatinib in a patient with chronic myeloid leukemia who previously experienced imatinib mesylate induced pneumonitis. Tuberc Respir Dis (Seoul). 2013;75(6):256–9. https://doi.org/10.4046/trd.2013.75.6.256.
9. Li J, Wang M, Zhang B, Wu X, Lin TL, Liu XF, Zhou Y, Zhang XH, Xu H, Shen LJ, Zou J, Lu P, Zhang D, Gu WJ, Zhang MX, Pan J, Cao H, Chinese Society of Surgeons for Gastrointestinal Stromal Tumor of the Chinese Medical Doctor Association. Chinese consensus on management of tyrosine kinase inhibitor-associated side effects in gastrointestinal stromal tumors. World J Gastroenterol. 2018;24(46):5189–202. https://doi.org/10.3748/wjg.v24.i46.5189.

Part VI

Management of Patients with Special Gastrointestinal Stromal Tumors

Senile Gastrointestinal Stromal Tumors with Coronary Heart Disease

27

Chun Zhuang, Tianlong Ling, and Guoqing Liao

Keywords

Gastrointestinal stromal tumor · Advanced age · Coronary artery bypass grafting · Surgery

27.1 Case 37 An 83-Year-Old Man with Gastric GIST with Simultaneous Gastrointestinal Bleeding and Coronary Three-Vessel Disease

Chun Zhuang and Tianlong Ling

27.1.1 Introduction

With the increase in the elderly population year by year, population aging has become an increasingly serious social problem in China. Often, GISTs are diagnosed in middle-aged and elderly people. The clinical characteristics and treatment for elderly patients with GIST have certain particularity, which needs close attention from clinicians. Due to the common delay of treatment in elderly patients with GIST, the symptoms are often obvious, and the tumor stage is late. In addition, elderly patients are often complicated by various chronic diseases or organ dysfunction, which makes treatment more difficult. For some elderly patients with GIST and significant visceral insufficiency, it is necessary to carry out diagnosis and treatment through multidisciplinary cooperation (i.e., with a MDT).

C. Zhuang · T. Ling (✉)
Department of Gastrointestinal Surgery, Renji Hospital, Shanghai Jiaotong University School of Medicine, Shanghai, China

G. Liao
Department of Gastrointestinal Surgery, Xiangya Hospital, Central South University, Changsha, China
e-mail: liaoguoqing@medmail.com.cn

27.1.2 Case Background

The patient, an 83-year-old man, was admitted to the local hospital on May 11, 2016, for investigation of repeated black stool for 2 months with dizziness and fatigue. Gastroscopy revealed possible GIST and the patient was admitted to the hospital for surgery. Preoperative coronary CT angiography showed coronary atherosclerosis, limited occlusion of the proximal part of the left anterior descending artery, severe stenosis of the local lumen of the proximal part of the right coronary artery, and multiple mild stenosis of the remaining lumen. The attending physician considered that there was high risk for surgery and did not recommend surgical treatment at that time. On July 27, 2016, the patient visited Renji Hospital Affiliated to Shanghai Jiaotong University School of Medicine and underwent coronary angiography, which indicated coronary heart disease and serious lesions of three coronary arteries. Because the patient had serious lesions in three coronary arteries and gastric GIST with chronic bleeding, after MDT discussion, the patient decided to have surgery for both conditions at the same time and was admitted to the hospital.

27.1.2.1 Past History and Family History

The patient had a >20-year history of hypertension which was controlled with drugs. The patient reported no history of drug allergies, their parents were deceased, and there was no similar medical history in the family.

27.1.2.2 Physical Examination

The patient's vital signs were stable, the patient exhibited apparent anemia, and the skin and mucous membrane were free of yellow staining. The abdomen was flat and soft, with no tenderness, rebound tenderness, palpable abdominal mass, or guarding. The bowel sounds were normal.

27.1.2.3 Auxiliary Examination

Gastroscopy A 4.0 cm × 4.0 cm lesion from the lesser curvature of the stomach protruded intraluminally. The top of

K. Tao, H. Cao (eds.), *Clinical Management of Gastrointestinal Stromal Tumor*, https://doi.org/10.1007/978-981-99-9392-5_27

the lesion was ulcerated, and covered with dirty moss, the mucosa was fragile, and bled easily. Gastroendoscopic diagnosis: Gastric tumor, possible GIST.

Enhanced CT of Upper and Lower Abdomen Soft tissue mass, possible GIST, on the lesser curvature of stomach, 3.5 cm × 3.2 cm in size, accompanied by enlargement of surrounding lymph nodes, gallstones, and cholecystitis (Fig. 27.1).

Cardiac Doppler Color Ultrasound The result revealed left atrial enlargement, thickening of the basal segment of the ventricular septum, calcification of the mitral and aortic valves, normal left ventricular systolic function, decreased left ventricular diastolic function, and left ventricular ejection fraction (LVEF): 63%.

Coronary Angiography The result revealed coronary heart disease, serious lesions of three coronary arteries, posterior occlusion of the first diagonal branch in the middle of the anterior descending branch, posterior occlusion of the first blunt marginal branch in the middle of the circumflex branch, and 95% stenosis at the opening of the right coronary artery (Fig. 27.2).

27.1.2.4 Preliminary Diagnosis

1. Soft tissue tumor on the lesser curvature of the stomach: likely GIST
2. Coronary atherosclerotic multi-vessel disease
3. Hypertension, grade 3, very high risk
4. Gallstones

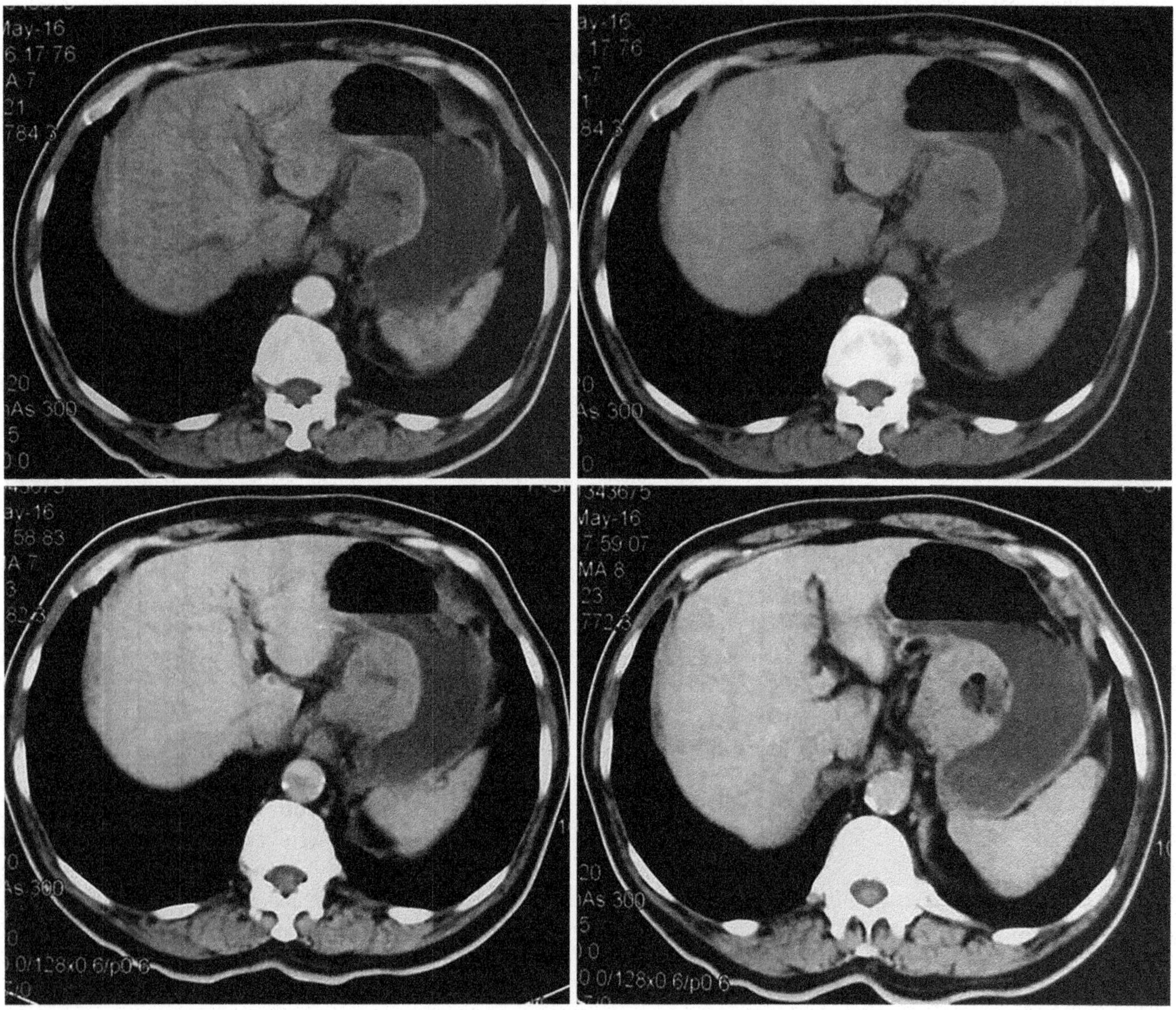

Fig. 27.1 Abdominal CT revealed a soft tissue mass on the lesser curvature of the stomach

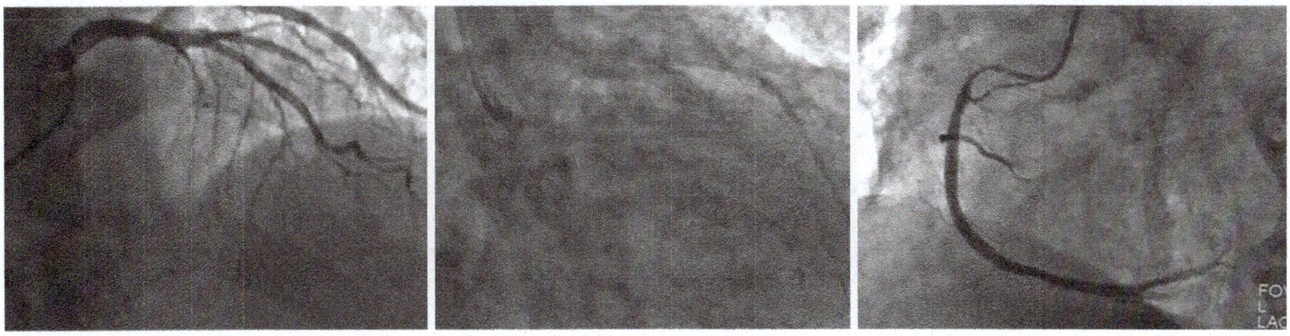

Fig. 27.2 Coronary angiography showed severe lesions in the three coronary arteries

27.1.3 Therapy

27.1.3.1 Case Analysis

The patient was an elderly man who was treated for gastrointestinal bleeding. Gastroscopy and imaging showed GIST on the lesser curvature of the stomach, and the surgical indication was clear. However, the general health of the patient was poor, the three branches of the coronary artery were seriously diseased, and the operation risk was very high. The MDT discussions suggested that postoperative anticoagulant therapy following coronary stent implantation could worsen gastrointestinal bleeding. Simultaneous coronary artery bypass grafting and gastric GIST resection was, therefore, considered. Due to the high risk of general anesthesia and operation, close monitoring would be required during the perioperative period.

27.1.3.2 Treatment

On August 15, 2016, non-stop coronary artery bypass grafting was performed under general anesthesia. The appearance of coronary lesions was consistent with the preoperative angiography. Aortic calcification was severe. The operation was performed routinely, and the left internal mammary artery (LIMA) was abandoned due to poor blood flow. With the help of easy buckle, shunt bolt and non-stop jumping bypass fixator, coronary artery by-pass surgery was performed. Subsequently, partial gastrectomy was performed for GIST removal. Intraoperatively, the tumor was found on the small curvature of the stomach below the gastric cardia, with a diameter of 4.5 cm and ulceration with bleeding on the surface. The gastric body was separated along the greater curvature of the gastric fundus, the left side of the cardia was freed, and the hepatogastric ligament was separated from the mass. The serosa of the gastric wall was incised on the lesser curvature, and the mass, with envelope, was completely removed. The gastric mucosa was continuously sutured with 2-0 absorbable suture, and the seromuscular layer was sutured intermittently. The operation was successful, and the patient was treated with antibiotics, cardiotonic agents, coronary dilation, and antiplatelet therapy (Fig. 27.3).

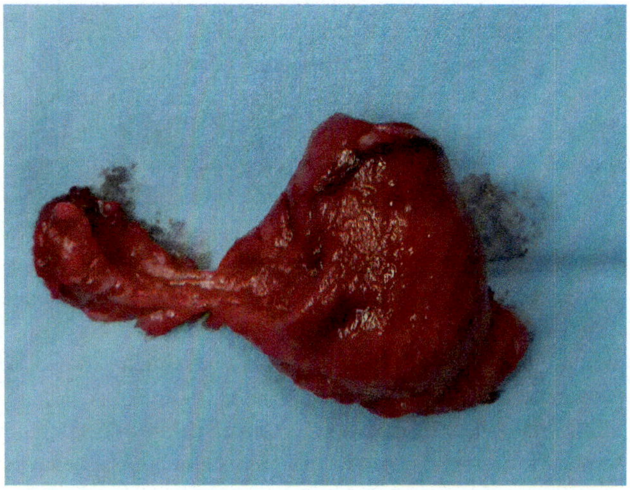

Fig. 27.3 The gross specimen of tumor specimens

27.1.3.3 Postoperative Pathology and Genetic Testing

Pathological Diagnosis Gastric GIST, 4.0 cm × 3.0 cm × 2.5 cm in size, mitotic count <2/50 HPF, classified as low risk according to the modified NIH criteria.

Immunohistochemistry CD117 (+), CD34 (+), DOG-1 (+), SMA (−), S-100 (−), Ki-67 (+), ALK (−), β-catenin (+).

Genetic Testing Mutations in exon 11 of *KIT*: a heterozygous mutation in codon 555, GTA>CCA, resulting in change of valine to proline; a heterozygous mutation in codon 556, CAG>CAT, change of glutamine to histidine; and a loss of codons 557–559, resulting in loss of coding amino acids tryptophan, lysine, and valine. Exons 9, 13 and 17 of *KIT* and exons 12 and 18 of *PDGFRA* were wild type.

27.1.4 Prognosis

The patient was given a semiliquid diet for 5 days after surgery and was discharged from the hospital 12 days after the operation. He did not receive postoperative imatinib adjuvant therapy. Until December 2018, outpatient and telephone follow-up showed that the patient had good quality of life and did not complain of obvious discomfort.

27.1.5 Experience of Diagnosis and Therapy

The elderly patient in this case had been admitted to the local hospital and surgery for GIST was planned. The ejection fraction of preoperative color Doppler ultrasound was greater than 60%, which did not show clear surgical contraindications. However, during a preoperative evaluation, the anesthesiologist noted that the patient experienced chest pain when fatigued. Therefore, the attending physician suspended the operation and requested coronary computed tomography angiography, which revealed serious coronary lesions and led to the cancellation of the procedure. This highlights that if the preoperative evaluation is not detailed and comprehensive, the consequences may be severe and life-threatening.

There are an increasing number of cases of gastrointestinal malignancies with major comorbidities [1]. Malignant digestive tract tumors and coronary artery disease both require timely treatment. When the above two diseases coexist, which condition requires the highest priority treatment should be determined according to the actual situation. Coronary multi-branch lesions may lead to sudden cardiac death at any time, which should be treated first [2]. The biological behavior of GIST is relatively inert. If this patient had no ulcer bleeding related to the tumor, coronary stent implantation could have been performed first, and gastric tumor resection could be performed within a time limit after the heart condition was stable. However, this patient had gastrointestinal bleeding and the requirement for anticoagulant therapy after coronary stent implantation would aggravate gastrointestinal bleeding [3]. There were contradictions for treatment, which also presented difficulty in the treatment of this case. Finally, the results of investigations showed that simultaneous coronary artery bypass grafting and gastric tumor resection were reasonable treatment options for this case.

Focusing on the diagnosis and treatment plan of middle-aged and elderly patients in this case, the hospital organized MDT discussions before and after investigations. After the first discussion, it was decided to assess the severity of coronary artery disease by coronary angiography first, and at the second discussion, a consensus was reached to operate on both conditions at the same time according to the results of coronary angiography and formulate a specific implementation plan. Representatives from the gastrointestinal surgery, cardiology, cardiac surgery, anesthesiology, critical medicine, oncology, gastroenterology, clinical nutrition, and other relevant departments participated in the MDT collaborative diagnosis and treatment of this case. Through the whole treatment process, various disciplines worked seamlessly to carry out careful perioperative preparations for the treatment, ensuring the success of the treatment. Patients have the opportunity to get the best treatment choice from the MDT discussion, and a treatment plan jointly formulated by many experts also effectively reduces the medical risk.

In this case, the GIST was located on the lesser curvature below the cardia, with a diameter of about 4 cm. The final surgical scheme was to perform coronary artery bypass grafting first, followed by abdominal surgery. Abdominal surgery was performed using open gastrectomy with an incision of the gastric wall and complete resection along the outside of the tumor capsule. The following points should be considered in the selection of operation methods: (1) The risk of coronary artery bypass grafting is greater than that of abdominal surgery, and as it is aseptic surgery, needs to be performed first. Additionally, coronary artery bypass grafting should be carried out first to minimize the risk of cardiovascular accident during the operation; (2) Given the patient's advanced age and cardiopulmonary dysfunction, laparoscopic surgery was not recommended after coronary bypass. (3) Surgeons should choose the most direct and effective way of performing laparotomy to avoid prolonged operation time and the impact of excessive surgical trauma on patients.

27.2 Expert Comments

Guoqing Liao

The clinical manifestations of GIST are nonspecific. Elderly patients visit relatively late, and their condition is often complicated by diseases of the respiratory and circulatory systems, and the operative risk is relatively high [4]. Additionally, elderly patients often have poor nutritional status, which can slow postoperative recovery. At the same time, basic diseases also seriously affect the recovery of patients. Elderly patients often face challenges with quality of life and may struggle with treatment compliance, making regular follow-up challenging. Therefore, for elderly GIST patients, we should strive to improve the early diagnosis rate, make a clear diagnosis before operation, fully evaluate the operation risk, and actively carry out MDT consultation to reduce the surgical risk [5]. Reasonable and standardized comprehensive treatment should be given after operation to improve the prognosis of elderly patients with GIST.

References

1. Ogle KS, Swanson GM, Woods N, Azzouz F. Cancer and comorbidity: redefining chronic diseases. Cancer. 2000;88:653–63. https://doi.org/10.1002/(sici)1097-0142(20000201)88:3<653::aid-cncr24>3.0.co;2-1.
2. Wang Y, Liu J, Wang W, Wang M, Qi Y, Xie W, Li Y, Sun J, Liu J, Zhao D. Lifetime risk for cardiovascular disease in a Chinese population: the Chinese Multi-Provincial Cohort Study. Eur J Prev Cardiol. 2015;22(3):380–8. https://doi.org/10.1177/2047487313516563.
3. Lanas-Gimeno A, Lanas A. Risk of gastrointestinal bleeding during anticoagulant treatment. Expert Opin Drug Saf. 2017;16(6):673–85. https://doi.org/10.1080/14740338.2017.1325870.
4. Tham CK, Poon DY, Li HH, Tan MH, Choo SP, Foo KF. Gastrointestinal stromal tumour in the elderly. Crit Rev Oncol Hematol. 2009;70(3):256–61. https://doi.org/10.1016/j.critrevonc.2008.09.007.
5. Extermann M, Hurria A. Comprehensive geriatric assessment for older patients with cancer. J Clin Oncol. 2007;25(14):1824–31. https://doi.org/10.1200/JCO.2007.10.6559.

Gastric Gastrointestinal Stromal Tumors with Gastroparesis After Surgery

28

Lin Tu, Peng Zhang, and Junbo Hu

Keywords

Gastrointestinal stromal tumor · Surgery · Complication · Gastroparesis

28.1 Case 38 A 69-Year-Old Woman with GIST and Postoperative Gastroparesis

Lin Tu and Peng Zhang

28.1.1 Introduction

Gastroparesis refers to a gastric motility disorder syndrome, clinically mainly manifested as gastric emptying disorder, which is caused by non-mechanical obstructive factors secondary to abdominal surgery. Gastroparesis is one of the common complications of abdominal surgery, especially gastroduodenal surgery. Once gastroparesis occurs, it often lasts for several weeks or even longer, and there is not an effective therapy at present. Since the surgical treatment principle of gastric GIST does not require excessive gastrectomy and lymph node dissection, partial gastrectomy or wedge resection is generally adopted, and radical resection can be achieved by obtaining a negative margin. There is a possibility of gastroparesis occurring after surgery for gastric GIST, but the mechanism warrants further investigation.

L. Tu
Department of Gastrointestinal Surgery, Renji Hospital, Shanghai Jiaotong University School of Medicine, Shanghai, China

P. Zhang (✉)
Department of Gastrointestinal Surgery, Union Hospital, Tongji Medical College, Huazhong University of Science and Technology, Wuhan, China
e-mail: zhangpengwh@hust.edu.cn

J. Hu
Department of Gastrointestinal Surgery, Tongji Hospital, Tongji Medical College, Huazhong University of Science and Technology University, Wuhan, China
e-mail: jbhu@tjh.tjmu.edu.cn

28.1.2 Case Background

The patient, a 69-year-old woman, felt pain and discomfort in the upper abdomen with no obvious causes on April 20, 2014. The pain was accompanied by acid reflux and belching, but no nausea, vomiting, hematemesis, melena, or other symptoms, and the pain was relieved after meals. A CT scan was performed by the local hospital and showed a space-occupying lesion in the pylorus of stomach. The patient visited to the Outpatient Department of Gastrointestinal Surgery, Union Hospital, Tongji Medical School, Huazhong University of Science and Technology for further treatment, and was admitted to the hospital for treatment of a pyloric space-occupying lesion.

28.1.2.1 Past History and Family History

The patient was previously healthy, with a >2-year history of hypertension, the highest reported blood pressure was 160/90 mmHg, and blood pressure was well controlled by oral medications at present. Hysterectomy, which required an intraoperative blood transfusion, was performed in 1991. The patient reported no history of hepatitis, tuberculosis or other infectious diseases, and no drug or food allergies. There was no similar medical history in the family.

28.1.2.2 Physical Examination

The abdomen was flat, and no gastrointestinal or peristaltic waves were seen. No obvious abnormalities were observed by abdominal palpation. There was no tenderness or rebound tenderness, no masses were palpable, and the liver and spleen were not palpable below the costal margin. There was no shifting dullness detected by abdominal percussion. The bowel sounds were normal.

K. Tao, H. Cao (eds.), *Clinical Management of Gastrointestinal Stromal Tumor*, https://doi.org/10.1007/978-981-99-9392-5_28

28.1.2.3 Auxiliary Examination

Blood Routine WBC 4.11 × 10^9/L, RBC 4.13 × 10^{12}/L, Hb 126 g/L, PLT 111 × 10^9/L, NEUT% 57.34%, LY% 28.4%.

Blood Biochemistry TBil 45.3 mol/L, DBil 29.3 mol/L, ALT 32 U/L, AST 133 U/L, TP 70.0 g/L↓, ALB 40.0 g/L, Cre 54.8 mol/L, BUN 3.5 mmol/L, Na^+ 140.0 mmol/L, K^+ 3.40 mmol/L, Cl^- 108.0 mmol/L.

Tumor Markers Normal.

Electronic Gastroscopy A huge gourd-shaped bulge protruded into the stomach at the lesser curvature of the gastric antrum with a smooth surface. Ultrasound indicated that the bulge originated from the muscularis propria, was approximately 4.8 cm × 2.5 cm in size, and no obvious enlarged lymph nodes were seen outside the stomach (Fig. 28.1).

Stomach, Lower Abdomen, and Pelvic Cavity CT Scan with Enhancement (1) Gastric pylorus space-occupying lesion, partly protruding into the duodenal bulb, slightly dumbbell-shaped, with clear borders, approximately 5.1 cm × 3.6 cm in size. Consistent with mesenchymal tumor (GIST possible); (2). No abnormalities in the liver, pancreas, or kidneys (Fig. 28.2).

28.1.2.4 Preliminary Diagnosis

1. Gastric space-occupying lesion (possible GIST)
2. Hypertension, Grade 2, High Risk

28.1.3 Therapy

28.1.3.1 Case Analysis

The patient was an elderly woman, who visited the doctor because of pain and discomfort in the upper abdomen. Electronic gastroscopy and abdominal CT scan indicated a neoplastic lesion in the stomach, with a strong possibility of GIST. The preoperative examination showed poor liver function and low levels of total protein. The liver function improved after liver protecting treatment. The primary tumor was located in the pylorus of the stomach, approximately 5 cm × 3 cm in size, it was estimated to be resectable and should be treated with surgery. Postoperative pathological examination should be performed to determine the nature of the tumor and guide postoperative treatment.

28.1.3.2 Treatment

Surgery was performed on May 23, 2014. Intraoperatively, a hard mass, approximately 5 cm × 3 cm in size, was seen in the pylorus of stomach, protruding from the mucosal surface, with good mobility, the boundary with surrounding tissue was clear, and no enlarged lymph nodes were seen. Laparoscopic partial gastrectomy with pylorus preservation was performed under the premise of ensuring radical resection, and the operation was performed smoothly (Fig. 28.3).

28.1.3.3 Postoperative Pathology

Postoperative Pathology Gastric GIST, approximately 5.3 cm × 2.8 cm in size, mitotic count <5/50 HPF, intermediate risk by the modified NIH recurrence risk classification. No metastasis was seen on the slices of three lymph nodes

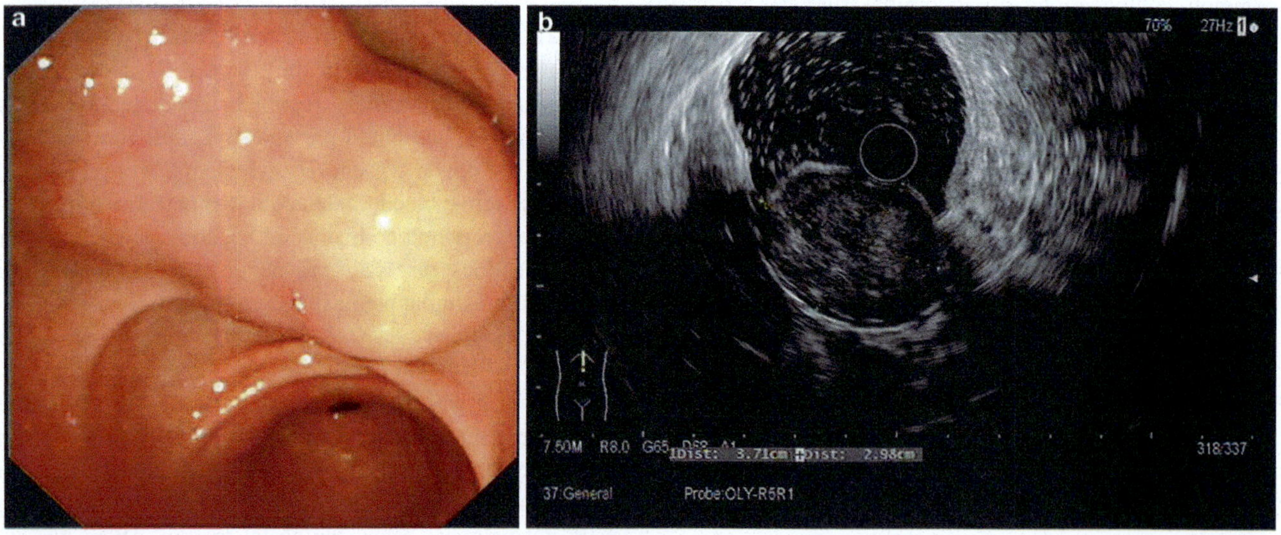

Fig. 28.1 Preoperative gastroscope showed a mass in the lesser curvature of the gastric antrum. **a** A bulge in the lesser curvature of gastric antrum. **b** Ultrasound showed that the bulge originated from the muscularis propria

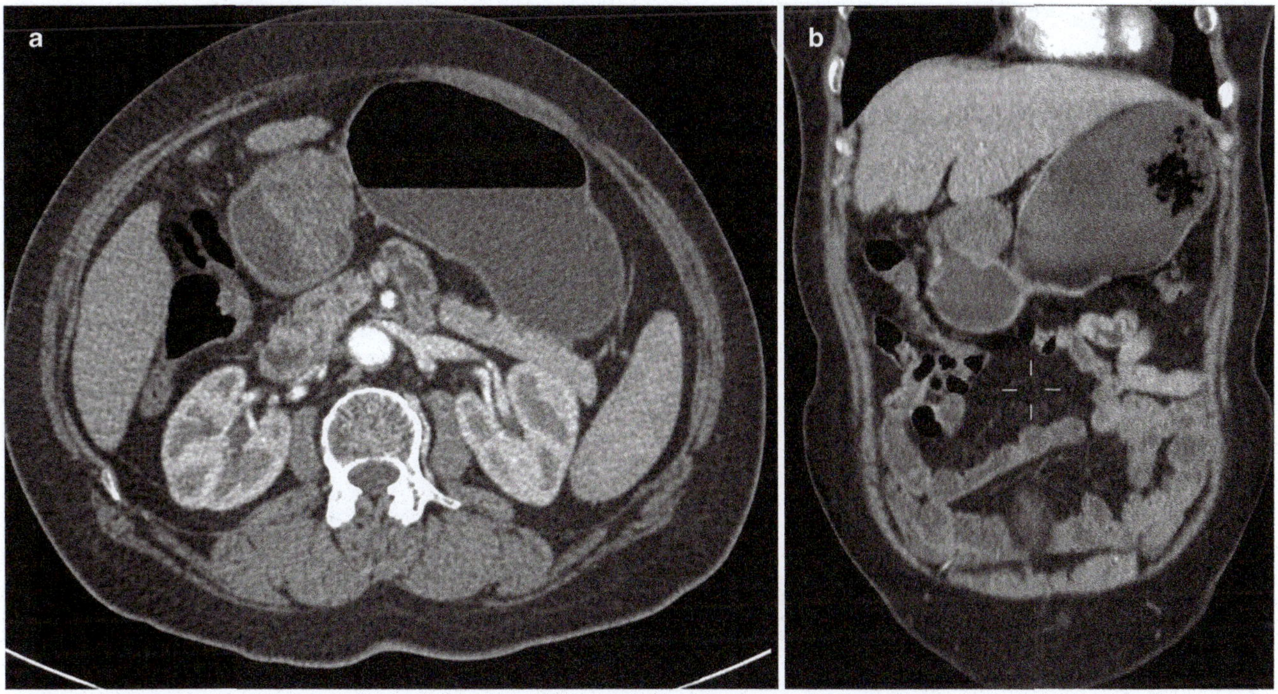

Fig. 28.2 CT showed gastric pyloric space-occupying lesion. **a** Cross-section. **b** Coronal plane

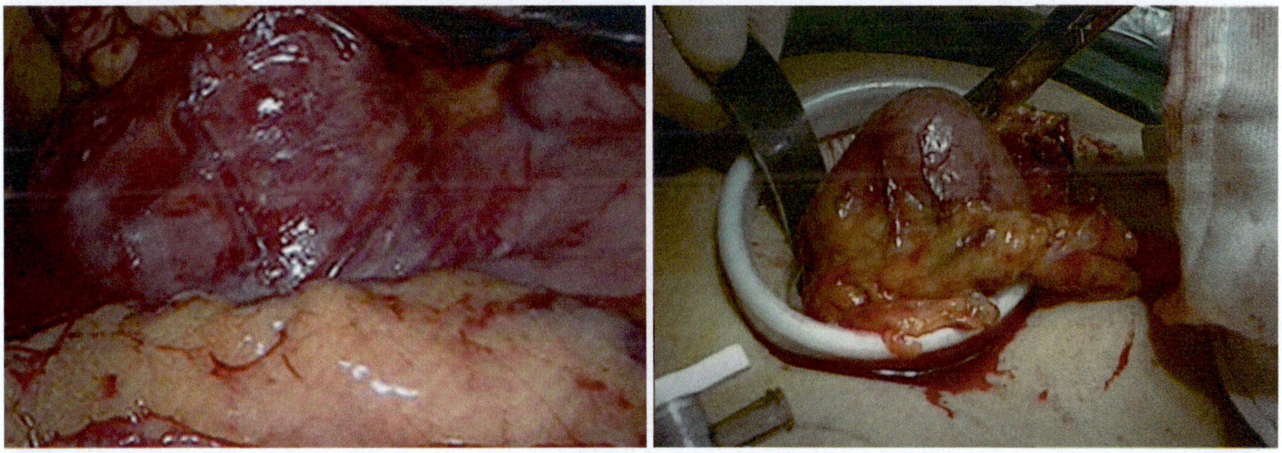

Fig. 28.3 Intraoperative findings

from the greater curvature, and surgical margins on both sides were free of tumor.

Immunohistochemistry CD117 (+), CD34 (+), DOG-1 (+), SMA (−), S-100 (−), Ki-67 (Li: 2%).

Genetic Testing The patient refused genetic testing for financial reasons.

28.1.4 Prognosis

The patient was discharged from the hospital 7 days after the operation, and no targeted therapy was performed for economic reasons. The patient developed vomiting after meals 10 days postoperatively, accompanied by abdominal distension, acid reflux, and belching. Upper gastrointestinal iodine radiography showed that the stomach was hook-shaped, the gastric antrum-pylorus was obstructed, the edge of the obstruction was rough, and the iodine was difficult to pass through the obstruction. No obvious abnormalities were seen in the proximal stomach. Considering postoperative gastroparesis (Fig. 28.4), the patient was readmitted to the hospital. To alleviate discomfort, a three-chamber gastric tube was used for gastrointestinal decompression and nasal feeding, and enteral nutrition was administered. In addition, gastrointestinal motility drugs were given to promote gastric peristalsis, the patient fasted from food and water, and disorders of water-electrolyte acid-base balance were corrected. After one and a half months of comprehen-

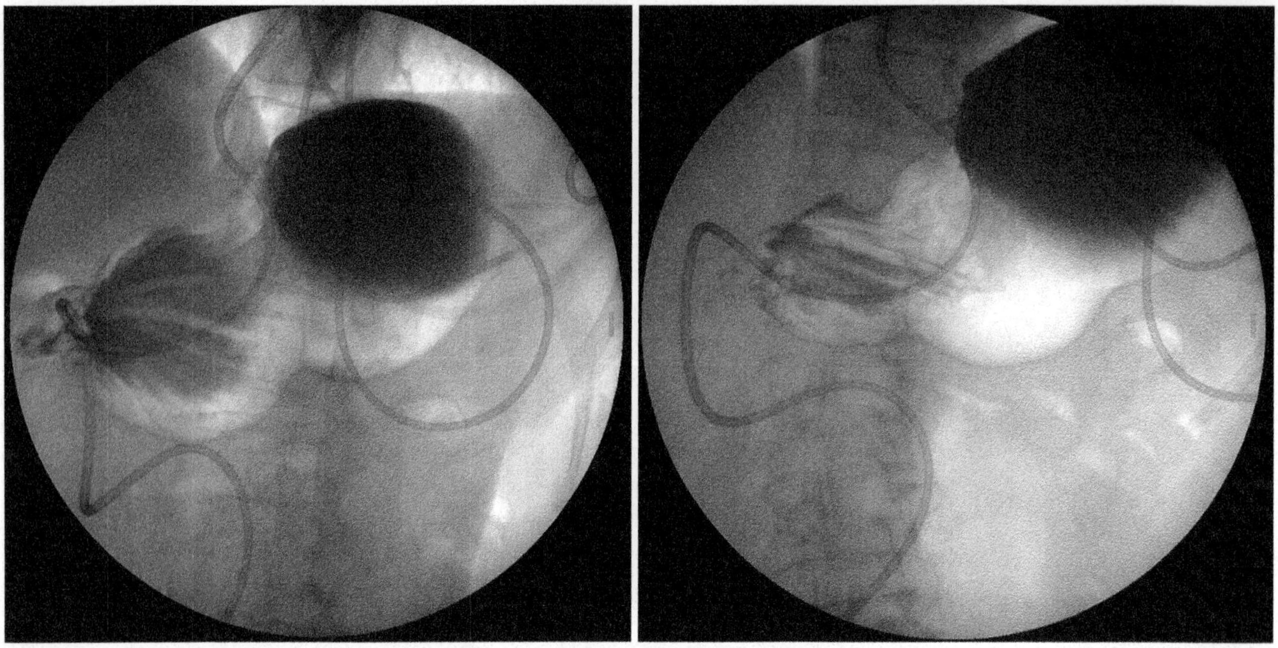

Fig. 28.4 The upper gastrointestinal radiography indicated gastroparesis 10 days after surgery

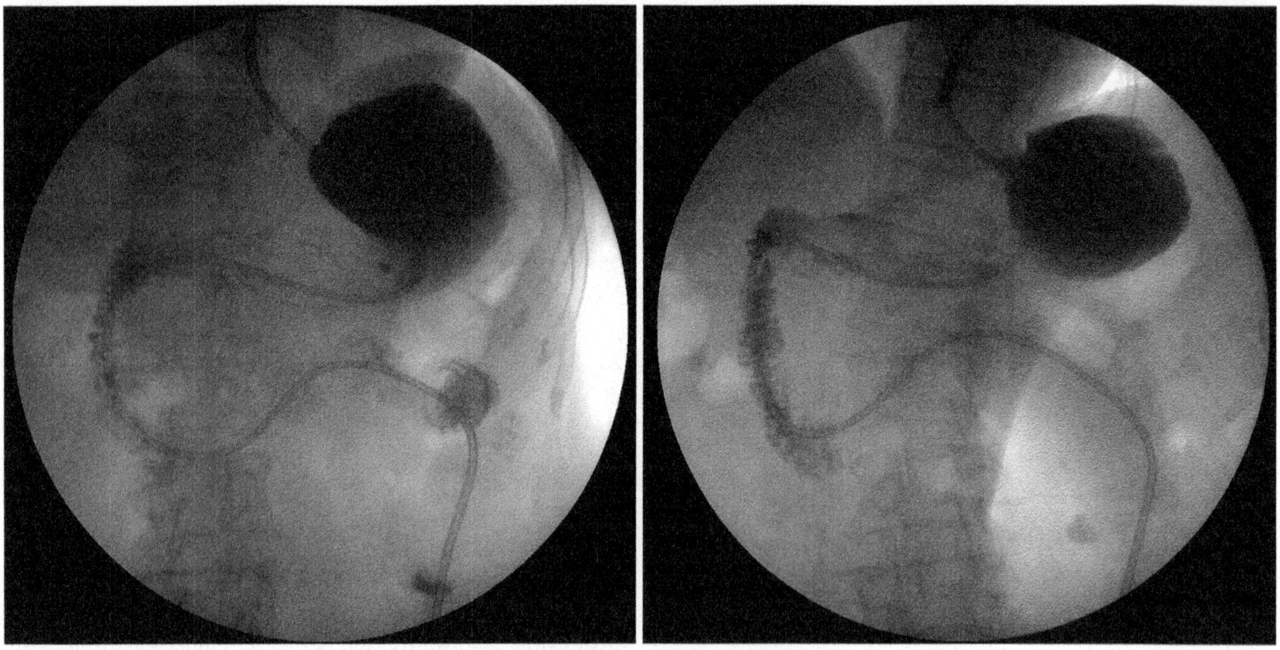

Fig. 28.5 Re-examination of upper gastrointestinal radiography 2 months after surgery

sive treatment, symptoms of gastroparesis improved significantly, and the patient gradually returned to a liquid diet. Re-examination of the upper gastrointestinal tract in August 2014 indicated postoperative partial gastrectomy, no obvious stenosis or fistula in the anastomosis, no fluid retention in the remnant stomach, and intermediate tension of stomach (Fig. 28.5). The patient survived disease free for 49 months of follow-up to June 2018.

28.1.5 Experience of Diagnosis and Therapy

28.1.5.1 What Are the Factors that Cause Gastroparesis After Gastric Surgery?

In this case, the patient's tumor was located in the pylorus with a size of approximately 5 cm × 3 cm. To protect the function of the pylorus and ensure complete resection of the tumor, pylorus-preserving gastrectomy with Billroth I anastomosis was performed [1]. However, the patient still developed gastroparesis after surgery, which may be related to an injury of the vagus nerve during the operation, thus changing the regulation of neural and myogenic hormones on gastric emptying [2]. If this was the case, the activity of gastric sympathetic nerves would have a stronger effect on inhibiting the myoelectric activity of the stomach, leading to delay in gastric emptying. In addition, the patient consumed semi-liquid food prematurely after operation, which may have increased the intragastric pressure and might also have caused gastroparesis. The basic physical condition of the patient, surgical injury, postoperative hypoalbuminemia, hyperglycemia, analgesia and anesthesia use, mental factors, and improper dietary order after surgery are all important factors that may cause gastroparesis after gastric surgery. Therefore, clinicians must prepare adequately before surgery, evaluate the risks of surgery, select appropriate surgical methods, and carry out nutritional support and anti-infective treatment actively after surgery. For patients with postoperative complications of gastroparesis, we must consider all aspects comprehensively, and perform etiological and symptomatic treatment after clarifying the cause.

28.1.5.2 What Are the Clinical Manifestations and Treatment of Gastroparesis After Gastrointestinal Surgery?

Gastroparesis is a common complication after abdominal surgery, especially radical gastric cancer surgery and pancreaticoduodenectomy [3, 4]. Once gastroparesis occurs, it often lasts for several weeks or even longer. It is manifested as dietary intolerance, such as abdominal distension, nausea, or vomiting, after meals. Often gastrointestinal decompression is more than 80 mL/d, the upper abdomen is full with light tenderness, a vibrating sound can be heard, and abdominal CT and other imaging examinations show stomach dilation and retention. This disease is a functional disease rather than a mechanical obstruction, and non-surgical treatment is mainly used once it is diagnosed. In this case enteral nutrition was given, sufficient protein, energy, and vitamins were supplemented, fluid infusions were performed to maintain the water, electrolyte and acid-base balances, and gastrointestinal motility drugs were given. In addition, the patient was educated to alleviate anxiety and was entrusted to increase the amount of everyday activity. Following treatment, symptoms of gastroparesis improved significantly. It should be noted that once the diagnosis of gastroparesis is clear, the gastric tube should not be removed without good reason and it is best to remove the tube after symptoms are relieved; otherwise, the recovery time may be prolonged. At the same time, hypertonic warm saline or procaine gastric lavage can reduce anastomotic edema. In addition, gastrointestinal motility drugs, such as metoclopramide, domperidone, and cisapride, can also be used to treat gastroparesis.

Laparoscopic pyloroplasty, which treats gastroparesis mainly through expanding the pyloric passage, is considered to be a safe and effective therapy for gastroparesis where medical treatment has been ineffective [5]. In recent years, gastric peroral endoscopic myotomy has also become more popular. In general, we should pay attention to establishing the concept of rapid recovery in the treatment of postoperative gastroparesis.

28.2 Expert Comments

Junbo Hu

The pathogenesis of gastroparesis is currently unclear, but the known possible factors related to gastroparesis include gastric retention, inflammation, vagus nerve injury, anastomotic edema, water and electrolyte disorders, improper diet, and mental factors. These factors would lead to both structural and functional disability, and nerve injury may be a primary cause. Therefore, the gastric nerves must be carefully identified and protected during gastric surgery, especially the preservation of the nerve trunk, which is of great significance for preventing postoperative gastroparesis.

The treatment for gastroparesis is based on conservative treatment, which requires routine continuous gastrointestinal decompression and gastric lavage. Strengthening nutritional support and maintaining water and electrolyte balance are the most critical measures. At the same time, it is also important to help patients maintain a good attitude. Early enteral nutrition, mainly using nasointestinal tube feeding, is of great significance to quickly improve the nutritional status of patients and promote the recovery of gastroparesis. Enteral nutrition can avoid complications caused by long-term parenteral nutrition, and enteral nutrition contains a variety of dietary fibers, which can not only meet the body's energy requirements, supplement water intake, and maintain electrolyte balance, but also plays an important role in maintaining the shape of the intestine, and promoting gastrointestinal peristalsis and nutrient absorption, which can promote the growth and cell proliferation of small intestinal and colonic mucosa, and help in the recovery of normal gastric emptying [6]. In addition, the application of gastrointestinal motility drugs also has certain effects [7].

The course of gastroparesis can be short as 1 week, and long as 6–8 weeks. After modern nutritional support and treatment, patients generally recover within 2 weeks. For patients with a difficult recovery course, it is necessary to look for reasons actively, including whether there are hidden infections and inflammatory lesions, and whether nutritional support meets the required standard [8]. On this basis, patients should be encouraged to exercise appropriately, which will also relieve patient anxiety. If necessary, the neurology department should be consulted to determine whether drug intervention is needed.

References

1. Li J, Ye Y, Wang J, Zhang B, Qin S, Shi Y, He Y, Liang X, Liu X, Zhou Y, Wu X, Zhang X, Wang M, Gao Z, Lin T, Cao H, Shen L, Chinese Society of Clinical Oncology Csco Expert Committee on Gastrointestinal Stromal Tumor. Chinese consensus guidelines for diagnosis and management of gastrointestinal stromal tumor. Chin J Cancer Res. 2017;29(4):281–93. https://doi.org/10.21147/j.issn.1000-9604.2017.04.01.
2. Gottfried-Blackmore A, Adler EP, Fernandez-Becker N, Clarke J, Habtezion A, Nguyen L. Open-label pilot study: non-invasive vagal nerve stimulation improves symptoms and gastric emptying in patients with idiopathic gastroparesis. Neurogastroenterol Motil. 2020;32(4):e13769. https://doi.org/10.1111/nmo.13769.
3. Sugase T, Takahashi T, Nakajima K, Hirota S, Masuzawa T, Nishida T, Kimura Y, Miyazaki Y, Makino T, Kurokawa Y, Yamasaki M, Takiguchi S, Mori M, Doki Y. Clinicopathological characteristics, surgery and survival outcomes of patients with duodenal gastrointestinal stromal tumors. Digestion. 2016;94(1):30–6. https://doi.org/10.1159/000447665.
4. Camilleri M, Sanders KM. Gastroparesis. Gastroenterology. 2022;162(1):68–87. e1. https://doi.org/10.1053/j.gastro.2021.10.028.
5. Jia LW, Lai SY, Wu JH. Comparison of the clinical efficacy of laparoscopic wedge resection and open wedge resection for the treatment of gastrointestinal stromal tumor. Zhonghua Zhong Liu Za Zhi. 2016;38(7):543–7. In Chinese. https://doi.org/10.3760/cma.j.issn.0253-3766.2016.07.012.
6. Limketkai BN, LeBrett W, Lin L, Shah ND. Nutritional approaches for gastroparesis. Lancet Gastroenterol Hepatol. 2020;5(11):1017–26. https://doi.org/10.1016/S2468-1253(20)30078-9.
7. Camilleri M, Parkman HP, Shafi MA, Abell TL, Gerson L, American College of Gastroenterology. Clinical guideline: management of gastroparesis. Am J Gastroenterol. 2013;108(1):18–37. https://doi.org/10.1038/ajg.2012.373.
8. Sullivan A, Temperley L, Ruban A. Pathophysiology, aetiology and treatment of gastroparesis. Dig Dis Sci. 2020;65(6):1615–31. https://doi.org/10.1007/s10620-020-06287-2.

Gastrointestinal Stromal Tumors with Brain Metastases

29

Lin Tu, Tao Chen, and Zhigang Jie

Keywords

Gastrointestinal stromal tumor · Wild type · Brain metastasis · Sunitinib

29.1 Case 39 A 56-Year-Old Woman with GIST and Brain Metastases

Lin Tu and Tao Chen

29.1.1 Introduction

GIST metastases are generally found in the liver and abdominal cavity, and metastases in the brain are extremely rare. So far only a few cases of GIST brain metastases have been reported. It is reported that sunitinib can penetrate the blood-brain barrier and has some effect on the treatment of brain metastases. This case describes the characteristics, therapy, and prognosis of a patient with wild-type GIST with brain metastases and discusses and analyzes the diagnosis and treatment.

29.1.2 Case Background

The patient, a 56-year-old woman, presented to the local hospital for investigation of upper abdominal discomfort for 1 week in January 2015. She was considered to have gastritis and was treated with oral traditional Chinese medicine. The above symptoms were relieved. The patient went to the Nanfang Hospital of Southern Medical University on March 3, 2015, due to dysphagia without obvious causes, especially when eating cooked rice and steamed buns. There were no chills, fever, heart palpitations, abdominal pain, black stool, or other symptoms. The preliminary report of gastroscopy in the outpatient clinic indicated a malignant tumor in the esophagus and cardia. After being admitted to the gastroenterology department, an ultrasound gastroscopy and biopsy were performed with a diagnosis of GIST in the esophagus and cardia. A PET-CT on March 5, 2015, identified multiple metastases in the abdominal cavity, retroperitoneum, and both lungs. The patient was treated with imatinib 400 mg/d and discharged from the hospital on March 12, 2015. After discharge from the hospital, she suffered sudden sensory and motor disorders in her left upper and lower limbs on March 24, 2015. A CT scan at the local hospital showed a space-occupying lesion on the right frontal lobe. The right frontal lobe tumor was resected under general anesthesia on March 25, 2015, and the postoperative pathology confirmed brain metastasis of GIST. On April 1, 2015, the patient came to Nanfang Hospital of Southern Medical University for further therapy and was admitted into the hospital for further treatment of a malignant GIST in the fundus and esophagus with brain metastasis.

29.1.2.1 Past History and Family History

The patient had a 1-year history of hypertension, took sustained release nifedipine 30 mg/d, and the blood pressure was controlled well. A total hysterectomy was performed at a local hospital for endometrial precancerous lesions in 2008. There was a history of allergy to "sulfa" drugs and she reported no family history of genetic disease.

29.1.2.2 Physical Examination

The patient's vital signs were stable, and the skin and mucous membranes were not yellowish or pale. The abdomen was

L. Tu
Department of Gastrointestinal Surgery, Renji Hospital, Shanghai Jiaotong University School of Medicine, Shanghai, China

T. Chen (✉)
Department of General Surgery, Nanfang Hospital, Southern Medical University, Guangzhou, China

Z. Jie
Department of General Surgery, The First Affiliated Hospital of Nanchang University, Nanchang, China

K. Tao, H. Cao (eds.), *Clinical Management of Gastrointestinal Stromal Tumor*, https://doi.org/10.1007/978-981-99-9392-5_29

flat, with no gastrointestinal or peristaltic wave, and no abdominal wall varicosis. The abdomen was soft, with no tenderness, rebound tenderness, or guarding. The liver and spleen were not palpable below the costal margin. There was no shifting dullness or abnormal bowel sounds.

29.1.2.3 Auxiliary Examination

PET-CT (1) Large masses of high-metabolic lesions were seen in the lower esophagus, cardia, and fundus of the stomach, with full-thickness infiltration; (2) Multiple nodular and massive high-metabolic lesions were seen alongside the lesser curvature of stomach, in the posterior area of the upper abdominal peritoneum and left hilum, which were considered to be multiple lymph node metastases; (3) Nodular high-metabolic lesions were seen in the medial segment of the right middle lung and dorsal segment of right lower lung, which were considered to be metastases in the right lung; (4) Calcification of intracranial cerebral falx, bilateral inflammatory hyperplasia of multiple lymph nodes in the neck, thyroid isthmus cyst, small calcification in the left breast, small benign nodule in the anterior segment of right upper lung, fiber cord shadow in the medial segment of right middle lung, inflammatory hyperplasia of multiple lymph nodes in the right hilum and mediastinum; (5) Slightly low-density space-occupying lesion in the upper segment of the right posterior lobe of liver without increase in metabolism, which was considered benign (hemangioma possible); (6) Postoperative absence of uterus, a small amount of effusion in the pelvic cavity, intervertebral disc bulging of lumbar 3/4 and lumbar 4/5, hyperplasia of multiple vertebral body of thoracolumbar vertebrae; (7) No obvious abnormalities in other parts of the body (Fig. 29.1).

MRI (1) Postoperative changes after resection of mass in the right frontal lobe, with hemorrhage in the operation area; multiple space-occupying lesions in the right temporal lobe and bilateral frontal lobe, which were considered to be metastases with a small amount of bleeding after considering the history; (2) A small area of white matter degeneration under the left frontal parietal cortex; (3) Bilateral ethmoid sinus and sphenoid sinus inflammation (Fig. 29.2).

29.1.2.4 Preliminary Diagnosis

1. EGJ GIST with brain metastases
2. Hypertension, grade 2, High Risk
3. Postoperative hysterectomy

29.1.3 Therapy

29.1.3.1 Case Analysis

The patient was a middle-aged woman with a clear diagnosis of GIST at the gastroesophageal junction with brain metastasis. She had been treated with imatinib and the disease progressed after resection of the right frontal lobe tumor. Thus, the case was considered to be imatinib-refractory GIST and treatment with sunitinib was planned.

29.1.3.2 Treatment

At the time of the second admission, April 2, 2015, imatinib was increased to 600 mg/d. During the treatment, multiple brain metastases with bleeding were found. The patient received sunitinib 37.5 mg/d and whole brain radiotherapy on April 13. The intracranial hematomas in the bilateral frontal lobe were punctured and drained using stereotactic puncture on April 15th. Both sides were successfully punctured at

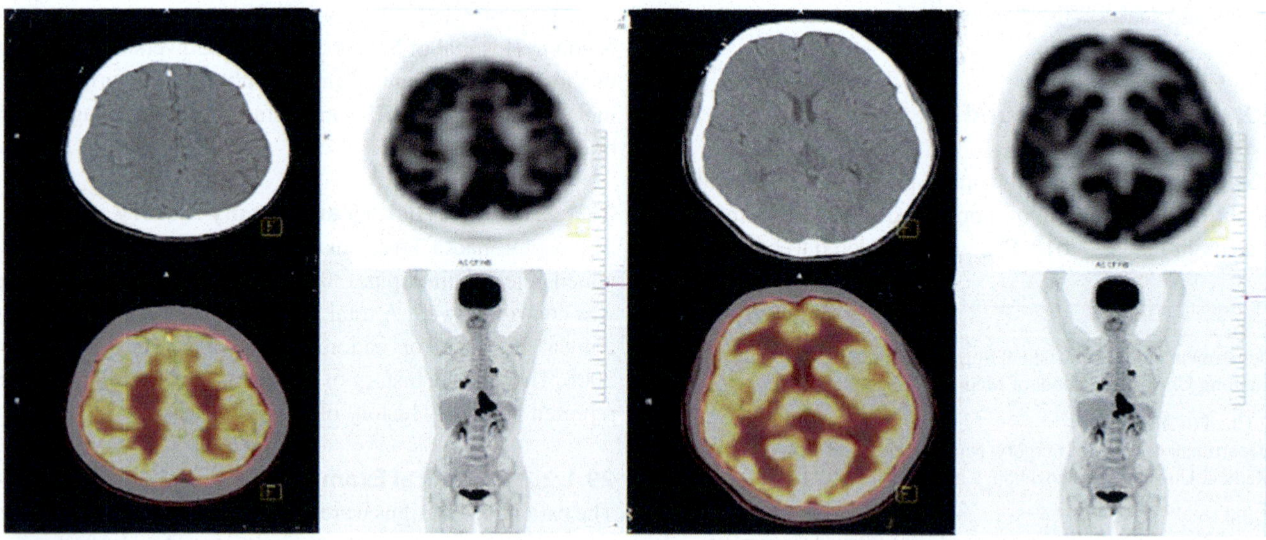

Fig. 29.1 Preoperative PET-CT image

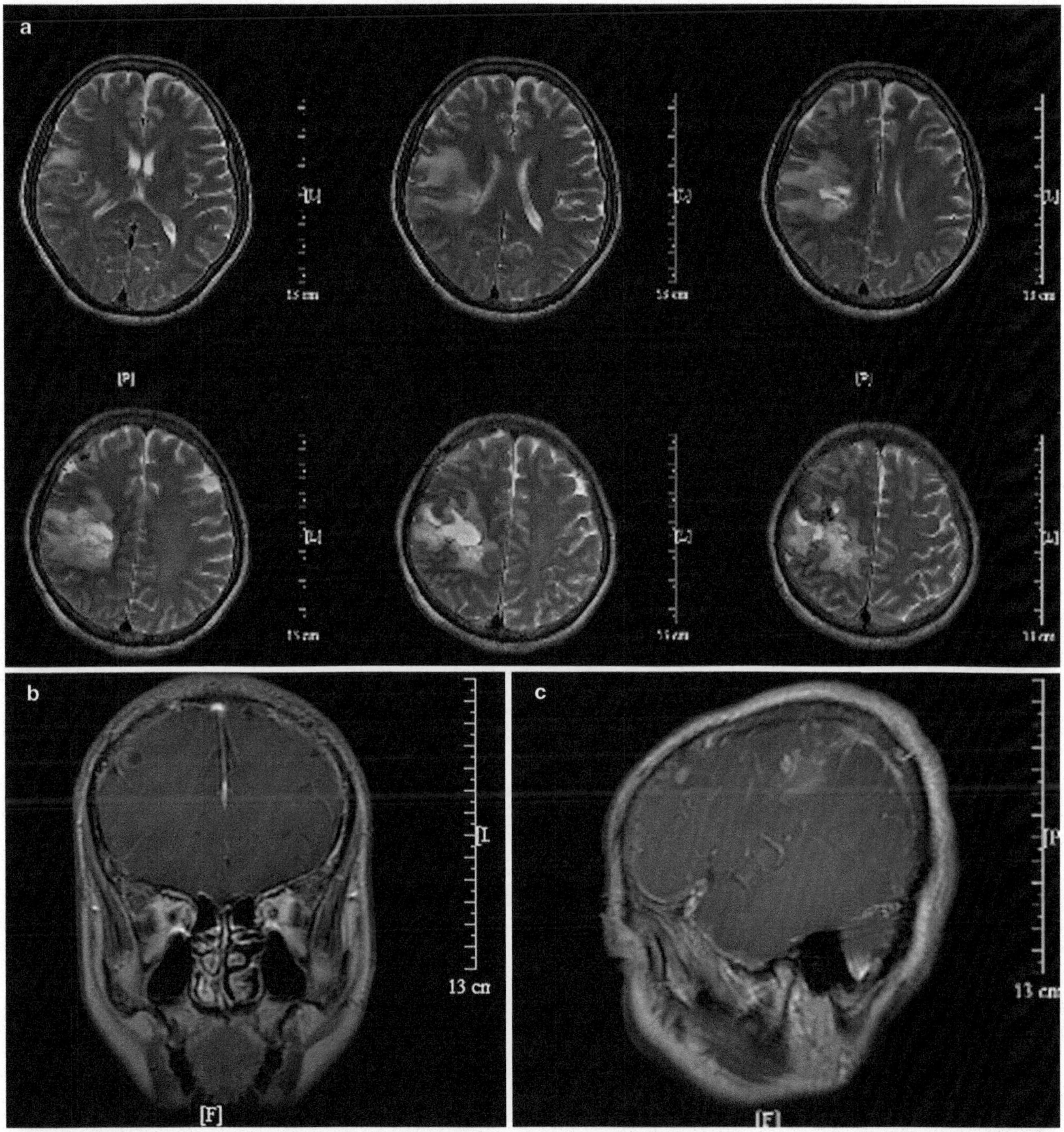

Fig. 29.2 Preoperative MRI image. **a** Transverse position; **b** Coronal position; **c** Sagittal position

one time, and 35 mL of non-coagulated blood was drained. The operation went smoothly. Sunitinib was increased to 50 mg/d after surgery.

29.1.3.3 Postoperative Pathology and Genetic Testing

Postoperative Pathology Malignant GIST, mild chronic superficial gastritis with erosion (Fig. 29.3).

Immunohistochemistry CK5/6 (−), P63 (−), Syn (−), CgA (−), Ki-67 (Li: 80%), CK (−), S-100 (−), HMB45 (−), MelanA (−), CD3 (−), CD20 (−), MPO (−), Vim (+), CD99 (+), CD56 (−), CD34 (−), CD117 (+), DOG-1 (−), desmin (−), myogenin (−), CD31 (−), WT-1 (+).

Pathology of Brain Tissue The results were consistent with metastatic GIST (Fig. 29.4).

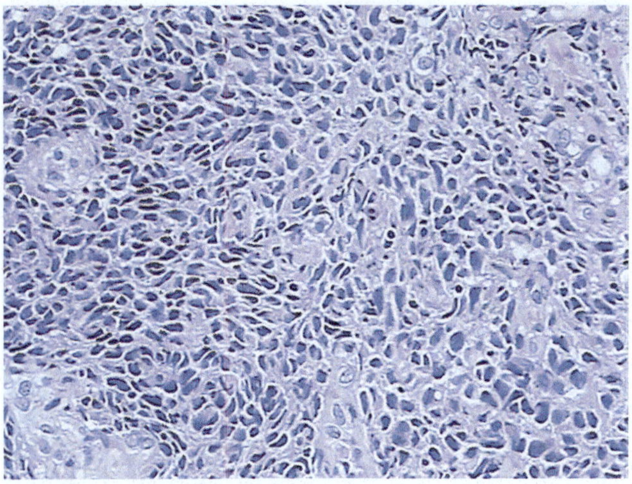

Fig. 29.3 H&E staining of gastric tissue

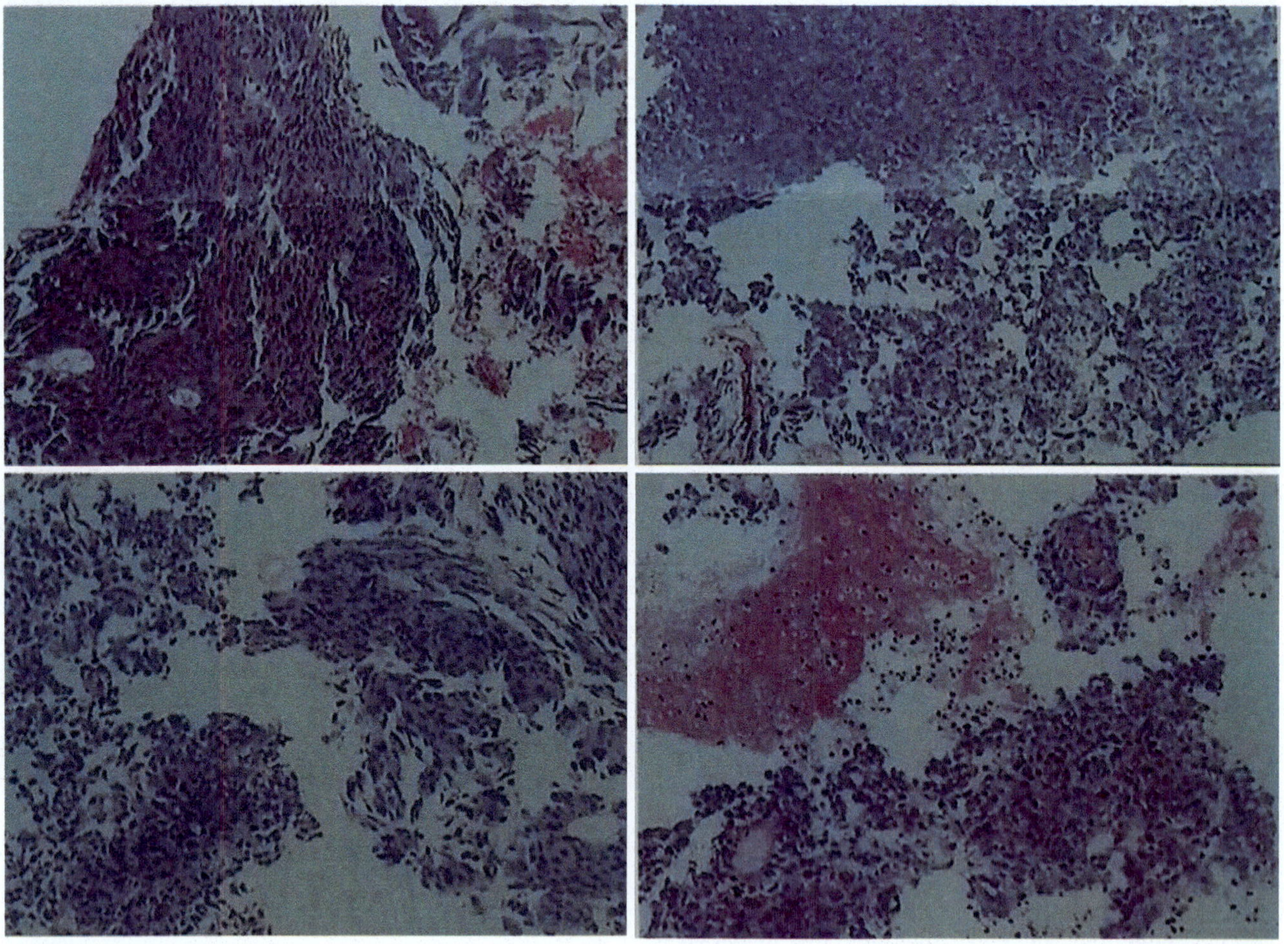

Fig. 29.4 H&E staining of brain tissue

Immunohistochemistry CD117 (+), CD34 (−), DOG-1 (−).

Genetic Testing No mutations in the exons 9, 11, 13 and 17 of *KIT*, synonymous mutation in exon 12 of *PDGFRA*, no mutations in exon 18 of *PDGFRA*.

29.1.4 Prognosis

Postoperative CT scan of the head on April 20 showed that the intracranial metastases were stable, and the edema and bleeding had been absorbed. A third PET-CT was performed on April 29, and it was found that the tumor had reduced in size, the metabolism of the intracranial lesion was significantly reduced, the bleeding in the lesion was largely absorbed, and no new bleeding was observed. A repeat CT scan on May 8 revealed that the intracranial metastases had shrunk and the hematoma had absorbed further since the previous scan. The patient developed systemic edema and renal insufficiency during subsequent therapy, so the dose of sunitinib was reduced to 25 mg/d, but the symptoms did not improve significantly. Regorafenib treatment was initiated at 160 mg/d on July 25. A PET-CT following the withdrawal of regorafinib on August 13 indicated that the primary lesion was progressing. Sunitinib treatment was restarted on August 18, and the patient relapsed with systemic edema and renal insufficiency. Sunitinib was discontinued on September 1, and the edema was relieved. A CT scan on September 2 revealed a new lesion on the brain. The patient died from cachexia on October 29.

29.1.5 Experience of Diagnosis and Therapy

Brain metastasis of GIST is very rare. There are only a few reports of such cases at present, but once brain metastases occur, the disease is often critical, and the prognosis is poor [1, 2]. Twenty days after the discovery of intracrania metastases and craniotomy, the patient was again found to have multiple brain metastases with hemorrhage, which showed rapid progression of the disease. In a case report by Doniel et al., it was mentioned that the average survival time of patients who died from GIST brain metastasis was 14.3 months, and the survival time of a patient who received only surgical treatment was just 7 months [3].

This patient's disease developed rapidly and increasing the dose of imatinib did not control the disease effectively, which may be related to the genetic type of the tumor. According to the results of postoperative genetic testing, the tumor could be judged as wild-type GIST. Wild-type GIST can be roughly divided into succinate dehydrogenase (SDH)-deficient GIST and non-SDH-deficient GIST [4]. This patient was not tested for SDH, so it is not possible to determine the subtype. The targets of TKIs currently used for treating GIST are those with *KIT* and *PDGFRA* mutations, while wild-type GIST does not carry genetic mutations, resulting in tumors being insensitive to traditional TKIs [5]. According to statistics, the effective rate of imatinib against wild-type GIST is 14%, while the overall effective rate against GIST is as high as 60–80%. Therefore, it is not difficult to understand why the patient's disease could not be effectively controlled with preliminary treatment.

The blood-brain barrier permeability of imatinib is only 10%, so its therapeutic effect for brain metastases is poor. Sunitinib, another TKI, has a blood-brain barrier permeability of 40% and has effective anti-angiogenesis and anti-tumor activities [6]. Sunitinib currently has approval for use in the treatment of advanced renal cell carcinoma, imatinib refractory GIST, and advanced pancreatic neuroendocrine tumors [7]. In this case, the disease could not be controlled with an increasing dose of imatinib after brain metastasis. However, the lesions shrank significantly after sunitinib treatment, confirming the therapeutic effect of sunitinib. However, attention should also be paid to the adverse effects associated with sunitinib. Common adverse effects include hand-foot syndrome, stomatitis, and other skin toxicities. In severe cases, cerebral hemorrhage may occur, especially in patients with hypertension [8]. In this case, the patient developed systemic edema and renal insufficiency after using sunitinib, and the edema was relieved after withdrawal of the drug. Therefore, although sunitinib is effective in the treatment of brain metastatic GIST, further exploration on how to balance safety and efficacy is warranted.

29.2 Expert Comments

Zhigang Jie

While GIST metastasis to the liver and peritoneum is common, metastasis outside the abdomen is rare, and brain metastasis is very rare. At present, there are only a few reports of such cases. In the early stage of brain metastasis, in addition to symptoms of the digestive system, the symptoms of the nervous system, such as signs of intracranial hypertension, are often not obvious. Once there are nervous system symptoms, it indicates that the tumor focus is large, compressing nerves and blood vessels, presents with symptoms such as intracranial hypertension, and the disease develops rapidly. At this time, craniotomy may be required to remove the tumor. In terms of drug treatment, it is difficult for the first-line treatment drug, imatinib, to pass through the blood-brain barrier. Therefore, the efficacy of imatinib in brain metastasis is insufficient. Sunitinib, another TKI, has a blood-brain barrier permeability of 40%. In one study, sunitinib was given to patients with brain metastasis. The results showed that the response lasted for more than 4 weeks, indicating that sunitinib has a certain therapeutic effect in controlling GIST brain metastasis. However, due to the low incidence rate and the small number of cases, there is no systematic study on epidemiology, clinical, and therapeutic results. The specific treatment plan after GIST brain metastasis still needs more in-depth clinical exploration. At present, it is considered that the application of the second-line drug sunitinib is an appropriate treatment option.

References

1. Takeuchi H, Koike H, Fujita T, Tsujino H, Iwamoto Y. Sunitinib treatment for multiple brain metastases from jejunal gastrointestinal stromal tumor: case report. Neurol Med Chir (Tokyo). 2014;54(8):664–9. https://doi.org/10.2176/nmc.cr2012-0426.
2. Prablek M, Srinivasan VM, Srivatsan A, Holdener S, Oneissi M, Heck KA, Jalali A, Mandel J, Viswanathan A, Patel AJ. Gastrointestinal stromal tumor with intracranial metastasis: case presentation and systematic review of literature. BMC Cancer. 2019;19(1):1119. https://doi.org/10.1186/s12885-019-6316-7.
3. Drazin D, Spitler K, Jeswani S, Shirzadi A, Bannykh S, Patil C. Multiple intracranial metastases from a gastric gastrointestinal stromal tumor. J Clin Neurosci. 2013;20(3):471–3. https://doi.org/10.1016/j.jocn.2012.02.037.
4. Wada R, Arai H, Kure S, Peng WX, Naito Z. "Wild type" GIST: clinicopathological features and clinical practice. Pathol Int. 2016;66(8):431–7. https://doi.org/10.1111/pin.12431.
5. Klug LR, Khosroyani HM, Kent JD, Heinrich MC. New treatment strategies for advanced-stage gastrointestinal stromal tumours. Nat Rev Clin Oncol. 2022;19(5):328–41. https://doi.org/10.1038/s41571-022-00606-4.
6. Soria JC, Blay JY, Spano JP, Pivot X, Coscas Y, Khayat D. Added value of molecular targeted agents in oncology. Ann Oncol. 2011;22(8):1703–16. https://doi.org/10.1093/annonc/mdq675.
7. Bose D, Meric-Bernstam F, Hofstetter W, Reardon DA, Flaherty KT, Ellis LM. Vascular endothelial growth factor targeted therapy in the perioperative setting: implications for patient care. Lancet Oncol. 2010;11(4):373–82. https://doi.org/10.1016/S1470-2045(09)70341-9.
8. Je Y, Schutz FA, Choueiri TK. Risk of bleeding with vascular endothelial growth factor receptor tyrosine-kinase inhibitors sunitinib and sorafenib: a systematic review and meta-analysis of clinical trials. Lancet Oncol. 2009;10(10):967–74. https://doi.org/10.1016/S1470-2045(09)70222-0.

30 Gastrointestinal Stromal Tumors with Giant Liver Metastases

Linxi Yang, Tianlong Ling, and Kaixiong Tao

Keywords

Gastrointestinal stromal tumor · ALPPS · Liver metastases · Imatinib

30.1 Case 40 A 49-Year-Old Woman with Advanced GIST Who Underwent ALPPS for Giant Liver Metastases

Linxi Yang and Tianlong Ling

30.1.1 Introduction

Targeted therapy is the main method for the treatment of recurrent and metastatic GIST. The value of surgery in the treatment of recurrent and metastatic GIST is still controversial, but a growing body of evidence-based science shows that cytoreductive surgery during the response to targeted drug therapy or localized progression may help to prolong patient survival.

30.1.2 Case Background

The patient, a 49-year-old woman, presented to local hospital due to abdominal pain. The enhanced abdominal CT scan showed a space-occupying lesion in the lesser curvature of the stomach (possible GIST). There were multiple space-occupying lesions in the liver, and metastasis was considered. The patient underwent needle biopsy of lesions in the right lobe of the liver. The biopsy showed GIST with less tissue, and the mitotic count could not be evaluated. Immunohistochemistry test results showed: CD117 (+), CD34 (+), DOG-1 (+), SMA (−), desmin (−), S100 (+), Ki67 (LI: 10%). Genetic testing was not performed due to insufficient tissue volume. The patient started imatinib treatment. The dose was 400 mg/d. The patient was regularly followed up until after 34 months, the latest abdominal enhanced CT scan showed that the maximum diameter of the primary gastric tumor increased from 2.8 to 3.0 cm; the largest metastatic tumor in the right lobe of liver increased from 6.1 to 7.2 cm; the number of metastases in the right lobe of the liver also increased. Considering the tumor progression and possible imatinib drug resistance, imatinib was discontinued and sunitinib 50 mg/d treatment was initiated. An enhanced abdominal CT 6 months later showed that the largest diameter of the primary gastric tumor had increased to 4.2 cm, and the largest metastatic tumor in the right lobe of the liver had increased to 12.2 cm. The patient was admitted to hospital for further treatment.

30.1.2.1 Past History and Family History

The patient was previously healthy and reported no history of drug allergies. The patient's parents were alive, and there was no similar medical history in the family.

30.1.2.2 Physical Examination

The patient's vital signs were stable, and the skin and mucous membranes were not yellowish or pale. The abdomen was flat, and no gastrointestinal or peristaltic wave was observed. The abdomen was soft, with right upper quadrant tenderness, and no palpable mass in the abdomen. The bowel sounds were normal.

30.1.2.3 Auxiliary Examination

Abdomen CT The space-occupying side of the lesser curvature of the stomach (GIST possible) was larger than before; there were multiple liver-occupying masses, considering the

L. Yang · T. Ling (✉)
Department of Gastrointestinal Surgery, Renji Hospital, Shanghai Jiaotong University School of Medicine, Shanghai, China

K. Tao
Department of Gastrointestinal Surgery, Union Hospital, Tongji Medical College, Huazhong University of Science and Technology University, Wuhan, China
e-mail: kaixiongtao@hust.edu.cn

K. Tao, H. Cao (eds.), *Clinical Management of Gastrointestinal Stromal Tumor*, https://doi.org/10.1007/978-981-99-9392-5_30

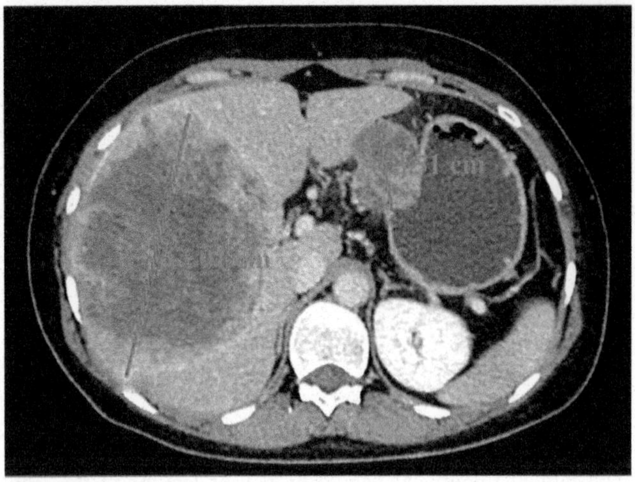

Fig. 30.1 CT showed obvious tumor progression

metastasis, and some lesions progressed significantly compared with the previous (Fig. 30.1).

30.1.3 Therapy

30.1.3.1 Case Analysis

A MDT discussion was held in our center to discuss the patient's condition. After joint discussion and evaluation by the departments of oncology, liver surgery, gastrointestinal surgery, and imaging, it was considered that the metastases in the right lobe of the patient's liver and the primary gastric tumor had progressed, although the other intrahepatic metastases were still stable. Surgical resection could be considered, and genetic mutation information could be obtained at the same time. The patient had no underlying liver disease. The future liver remnant (FLR) of the patient was estimated to be about 253 mL based on the enhanced abdominal CT, the standard liver volume (SLV) was about 1100 mL and the FLR/SLV was 23%. Therefore, associating liver partition and portal vein ligation for staged hepatectomy (ALPPS) could be considered. First, the primary gastric tumor was resected. The right portal vein and the liver parenchyma were ligated, and the liver parenchyma was severed. The patient was evaluated weekly after the operation. After the FLR/SLV was more than 30%, right hepatic trilobectomy was performed.

30.1.3.2 Treatment

The patient underwent partial gastrectomy and special hepatic segmentectomy (the first step of ALPPS) on April 29, 2021. A lobulated exophytic tumor 4 cm in diameter was located in the middle of the lesser curvature of the stomach, with abundant blood supply. The right liver was occupied by a huge tumor with a diameter of about 15 cm. There were several metastatic nodules in the left liver, ranging in diameter from 1 to 3 cm, showing post-treatment changes (hyalinization) (Fig. 30.2). The patient recovered well after the operation. Two weeks after the operation, the CT scan showed that the multiple nodules in the liver were a similar size to the previous scan. The FLR increased to 412 mL, and the FLR/SLV was 37%. The patient underwent right hepatic trilobectomy on May 17, 2021. The omentum and liver sections were densely adhered, and the right liver was ischemic and necrotic, with dark green effusion in the necrotic lesions; the left liver displayed compensatory hyperplasia (Fig. 30.3).

30.1.3.3 Postoperative Pathology and Genetic Testing

Pathological Diagnosis Gastric GIST, 4.5 cm × 4 cm × 3 cm in size, mitotic count 30/50 HPF. Liver GIST, 19 cm × 16 cm × 10 cm in size, mitotic count 40/50 HPF.

Immunohistochemistry CD117 (+), DOG-1 (+), CD34 (+), S-100 (−), Ki-67 (Li: 40%), SDHB (+).

Genetic Testing Heterozygous mutations in exon 11 of *KIT*, 553–558 deletion, cause the deletion of the encoded amino acids tyrosine, glutamic acid, valine, glutamine, tryptophan, and lysine. Exons 9, 13 and 17 of *KIT* and exons 12 and 18 of *PDGFRA* were all wild type.

30.1.4 Prognosis

The patient recovered well after the operation and resumed imatinib 400 mg/d treatment after discharge. As of December 2021 follow-up, there were no new metastasis in the abdominal cavity or liver (Fig. 30.4).

30.1.5 Experience of Diagnosis and Therapy

30.1.5.1 The Role of Cytoreductive Surgery in Delaying Tumor Progression After Secondary Resistance to TKIs

Previous studies have demonstrated that R0/R1 cytoreduction in patients who have not progressed on targeted drug therapy can prolong PFS in patients with advanced GIST [1]. At the same time, in some patients with advanced GIST with focal progression, complete resection of imatinib-resistant lesions can also lead to longer disease control time [2–5]. At present, it is believed that for the evaluation of resectable focal recurrence and metastasis and liver metastasis of recurrent and metastatic GIST, surgical resection combined with targeted drug therapy can bring survival benefits to patients with advanced GIST, and the 2021 Chinese Society of Clinical Oncology GIST diagnosis and treatment guidelines also recommend cytoreductive surgery as a grade II suggestion [6].

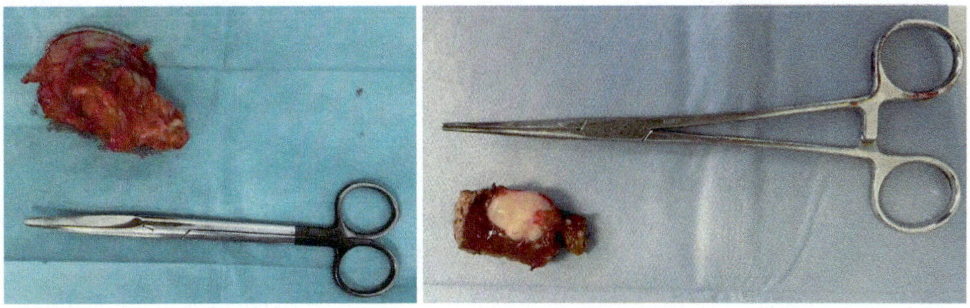

Fig. 30.2 Isolated liver tumor and gastric tumor specimens in the first step of ALPPS

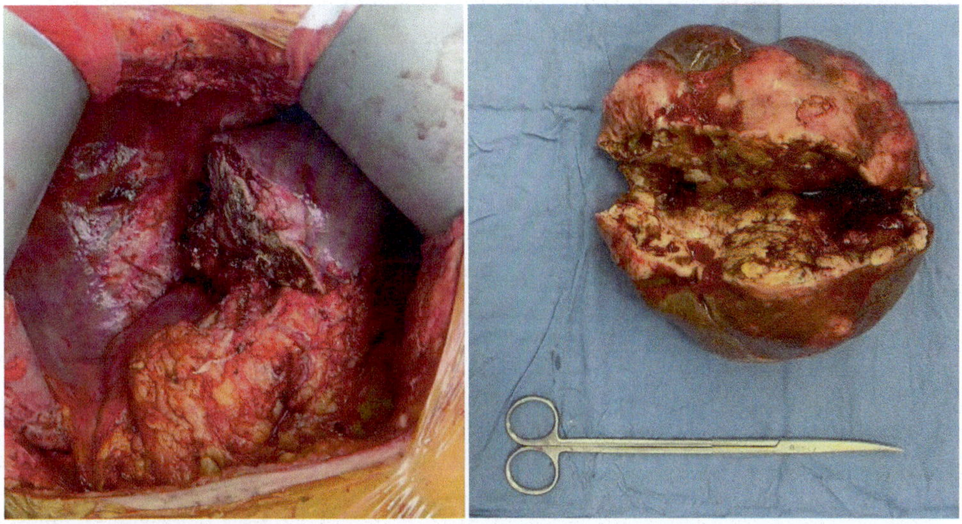

Fig. 30.3 Intraoperative liver in the second step of ALPPS and isolated liver tumor specimens

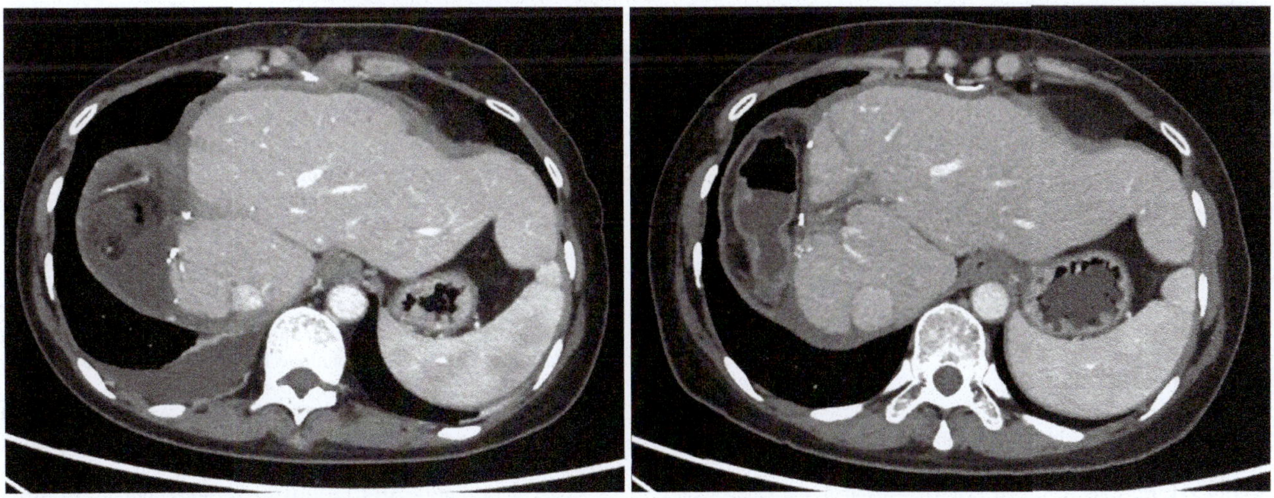

Fig. 30.4 CT results 2 weeks and 6 months after surgery

30.1.5.2 Treatment Options for Advanced GIST with Liver Metastases

Patients with advanced GIST and liver metastases are not uncommon. In addition to drug therapy, the treatment modes for patients with liver metastases include RFA, TACE, and surgery. Surgical resection is usually reserved for patients with resectable metastases and adequate residual liver volume. Surgery was previously considered inappropriate for patients who would have insufficient remaining liver volume. Since ALPPS was first reported in 2007, it has been mostly used to treat large liver lesions with a high risk of post-resection liver failure due to insufficient residual liver volume. It is mainly used to treat liver metastases from colorectal cancer, hepatocellular carcinoma, and hilar cholangiocarcinoma, and fewer than ten cases of ALPPS have been reported for liver metastases from GIST [7, 8]. Among the three patients with GIST who received ALPPS with follow-up, two patients had no metastasis at 17 months and

37 months after surgery, and one patient had recurrence 6 months after surgery [9–11].

The total course of the patient's disease was nearly 4 years, she received first- and second-line drug treatments, and disease progression was observed during both treatments. The first-line drug, imatinib, brought nearly 3 years of disease control, and the second-line drug sunitinib only provided PFS for less than 6 months. According to previous studies, if patients receive third-line regorafenib therapy, gastric primary tumors and liver metastases may continue to progress. Fortunately, the patient's metastatic lesions were limited to the liver, and the left liver lesions were all stable. The progressive lesions were limited to the right half of the liver, and there was no metastatic lesion in the abdominal cavity, which just met the requirements for ALPPS. The patient achieved disease control for half a year, and all the liver metastases which were previously well controlled by imatinib did not progressed. No new lesions had appeared. The left liver had satisfactory compensatory hyperplasia, with no abnormal liver function and good quality of life.

30.2 Expert Comments

Kaixiong Tao

This case introduces the experience of surgical resection of a localized progressive lesion during targeted drug therapy. The 2-staged hepatectomy used in this case is suitable for liver lesions with large volume. The advantage is that the volume and function of residual liver can be ensured and the risk of liver failure can be reduced. However, this technology is difficult and is not suitable for cases with other metastatic lesions in the residual liver or the abdominal cavity. The MDT cooperation for diagnosis and treatment is necessary to guarantee success for such surgery.

References

1. Bauer S, Rutkowski P, Hohenberger P, Miceli R, Fumagalli E, Siedlecki JA, Nguyen BP, Kerst M, Fiore M, Nyckowski P, Hoiczyk M, Cats A, Casali PG, Treckmann J, van Coevorden F, Gronchi A. Long-term follow-up of patients with GIST undergoing metastasectomy in the era of imatinib – analysis of prognostic factors (EORTC-STBSG collaborative study). Eur J Surg Oncol. 2014;40(4):412–9. https://doi.org/10.1016/j.ejso.2013.12.020.
2. Park SJ, Ryu MH, Ryoo BY, Park YS, Sohn BS, Kim HJ, Kim CW, Kim KH, Yu CS, Yook JH, Kim BS, Kang YK. The role of surgical resection following imatinib treatment in patients with recurrent or metastatic gastrointestinal stromal tumors: results of propensity score analyses. Ann Surg Oncol. 2014;21(13):4211–7. https://doi.org/10.1245/s10434-014-3866-4.
3. Raut CP, Posner M, Desai J, Morgan JA, George S, Zahrieh D, Fletcher CD, Demetri GD, Bertagnolli MM. Surgical management of advanced gastrointestinal stromal tumors after treatment with targeted systemic therapy using kinase inhibitors. J Clin Oncol. 2006;24(15):2325–31. https://doi.org/10.1200/JCO.2005.05.3439.
4. Yeh CN, Chen TW, Tseng JH, Liu YY, Wang SY, Tsai CY, Chiang KC, Hwang TL, Jan YY, Chen MF. Surgical management in metastatic gastrointestinal stromal tumor (GIST) patients after imatinib mesylate treatment. J Surg Oncol. 2010;102(6):599–603. https://doi.org/10.1002/jso.21630.
5. Fairweather M, Balachandran VP, Li GZ, Bertagnolli MM, Antonescu C, Tap W, Singer S, DeMatteo RP, Raut CP. Cytoreductive surgery for metastatic gastrointestinal stromal tumors treated with tyrosine kinase inhibitors: a 2-institutional analysis. Ann Surg. 2018;268(2):296–302. https://doi.org/10.1097/SLA.0000000000002281.
6. Li J, Ye Y, Wang J, Zhang B, Qin S, Shi Y, He Y, Liang X, Liu X, Zhou Y, Wu X, Zhang X, Wang M, Gao Z, Lin T, Cao H, Shen L, Chinese Society of Clinical Oncology Csco Expert Committee on Gastrointestinal Stromal Tumor. Chinese consensus guidelines for diagnosis and management of gastrointestinal stromal tumor. Chin J Cancer Res. 2017;29(4):281–93. https://doi.org/10.21147/j.issn.1000-9604.2017.04.01.
7. Lang H, Baumgart J, Mittler J. Associated liver partition and portal vein ligation for staged hepatectomy (ALPPS) registry: what have we learned? Gut Liver. 2020;14(6):699–706. https://doi.org/10.5009/gnl19233.
8. Lai Q, Mennini G, Larghi Laureiro Z, Rossi M. Uncommon indications for associating liver partition and portal vein ligation for staged hepatectomy: a systematic review. Hepatobiliary Surg Nutr. 2021;10(2):210–25. https://doi.org/10.21037/hbsn-20-355.
9. Liu J, Zhang C, Hong D, Shang M, Yao W, Chen Y. Percutaneous microwave ablation liver partition and portal vein embolization for planned hepatectomy due to large gastrointestinal stromal tumor metastases: a case report. Medicine (Baltimore). 2017;96(42):e8271. https://doi.org/10.1097/MD.0000000000008271.
10. Sanei B, Sheikhbahaei S, Sanei MH, Bahreini A, Jafari HR. Associating liver partition and portal vein ligation for staged hepatectomy: a surgical technique for liver resections. J Res Med Sci. 2017;22:52. https://doi.org/10.4103/jrms.JRMS_829_16.
11. Troja A, Khatib-Chahidi K, El-Sourani N, Antolovic D, Raab HR. ALPPS and similar resection procedures in treating extensive hepatic metastases: our own experiences and critical discussion. Int J Surg. 2014;12(9):1020–2. https://doi.org/10.1016/j.ijsu.2014.07.006.

Part VII

Management of Misdiagnosed Gastrointestinal Stromal Tumors

31 Small Intestine Gastrointestinal Stromal Tumor Misdiagnosed as Gynecological Tumor

Lin Tu, Youwei Kou, and Jinbo Gao

Keywords

Gastrointestinal stromal tumor · Gynecological tumor
Secondary resistance

31.1 Case 41 A 56-Year-Old Woman with Small Intestine GIST Misdiagnosed as a Gynecological Tumor

Lin Tu and Youwei Kou

31.1.1 Introduction

Due to the relatively fixed location of giant small intestinal GIST, especially small intestine GIST in the pelvic cavity, which move poorly and adhere to the uterus and appendages, it is difficult to distinguish from gynecological tumors and is often misdiagnosed as ovarian tumors or uterine fibroids. Incorrect diagnosis and treatment may lead to iatrogenic dissemination of tumors, thereby affecting patient prognosis.

L. Tu
Department of Gastrointestinal Surgery, Renji Hospital, Shanghai Jiaotong University School of Medicine, Shanghai, China

Y. Kou (✉)
Department of Gastrointestinal Surgery, Shengjing Hospital of China Medical University, Shenyang, China
e-mail: kouyw@sj-hospital.org

J. Gao
Department of Gastrointestinal Surgery, Union Hospital, Tongji Medical College, Huazhong University of Science and Technology University, Wuhan, China

31.1.2 Case Background

The patient, a 56-year-old woman, presented to the gynecology clinic of our hospital in June 2015. She reported that she had frequent urination for the past year, up to 10–13 times a day, with no abnormal vaginal bleeding or discharge, no urgent urination or odynuria, and no abdominal pain or fever. She developed distension and pain in the middle and lower abdomen 6 days previously. Ultrasonography was performed in another hospital and showed a space-occupying lesion in the right pelvic cavity, indicating an ovarian tumor. The patient came to our hospital for further diagnosis and treatment.

31.1.2.1 Past History and Family History

The patient had a 2-year history of hypertension, highest blood pressure of 175/95 mmHg, and took oral amlodipine, 1 tablet/day, which controlled the blood pressure at 120/85 mmHg. She reported no history of infectious diseases, such as hepatitis and tuberculosis, heart disease, diabetes, trauma, allergies to food and drug, or blood transfusions.

31.1.2.2 Physical Examination

The patient was conscious, with no yellowing of sclera, no appearance of anemia, clear breath sounds on both lungs, and a heart rate of 80 beats/min. The abdomen was soft, with slight tenderness in the lower abdomen, and no rebound tenderness or guarding. The liver and spleen were not palpable below the costal margin, there were no bowel sounds, shifting dullness, or edema in the lower limbs, and the patient had normal movement of the limbs. Gynecological examination revealed normal vulva development, smooth vagina, no mucosal hyperemia, a small amount of secretion in the vagina, no peculiar smell. Cervical hypertrophy, center, anterior uterus, which was shrinking, hard, a slightly irregular shape, and movable. A 12 cm mass could be palpated in the right adnexal area, the mass was hard, with poor mobility, and tenderness. There were no obvious abnormalities in the left adnexa area.

K. Tao, H. Cao (eds.), *Clinical Management of Gastrointestinal Stromal Tumor*, https://doi.org/10.1007/978-981-99-9392-5_31

31.1.2.3 Auxiliary Examination

Blood Routine WBC 8.38 × 10^9/L, RBC 4.0 × 10^{12}/L, Hb 119 g/L, PLT 351 × 10^9/L↑, NEUT% 59.4%, LY% 32.6%.

Blood Biochemistry No abnormalities.

Tumor Marker CA125 21.85 U/mL.

Gynecological Color Doppler Ultrasound The uterus was about 3.7 cm × 3.5 cm × 3.2 cm in size with uniform echo, and the intima was 0.3 cm in thickness. The left ovary was unclear. A hypoechoic mass was seen in the right pelvic cavity, with a range of approximately 16.8 cm × 12.6 cm × 11.4 cm, irregular shape, unclear borders, and no capsule. Multiple irregular anechoic areas were seen inside of the mass, the largest one was 3.3 cm × 2.8 cm in size, the color blood flow was rich, and the arteriovenous frequency spectrum could be explored. A free anechoic space was seen in the pelvis, about 1.2 cm in depth. Ultrasound findings showed postmenopausal uterus, right pelvic space occupying lesion (Fig. 31.1).

31.1.2.4 Preliminary Diagnosis

1. Space-occupying lesion of right pelvic cavity: possible ovarian tumor
2. Hypertension, grade 2, Intermediate Risk

31.1.3 Therapy

31.1.3.1 Case Analysis

The patient was a middle-aged woman with abdominal distension for more than 1 week. Gynecological color Doppler ultrasound and CT of abdomen and pelvis revealed a huge mass in the right pelvic cavity, which was considered to be a gynecological tumor. In order to clarify the nature of the mass and guide the subsequent diagnosis and treatment, exploratory laparotomy was performed.

31.1.3.2 Treatment

After the patient was admitted to the hospital, active preoperative preparations were performed, and the patient underwent laparotomy. During the operation, a solid mass of 16 cm in diameter was observed in the right pelvic cavity. The surfaces of the liver, spleen, stomach, and diaphragm were smooth, and the greater omentum was normal. The mass originated from the small intestine and adhered to the appendix, colon, and abdominal wall. An abdomen opener was used, the intestinal tube was padded with a bowel guard, and, after loosening the adhesions, the mass was gradually removed. A frozen sample was sent for pathological analysis which revealed that the tumor was a small intestinal GIST. Following the diagnosis, a partial small bowel resection was performed.

31.1.3.3 Postoperative Pathology and Genetic Testing

Postoperative Pathology Small intestinal GIST, mitotic count 11/50 HPF, modified NIH recurrence risk classification: high risk.

Immunohistochemical Staining CD117 (+), CD34 (+), DOG-1 (+), SMA (−), S-100 (−), Ki67 (Li: 10%).

Genetic Testing Mutation in exon 11 of *KIT*, Exons 9, 13 and 17 of *KIT* and exons 12 and 18 of *PDGFRA* were all wild type.

31.1.4 Prognosis

The postoperative genetic test revealed a mutation in exon 11 of *KIT*, and the patient was treated with imatinib 400 mg/d and was reexamined regularly after surgery. The tumor recurred *in situ* 17 months postoperatively (Fig. 31.2), suggesting tumor resistance. The patient chose surgical treatment again after discussion with her family. Extensive adhesions between the greater omentum, peritoneum, and small intestine were seen and were carefully separated during the opera-

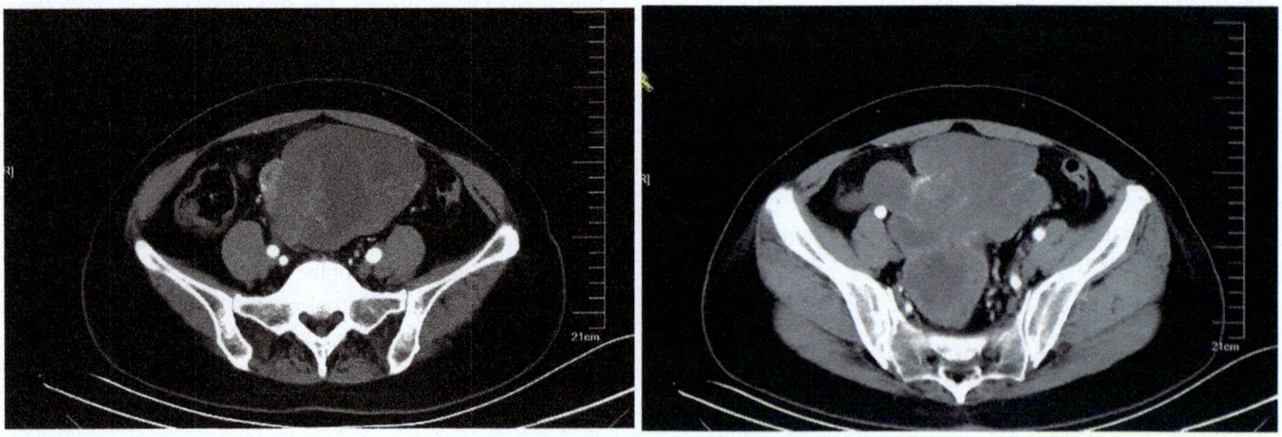

Fig. 31.1 Preoperative CT results

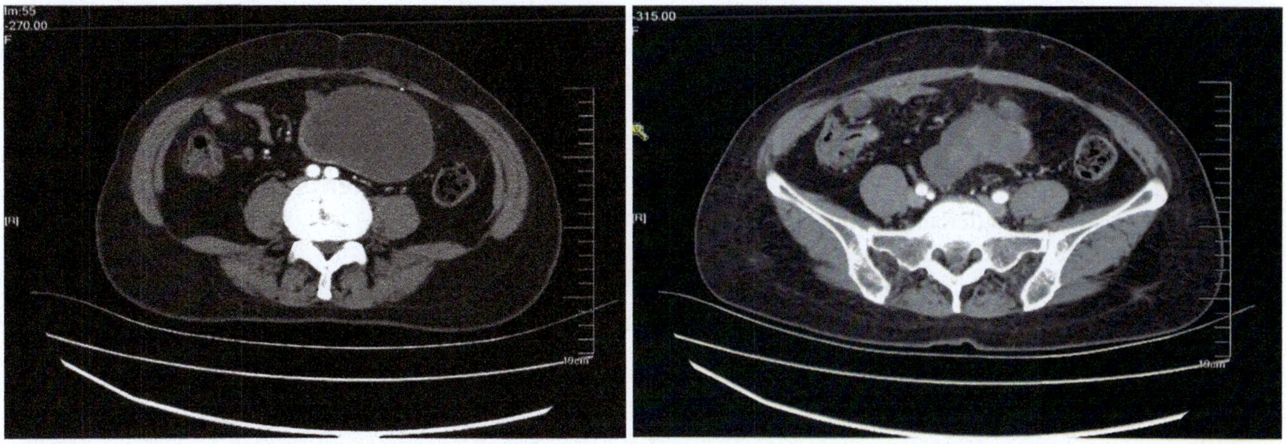

Fig. 31.2 Recurrence after 17 months of adjuvant treatment

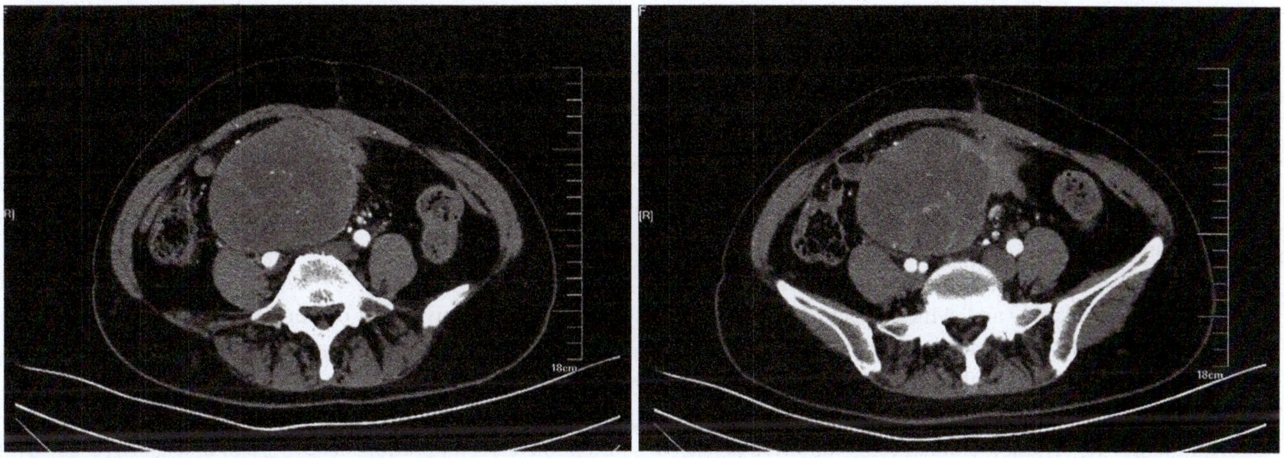

Fig. 31.3 Recurrence after the second surgery

tion. There was no ascites in the abdominal cavity, and no metastatic nodules in the pelvic cavity or peritoneum were seen. The tumor was located at the root of the mesentery with a diameter of about 10 cm and was mixed with cysts and solid masses. The peritoneum at the root of the mesentery where the mass was located was separated, and part of the peritoneum was removed to completely free the tumor. The tumor was removed, and the exploration continued. There were three additional localized nodules of different sizes, which were removed individually. Postoperative pathology indicated small intestinal GIST, and genetic testing showed exon 11 and 13 mutations of *KIT*, of which the exon 13 mutation was V654A. The patient continued to take imatinib 400 mg/d after surgery. The tumor recurred locally 3 months later (Fig. 31.3), and the patient was commenced on sunitinib 37.5 mg/d. The tumor shrank subsequently and the patient is still under close follow-up (Fig. 31.4).

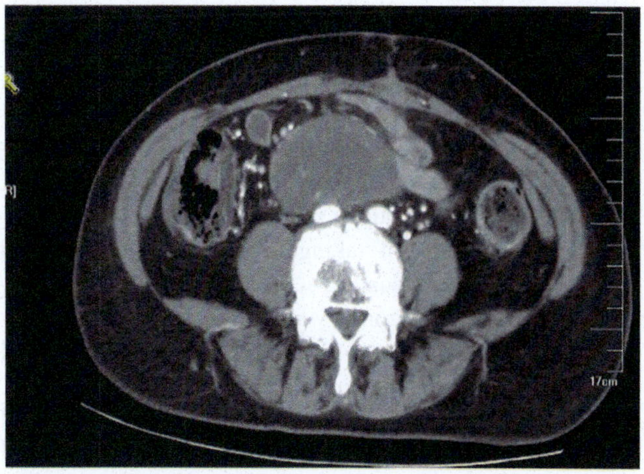

Fig. 31.4 Reexamination of CT 3 months of sunitinib therapy

31.1.5 Experience of Diagnosis and Therapy

This case was initially misdiagnosed as a gynecological tumor. Due to the limitations of CT and ultrasound, it is often difficult to determine the source of pelvic tumors [1]. Small bowel GIST are often misdiagnosed as ovarian masses or uterine fibroids. Due to different principles of surgery for gynecological uterine fibroids and surgical GIST, the gynecologist opened the abdomen for exploration and removed gynecological uterine fibroids while protecting the intestinal tract from damage as much as possible. However, most small intestinal GIST invade the entire layer of the small intestine; therefore, it is difficult to ensure that the tumor does not rupture and is completely removed while ensuring that the small intestine is not damaged. In this case, the tumor was first treated as a gynecological tumor and was removed. The pathological results indicated small intestine GIST, and intestinal resection was performed, which greatly affected the patient's prognosis. Therefore, if the pelvic mass was suspected of intestinal origins during the gynecological surgery, operation should be performed by gastrointestinal surgeons to remove both the mass and adjacent intestinal segments, which is better to avoid iatrogenic tumor rupture.

The preoperative CT scan showed a pelvic mass, which was large and lobulated, and which would be difficult to remove surgically. In such cases, a puncture biopsy can be conducted to obtain a clear pathological diagnosis before surgery. For GIST, preoperative target therapy can be administered, and tumor resection, including removal of the diseased intestinal segment, can be performed after the tumor has shrunk [2, 3]. Unfortunately, the correct diagnosis was not made for this patient before operation and the difficulty of the operation was incorrectly estimated, which also reminds us of the importance of MDT discussions. For patients with giant pelvic masses, MDT discussions, including clinicians from general surgery, urology, obstetrics and gynecology, oncology, radiology, and endoscopy disciplines, should be organized before surgery to develop individualized treatment plans and ensure that patients receive the best treatment.

After 17 months of taking imatinib, the patient had tumor recurrence, indicating secondary resistance of imatinib. Most cases of secondary resistance are caused by secondary genetic mutations [4]. Genetic testing of the second resected tumor showed exon 11 and 13 mutations of *KIT*, and the mutation of exon 13 was V654A, which is reported to result in drug-resistance [5]. The second-line drug should be taken as soon as possible according to the 2017 expert consensus. However, because the patient refused to use second-line treatment after the second operation, the tumor recurred rapidly after resection, which prompted the guiding role of genetic testing for the subsequent treatment of patients with secondary resistance. We should choose reasonable medications based on the results of genetic testing, so as to better improve the patients' relapse-free and overall survival times [6].

31.2 Expert Comments

Jinbo Gao

Large GIST and those that originate from the lower small intestine often fall into the pelvic cavity and adhere to the uterus or accessories. The symptoms and examination results are often similar to gynecological diseases, and are easily confused with some ovarian and uterine tumors, resulting in misdiagnosis. In this case, a mass approximately 12 cm in size could be felt in the region of the right appendix. Gynecological ultrasaound suggested a space occupying lesion in the right pelvic cavity, which was very easy to misdiagnose as a gynecological tumor. Therefore, GIST should be considered in the differential diagnosis of pelvic masses. If necessary, multiple ultrasound combined with CT and enteroscopy should be performed to clarify the nature of a pelvic mass and improve the preoperative diagnosis rate, so as to avoid misdiagnosis and miss the best treatment opportunity [7].

The retrospective data of our center showed that among the 38 GIST misdiagnosed as gynecological tumors in the past 13 years, 33 cases originated from the jejunum. They were all high-risk according to the modified NIH risk classification after operation. The 5-year disease-free survival rate and specific survival rate were 37.0% and 48.3%, respectively, which were significantly lower than other high-risk female GIST groups, suggesting that the malignant degree of such GIST was higher than that of ordinary high-risk female GIST. Therefore, appropriately prolonging the postoperative adjuvant treatment time of imatinib in this group of patients may be beneficial to their prognosis [8].

References

1. Boyle W, Phillips A, Vella J, Williams A, Ganesan R. Gastrointestinal stromal tumors (GISTs) as incidental findings in gynecological surgery. Int J Gynecol Pathol. 2022;41(2):186–90. https://doi.org/10.1097/PGP.0000000000000787.
2. Joensuu H, DeMatteo RP. The management of gastrointestinal stromal tumors: a model for targeted and multidisciplinary therapy of malignancy. Annu Rev Med. 2012;63:247–58. https://doi.org/10.1146/annurev-med-043010-091813.
3. von Mehren M, Joensuu H. Gastrointestinal stromal tumors. J Clin Oncol. 2018;36(2):136–43. https://doi.org/10.1200/JCO.2017.74.9705.
4. Hemming ML, Heinrich MC, Bauer S, George S. Translational insights into gastrointestinal stromal tumor and current clinical advances. Ann Oncol. 2018;29(10):2037–45. https://doi.org/10.1093/annonc/mdy309.

5. Gounder MM, Maki RG. Molecular basis for primary and secondary tyrosine kinase inhibitor resistance in gastrointestinal stromal tumor. Cancer Chemother Pharmacol. 2011;67:S25–43. https://doi.org/10.1007/s00280-010-1526-3.
6. Li J, Ye Y, Wang J, Zhang B, Qin S, Shi Y, He Y, Liang X, Liu X, Zhou Y, Wu X, Zhang X, Wang M, Gao Z, Lin T, Cao H, Shen L, Chinese Society of Clinical Oncology Csco Expert Committee on Gastrointestinal Stromal Tumor. Chinese consensus guidelines for diagnosis and management of gastrointestinal stromal tumor. Chin J Cancer Res. 2017;29(4):281–93. https://doi.org/10.21147/j.issn.1000-9604.2017.04.01.
7. Liu Y, Shahi M, Miller K, Meyer CF, Hung CF, Wu TC, Vang R, Xing D. Gastrointestinal stromal tumors mimicking gynecologic disease: clinicopathological analysis of 20 cases. Diagnostics (Basel). 2022;12(7):1563. https://doi.org/10.3390/diagnostics12071563.
8. Tao K, Zeng X, Liu W, Wang S, Gao J, Shuai X, Zhang P. Primary gastrointestinal stromal tumor mimicking as gynecologic mass: characteristics, management, and prognosis. J Surg Res. 2020;246:584–90. https://doi.org/10.1016/j.jss.2019.09.043.

32 Castleman Disease Misdiagnosed as Gastrointestinal Stromal Tumor

Chen Huang, Chun Zhuang, and Yulong He

Keywords

Gastrointestinal stromal tumor · Castleman disease · Misdiagnosis

32.1 Case 42 A 29-Year-Old Woman with Castleman Disease Misdiagnosed as Small Intestinal GIST

Chen Huang and Chun Zhuang

32.1.1 Introduction

GIST can occur at any age, but is more commonly found in middle-aged and elderly over 50 years of age, with no difference in the incidence between men and women. Additionally, GIST can occur anywhere in the gastrointestinal tract from the esophagus to the rectum. Some cases are found outside the GI tract, mainly in the omentum, mesentery and retroperitoneum, and have also been reported in the spleen, bladder, urethra and perineum. It is easy to misdiagnose GIST because of the variable sites of occurrence and the variety of imaging features. Surgeons should improve their knowledge of various rare diseases, consider the possibility of various diseases in their clinical work, and improve the accuracy of diagnosis through MDT discussion when necessary [1].

C. Huang · C. Zhuang (✉)
Department of Gastrointestinal Surgery, Renji Hospital, Shanghai Jiaotong University School of Medicine, Shanghai, China

Y. He
Digestive Diseases Center, The Seventh Affiliated Hospital of Sun Yat-sen University, Shenzhen, China
e-mail: heyulong@mail.sysu.edu.cn

32.1.2 Case Background

The patient, a 29-year-old woman, was admitted to the hospital in August 2017 for abdominal pain and bloating, with exhaustion and decreased defecation frequency. A CT scan of upper and lower abdomen showed a left mid-abdominal mass considered to be possible GIST. Gynecological ultrasound results showed no significant abnormalities. The patient came to hospital for further treatment and was admitted with an abdominal space-occupying lesion, possibly GIST.

32.1.2.1 Past History and Family History

The patient was previously healthy and reported no history of drug allergies. The patient's parents were alive, and there was no history of similar disease in the family.

32.1.2.2 Physical Examination

The patient's vital signs were stable, and the skin mucosa was not yellowish or pale. The abdomen was flat, and no gastrointestinal pattern or peristaltic waves were observed. The abdomen was slightly elevated, with mild tenderness, no rebound tenderness, and no muscle tension. A 5 cm diameter mass on the left side of the abdomen could be palpated, with medium firmness and moderate mobility. The bowel sounds were normal.

32.1.2.3 Auxiliary Examination

Enhanced Abdominal CT A left mid-abdominal mass was observed, 6.0 cm × 5.3 cm in size, considered to be possible GIST. Partial small bowel pneumatization and fluid accumulation, colon pneumatization, and stool accumulation were also observed (Fig. 32.1).

K. Tao, H. Cao (eds.), *Clinical Management of Gastrointestinal Stromal Tumor*, https://doi.org/10.1007/978-981-99-9392-5_32

32.1.2.4 Preliminary Diagnosis

Abdominal space-occupying lesions, possible GIST.

32.1.3 Therapy

32.1.3.1 Case Analysis

The patient was a young woman who presented with abdominal pain and distension for 4 days and CT revealed a possible abdominal GIST. The patient's general condition was good, and the tumor was evaluated to be resectable without metastasis. It was determined that surgical treatment should be performed, and postoperative treatment should be guided according to pathology and genetic test results.

32.1.3.2 Treatment

Laparoscopic resection of small bowel mesenteric tumor was performed under general anesthesia on August 21, 2017. Intraoperative findings revealed a 5 cm diameter spherical mass in the small intestine mesentery 30 cm below the flexor ligament with clear borders and medium texture. The intestinal wall was not involved, but the tumor was close to the small intestinal mesenteric margin, and the superior mesenteric arteriovenous trunk. Several abnormally large trophoblastic vessels could be seen on the surface of the tumor and several enlarged lymph nodes could be seen in the mesenteric root. No metastases were found in the liver, pelvis, or peritoneum, and no abnormalities were found in the uterus or bilateral adnexa. The uterus and bilateral adnexa did not show any abnormal occupancy (Figs. 32.2 and 32.3).

32.1.3.3 Postoperative Pathology and Genetic Testing

Pathological Diagnosis Small intestinal mesenteric *Castleman* disease (CD) proliferating cells.

Immunohistochemistry CD20 (+/−), CD79a (+/−), CD3 (+/−), CD5 (−), CD21 (dendritic cells, +), CD23 (dendritic cells, +), Bcl-2 (+), Bcl-6 (−), CyclinD1 (−), Ki-67 (Li: 30%), κ (+/−), λ (+/−), CD138 (+/−).

32.1.4 Prognosis

The patient was followed up regularly after surgery, and as of December 2021, no recurrence of metastasis was seen on CT review.

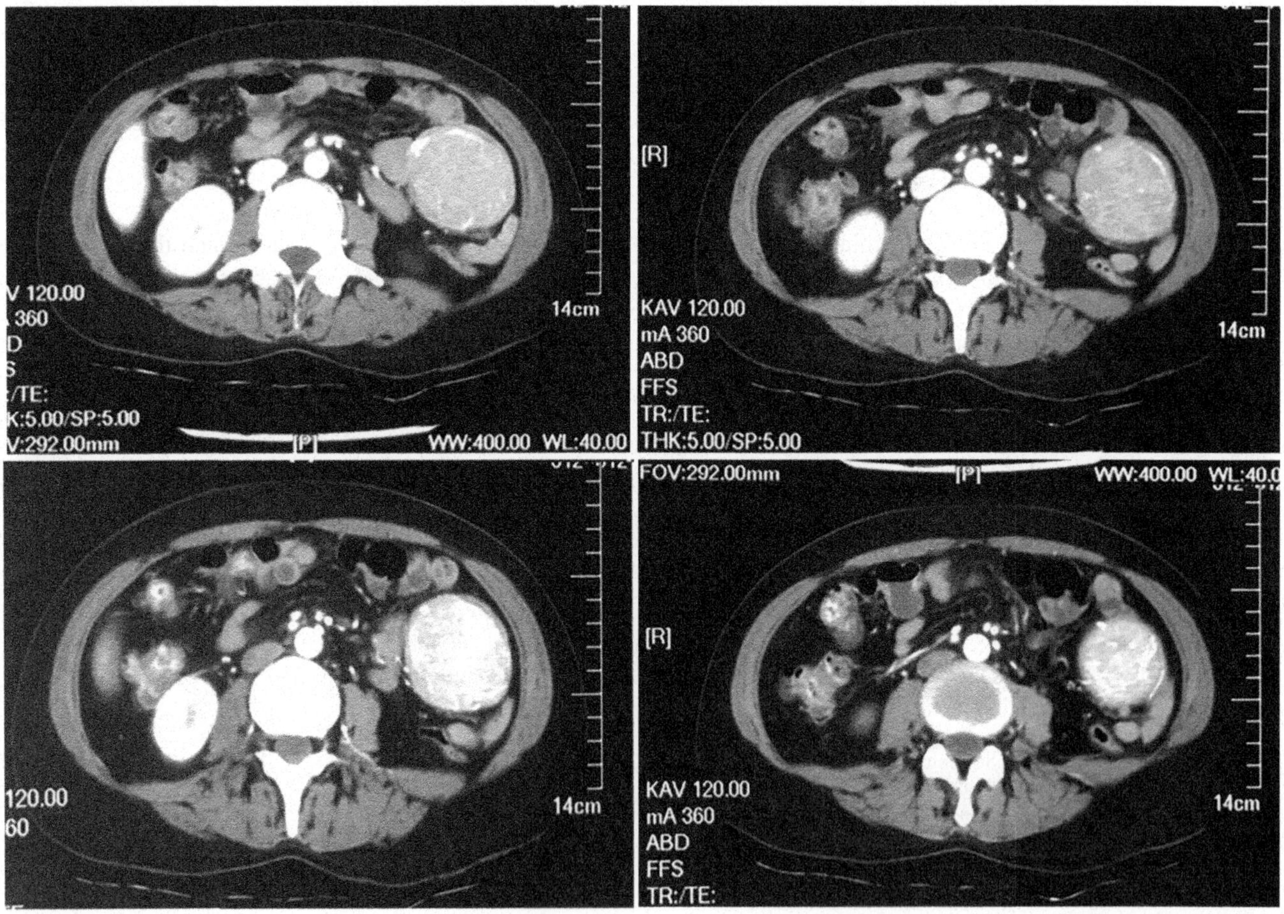

Fig. 32.1 CT showed a left mid-abdomen space-occupying lesion

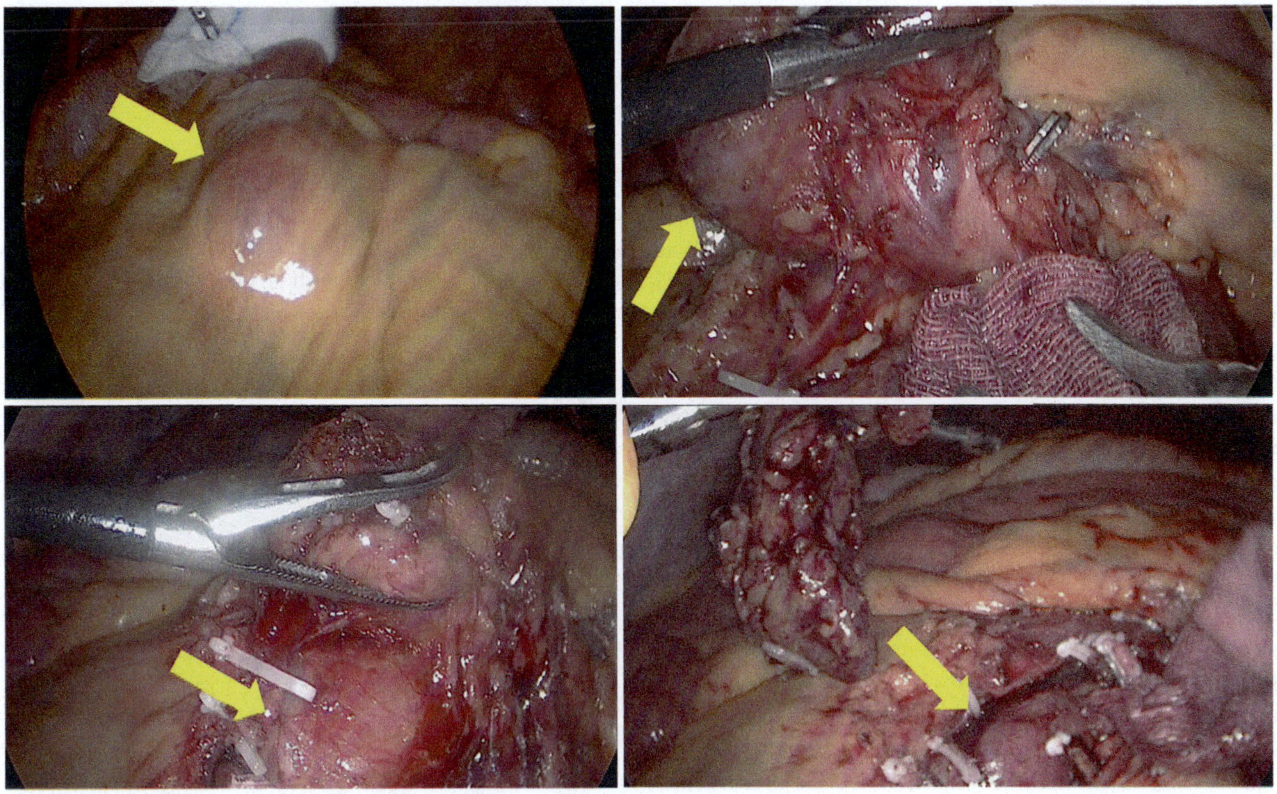

Fig. 32.2 Intraoperative laparoscopic exploration

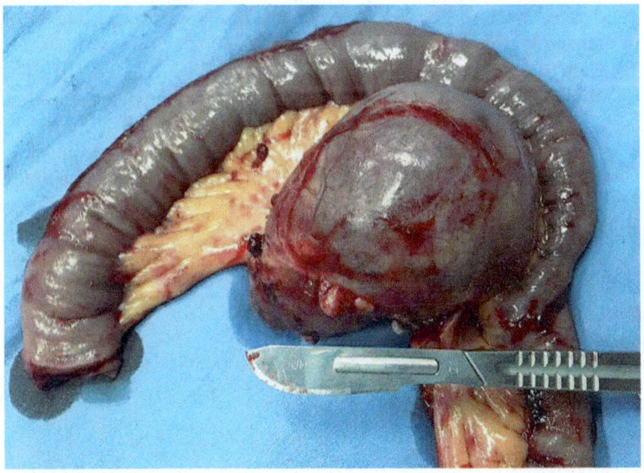

Fig. 32.3 The gross specimen

32.1.5 Experience of Diagnosis and Therapy

CD is a reactive lymphadenopathy of unknown origin and is relatively uncommon in clinical practice. The pathology is characterized by distinct lymphatic follicles, vascular and plasma cell hyperplasia of varying degrees, and significant enlargement of deep or superficial lymph nodes. Some cases of CD may be associated with systemic symptoms. In most cases, the results are good after surgical removal of the enlarged lymph nodes, and CD is clinically classified into focal and multicentric types [2].

1. Unicentric CD

The median age of onset is 20 years old. It can occur in any part of the lymphatic tissue, but mediastinal lymph nodes are the most common location, followed by cervical, axillary, and abdominal lymph nodes, and occasionally extra-nodal tissues, such as the larynx, vulva, pericardium, intracranial subcutaneous muscle, lung, and orbits. Most cases have no systemic symptoms, and masses can exist within the body for a long time, that is, they have a benign disease course.

2. Multicentric CD

Multicentric type CD is less common than the focal type, and the median age of onset is 57 years. Patients have enlarged lymph nodes in multiple locations and are prone to superficial lymph nodes. Multicentric type CD is associated with systemic symptoms (such as fever) and hepatosplenomegaly, and often manifests with multisystem involvement, such as nephrotic syndrome, amyloidosis, myasthenia gravis, peripheral neuropathy, temporal arteritis, Schegren's syndrome (dry syndrome), thrombotic thrombocytopenic purpura, and oral and corneal inflammatory reactions. Twenty to thirty percent of patients may develop Kaposi's sarcoma or B-cell lymphoma during the course of the disease. A few patients with concurrent polyneuropathy, organ enlargement (liver, spleen), endocrinopathy, serum monoclonal immunoglobulin, and skin lesions will constitute clinical signs of POEMS syndrome (polyneuropathy, organomegaly, endocrinopathy, M-protein, skin changes). In addition, the multicentric type often has an aggressive clinical course and is prone to concomitant infections [2–5].

Abdominal CD needs to be differentiated from a number of other tumors rich in blood supply, including GIST, paraganglioma, and nerve sheath tumors. GIST mostly originates from the gastrointestinal tract and show significant enhancement on enhanced CT. Paragangliomas are usually found in the para-aortic region of the sympathetic chain and exhibit moderate or significant enhancement on enhanced CT. Nerve sheath tumors are usually found in the retroperitoneal paraspinal sulcus and typically penetrate the intervertebral foramen with a dumbbell-like appearance. Cystic changes are more common, but calcification and hemorrhage are rare and can be significantly enhanced on enhanced CT; however, the degree of enhancement is lower than that of clear vascular CD.

The reason for the misdiagnosis in this case is the lack of awareness of rare diseases, and the first subjective preference for the most common disorder, GIST, after CT findings of interstitial lobar-derived masses, while ignoring some of the features that were not consistent with GIST in this case, such as age of onset, which was not consistent with GIST as this generally occurs in middle-aged and elderly; and multiple lymph node metastases, which rarely occur with GIST [2, 6–8].

32.2 Expert Comments

Yulong He

Castleman disease is a non-neoplastic lesion caused by proliferation of lymphoid tissue, also known as vascular follicular hyperplasia. When a tumor is located in the abdominal or pelvic cavities, it needs to be differentiated from GIST, lymphoma, and neurogenic tumors. In this case, preoperative CT suggested GIST, but preoperative cytological examination by fine needle aspiration was not performed, leading to misdiagnosis. The treatment of CD varies depending on the type of CD. For focal CD, surgery is preferred, and the prognosis is favorable, while multicentric and plasma cell CD are prone to recurrence and transformation into lymphoma, which should be treated with a combination of surgical resection and postoperative adjuvant chemotherapy.

References

1. Blay JY, Kang YK, Nishida T, von Mehren M. Gastrointestinal stromal tumours. Nat Rev Dis Primers. 2021;7(1):22. https://doi.org/10.1038/s41572-021-00254-5.
2. Hoffmann C, Hentrich M, Tiemann M, Rosenwald A, Weber F, Willenbacher W, Hubel K. Recent advances in Castleman disease. Oncol Res Treat. 2022;45(11):693–704. https://doi.org/10.1159/000526640.
3. Wu D, Lim MS, Jaffe ES. Pathology of Castleman disease. Hematol Oncol Clin North Am. 2018;32(1):37–52. https://doi.org/10.1016/j.hoc.2017.09.004.
4. Cronin DM, Warnke RA. Castleman disease: an update on classification and the spectrum of associated lesions. Adv Anat Pathol. 2009;16(4):236–46. https://doi.org/10.1097/PAP.0b013e3181a9d4d3.
5. Wang XQ, Zhong NN, Sun Q, Yan SC, Xu GC, Wang YG, Peng LW, Liu B, Bu LL. Comprehensive analysis of 65 patients with Castleman disease in a single center in China. Sci Rep. 2022;12(1):8694. https://doi.org/10.1038/s41598-022-12797-y.
6. Han SL, Chen XX, Zheng XF, Yan JY, Shen X, Zhu GB. The clinicopathological behaviour and surgical treatment of abdominal Castleman's disease. Singapore Med J. 2010;51(10):813–6.
7. Abramson JS. Diagnosis and management of Castleman disease. J Natl Compr Cancer Netw. 2019;17(11.5):1417–9. https://doi.org/10.6004/jnccn.2019.5037.
8. Dispenzieri A, Fajgenbaum DC. Overview of Castleman disease. Blood. 2020;135(16):1353–64. https://doi.org/10.1182/blood.2019000931.

Other Primary Malignant Tumors Misdiagnosed as Recurrent Gastrointestinal Stromal Tumor

33

Bo Ni, Lin Tu, Chen Huang, Xin Wu, Wenchang Yang, Weizhen Liu, and Hui Cao

Keywords

Abdominal mass · Recurrence · Gastrointestinal stromal tumor · Fibromatosis · Rhabdomyosarcoma · Misdiagnose

33.1 Case 43 A 53-Year-Old Man with Fibromatosis Misdiagnosed as Recurrent GIST

Bo Ni and Lin Tu

33.1.1 Introduction

The diagnosis of GIST mainly relies on histopathology and immunohistochemical staining [1, 2]. At present, the clinical protocol of diagnosis for GIST has been increasingly improved. However, it is common for GIST to be combined with other kinds of tumors, which is a challenge for clinical diagnosis and treatment [3, 4]. Especially for postoperative patients, recurrence and metastasis from primary GIST are difficult to distinguish from other tumors [5, 6]. These patients deserve more attention from clinicians to avoid misdiagnosis and mistreatment. Moreover, it is necessary to make full use of the combined MDT individualized treatment modeling, and devise an appropriate treatment and follow-up plan [7–9].

33.1.2 Case Background

In November 2015, the patient, a 53-year-old man, was diagnosed with fundic GIST by gastroscopy (Fig. 33.1) and underwent laparoscopic local resection. Postoperative pathological examination diagnosed a gastric GIST, 5.2 cm × 4.3 cm × 3.0 cm in size, mitotic count <5/50 HPF, and intermediate risk according to modified NIH risk classification. Genetic testing showed a heterozygous deletion mutation in exon 11 of *KIT* at codons 557–558, which encoded tryptophan and lysine amino acids. Adjuvant therapy with 400 mg/d imatinib was initiated 3 weeks after the operation. In May 2017, contrast-enhanced CT revealed possible postoperative changes in the stomach and an emerging mass in the mesogastric region of right lower abdomen with the possibility of metastases (Fig. 33.2). The patient then came to Renji Hospital Affiliated to Shanghai Jiaotong University School of Medicine for further treatment and was admitted with space-occupying lesions in the right lower abdomen following resection of gastric GIST.

33.1.2.1 Past History and Family History

The patient had a 10-year history of hypertension which was well controlled with medication, a 1-year history of coronary heart disease, and 50% stenosis in coronary angiography, identified 1 year earlier, controlled by oral aspirin. The patient reported no history of drug allergies or relevant family history.

33.1.2.2 Physical Examination

The patient had stable vital signs without any positive abdominal signs.

B. Ni · L. Tu (✉) · C. Huang · H. Cao
Department of Gastrointestinal Surgery, Renji Hospital, Shanghai Jiaotong University School of Medicine, Shanghai, China

X. Wu (✉)
Department of General Surgery, The First Medical Center, Chinese PLA General Hospital, Beijing, China

W. Yang · W. Liu (✉)
Department of Gastrointestinal Surgery, Union Hospital, Tongji Medical College, Huazhong University of Science and Technology, Wuhan, China
e-mail: yangwenchang@hust.edu.cn; liuweizhen@hust.edu.cn

K. Tao, H. Cao (eds.), *Clinical Management of Gastrointestinal Stromal Tumor*, https://doi.org/10.1007/978-981-99-9392-5_33

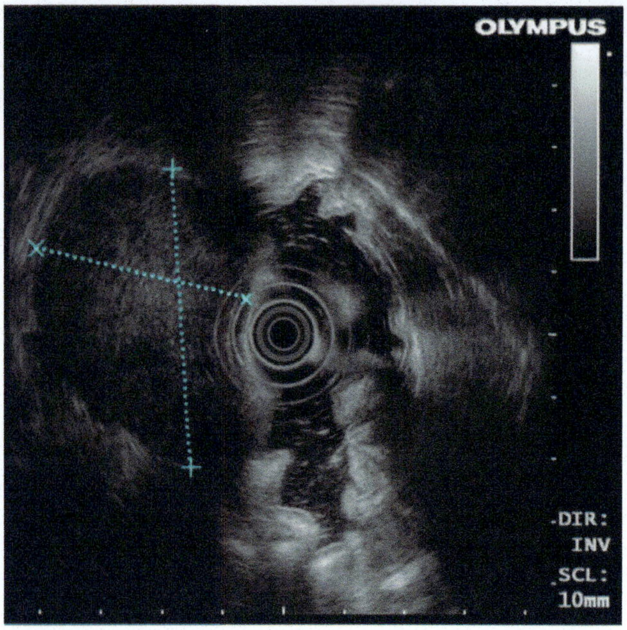

Fig. 33.1 Endoscopic Ultrasonography indicated the possible diagnosis of GIST

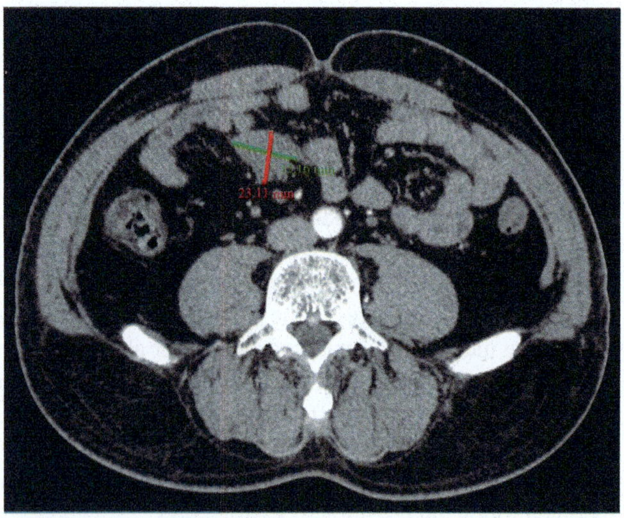

Fig. 33.2 Re-examination of enhanced CT before the secondary operation

33.1.2.3 Auxiliary Examination

Abdomen CT Postoperative changes of the stomach and an emerging mass in the mesogastric region of right lower abdomen with the possibility of GIST metastases.

33.1.2.4 Preliminary Diagnosis

1. Space-occupying lesions in abdominal cavity: possible recurrence and metastasis of GIST

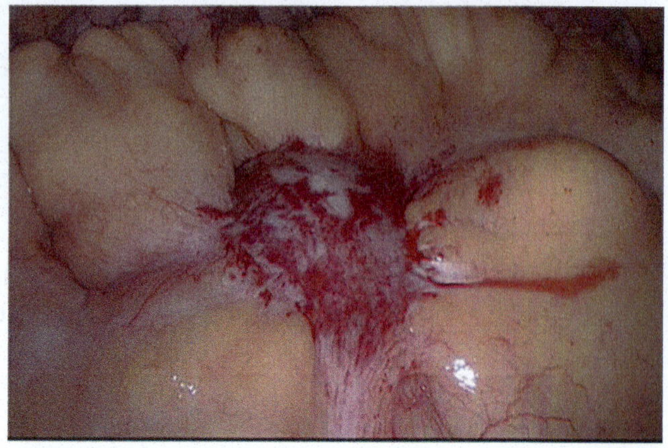

Fig. 33.3 Intraoperative exploration revealed an invasive tumor with a diameter of 3 cm at the mesentery of small intestine

2. Postoperative gastric GIST
3. Coronary heart disease
4. Hypertension grade 2, high-risk

33.1.3 Therapy

33.1.3.1 Case Analysis

The patient was a middle-aged man and had received resection of gastric GIST. The abdominal CT scan indicated a new mass possibly as recurrence. Considering this patient was generally in good health and the new tumor was resectable, it was determined that surgery should be performed. The postoperative targeted therapy should be scheduled based on the results of pathological examination.

33.1.3.2 Therapy

On July 24, 2017, laparoscopic exploration and resection of a small intestinal mesenteric tumor were performed under general anesthesia. During the operation, no obvious new mass was found at the resection site of the primary gastric tumor, but a 3 cm tumor was found in the mesentery of small intestine 2 m away from the ileocecal region. The tumor did not invade the intestinal wall of the small intestine, and there was not any relapse in the liver or peritoneum (Fig. 33.3).

33.1.3.3 Postoperative Pathology and Genetic Testing

Pathology The small intestinal mesenteric tumor was diagnosed as fibromatosis-like hyperplasia (4.0 cm × 3.5 cm × 2.0 cm, Fig. 33.4), with negative margin and negative regional lymph node.

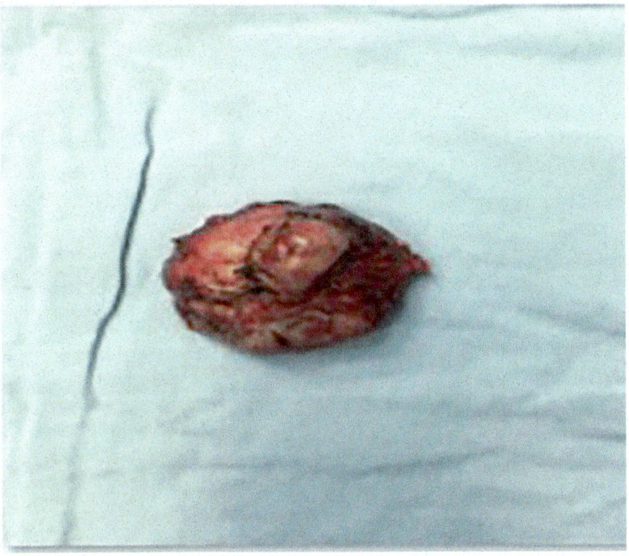

Fig. 33.4 The gross specimen

Immunohistochemistry β-catenin (+), SMA (+/−), CD117 (−), CD34 (−), DOG-1 (−), S-100 (−), Ki-67 (Li: <1%), P53 (+/−).

Genetic Testing Wild type *KIT* and *PDGFRA*.

Pathological Diagnosis Desmoid fibromatosis

33.1.4 Prognosis

The patient recovered smoothly and 400 mg/d imatinib was scheduled on the 7th day after surgery. Follow-up in December 2021 revealed no obvious tumor recurrence or metastasis.

33.2 Case 44 A 69-Year-Old Woman with Rhabdomyosarcoma Misdiagnosed as Recurrent GIST

Chen Huang and Xin Wu

33.2.1 Case Background

The patient, a 69-year-old woman, was admitted to our gynecology department in July 2017 for presentation of a pelvic mass with abdominal pain and distension for several months, 14 years after GIST. A PET-CT showed a right pelvic hypermetabolic lesion, which was considered malignant, and multiple hypermetabolic nodes in the right clavicular area, perihepatic and subperitoneal area, colonic splenic flexure, left parietal iliac vessels, and pelvic cavity, which were considered to have a high probability of being multiple metastatic lesions. Puncture biopsy of the pelvic mass revealed a spindle cell tumor, and immunohistochemistry showed CD117 (+), DOG-1 (+), CD34 (+), Ki-67 (Li: 15%), SMA (−), S-100 (−) (Fig. 33.5). Combined with the clinical history, the patient was considered to have multiple GIST metastases and Imatinib 600 mg/d was administered.

At the end of 2017, CT showed bilateral pleural effusion and increased abdominal effusion, and symptomatic support was given. In March 2018, she was treated in the emergency department for anemia, (Hb 60 g/L), and dyspnea, and CT revealed irregular pelvic and presacral masses with uneven density, consistent with GIST with necrosis and hemorrhage, and large abdominopelvic effusion. The patient was given a blood transfusion, drainage and symptomatic support and other treatments for symptom relief and started oral sunitinib 37.5 mg/d treatment. The patient was admitted to our hospital for further treatment in April 2018 when her abdominal symptoms worsened, and she developed intermittent fever.

33.2.1.1 Past History and Family History

Partial gastrectomy with pancreatic body and tail resection and splenectomy in August 2003 for gastric GIST. She reported no history of drug allergies. The parents were deceased, and there was no family history of similar disease.

33.2.1.2 Physical Examination

The patient's vital signs were stable, and she appeared anemic with visible emaciation and a lower abdominal bulge. A palpable mass, approximately 15 cm in size, was noted to be hard, with ill-defined borders, non-mobile, tender, without rebound tenderness, and normal bowel sounds were present.

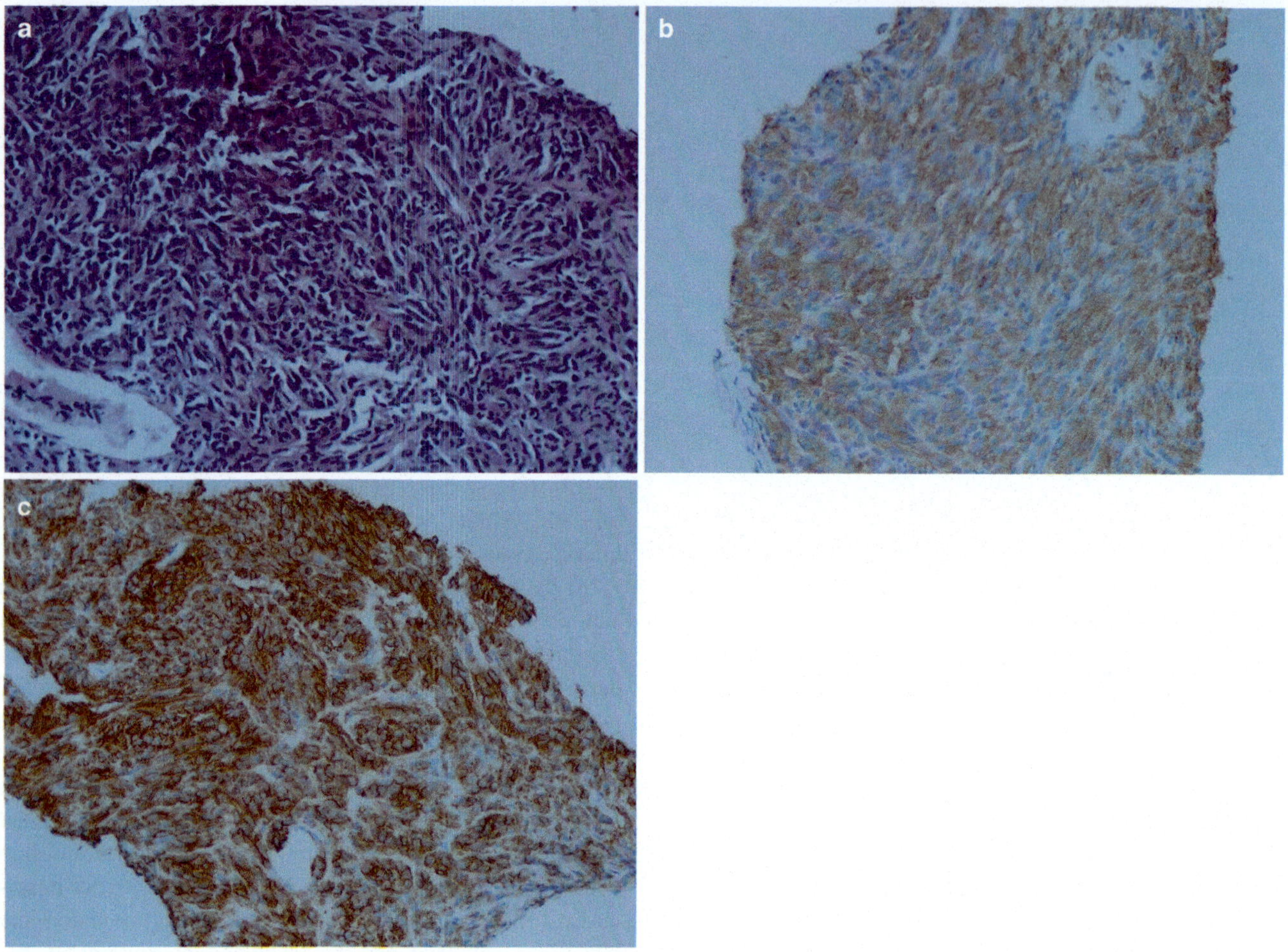

Fig. 33.5 Immunohistochemistry. **a** HE staining of the puncture specimen. **b** Positive CD117 staining. **c** Positive DOG-1 staining

33.2.1.3 Auxiliary Examination

Blood Routine Test Hb 90/L, no other abnormalities detected.

Biochemical and Tumor Markers ALB 31 g/L, CA125 1016 U/mL, the rest of the indicators were normal.

Enhanced Abdominal CT Diffuse occupancy of the abdominopelvic cavity with consideration of metastasis and abdominopelvic effusion (Fig. 33.6).

33.2.1.4 Preliminary Diagnosis

1. GIST abdominopelvic multiple metastases
2. Postoperative gastric GIST
3. Mild anemia
4. Abdominopelvic effusion

33.2.2 Therapy

33.2.2.1 Case Analysis

The patient was an elderly woman, who was previously treated with surgery for gastric GIST and received treatment with imatinib 400 mg/d for 14 years after surgery, with intermittent review and no tumor recurrence. One year ago, a pelvic mass with anemia was found, and a puncture biopsy confirmed the recurrence of GIST metastasis, and a higher imatinib dose and sunitinib were administered, but the tumor continued to increase in size, with rupture and bleeding. With symptomatic support and other treatments, the patient's condition was stable, and the tumor was evaluated for possible resection with indications for surgery and postoperative targeted therapy would be determined based on the results of genetic testing.

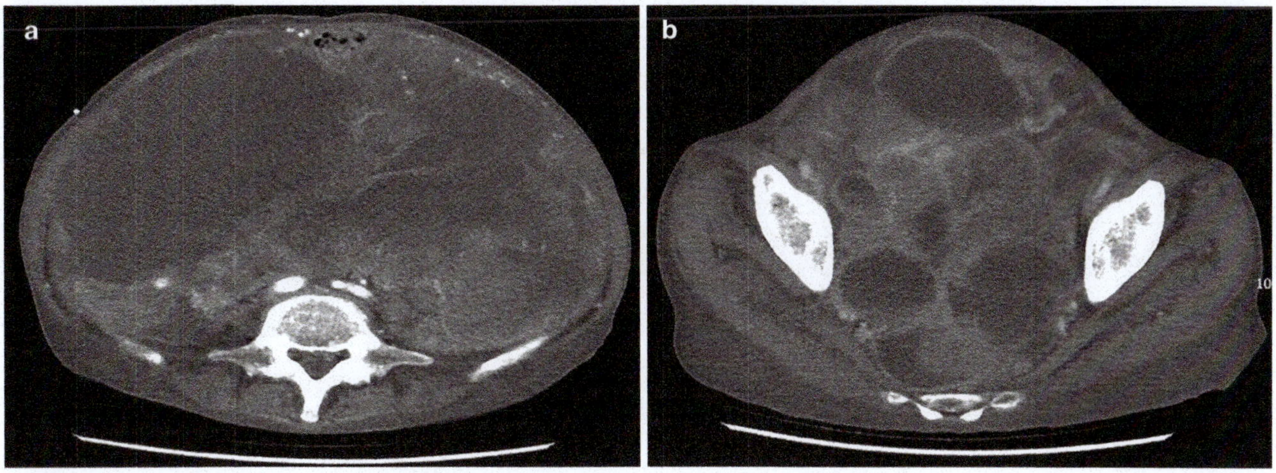

Fig. 33.6 Preoperative CT. **a** Abdominal cavity; **b** Pelvic cavity

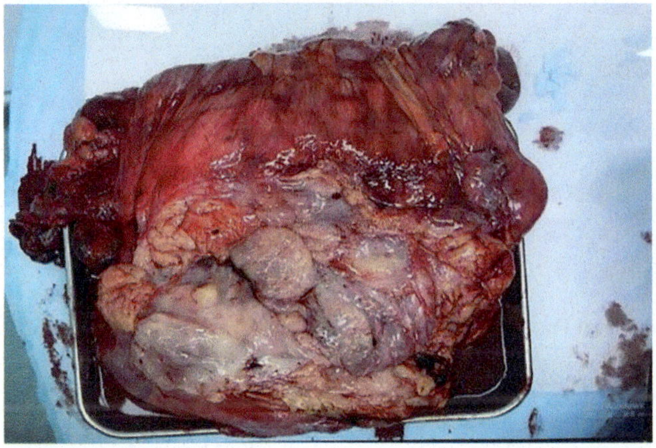

Fig. 33.7 The gross specimen

33.2.2.2 Treatment

A lumpectomy with multivisceral resection (uterus, bilateral adnexa, left hemi colon, sigmoid colon, part of rectum, greater omentum, appendix, and gallbladder), bilateral ureteral stent placement, transverse colon-rectal anastomosis with ileostomy were performed under general anesthesia on May 29, 2018. Intraoperative findings: clear and bright abdominal fluid of 1000 mL, multiple tumors of different sizes in the abdominopelvic cavity, the largest tumor in the main body was of the fusion type, with a diameter of more than 20 cm, spanning the abdominopelvic cavity (Fig. 33.7).

33.2.2.3 Postoperative Pathology and Genetic Testing

Pathological Diagnosis High-grade soft tissue sarcoma, considered together with immunohistochemistry, is consistent with rhabdomyosarcoma, histologically graded G3. The tumor invaded the plasma membrane of the uterus to the myometrium, the plasma layer of the colon and the greater omentum.

Immunohistochemistry CD117 (−), CD34 (−), DOG-1 (−), Ki-67 (Li:90%), S-100 (−), Vimentin (+), MyoD1 (+), Myoglobin (+), Myosin (focal +) (Fig. 33.8).

Genetic Testing No mutations in *KIT* or *PDGFRA*.

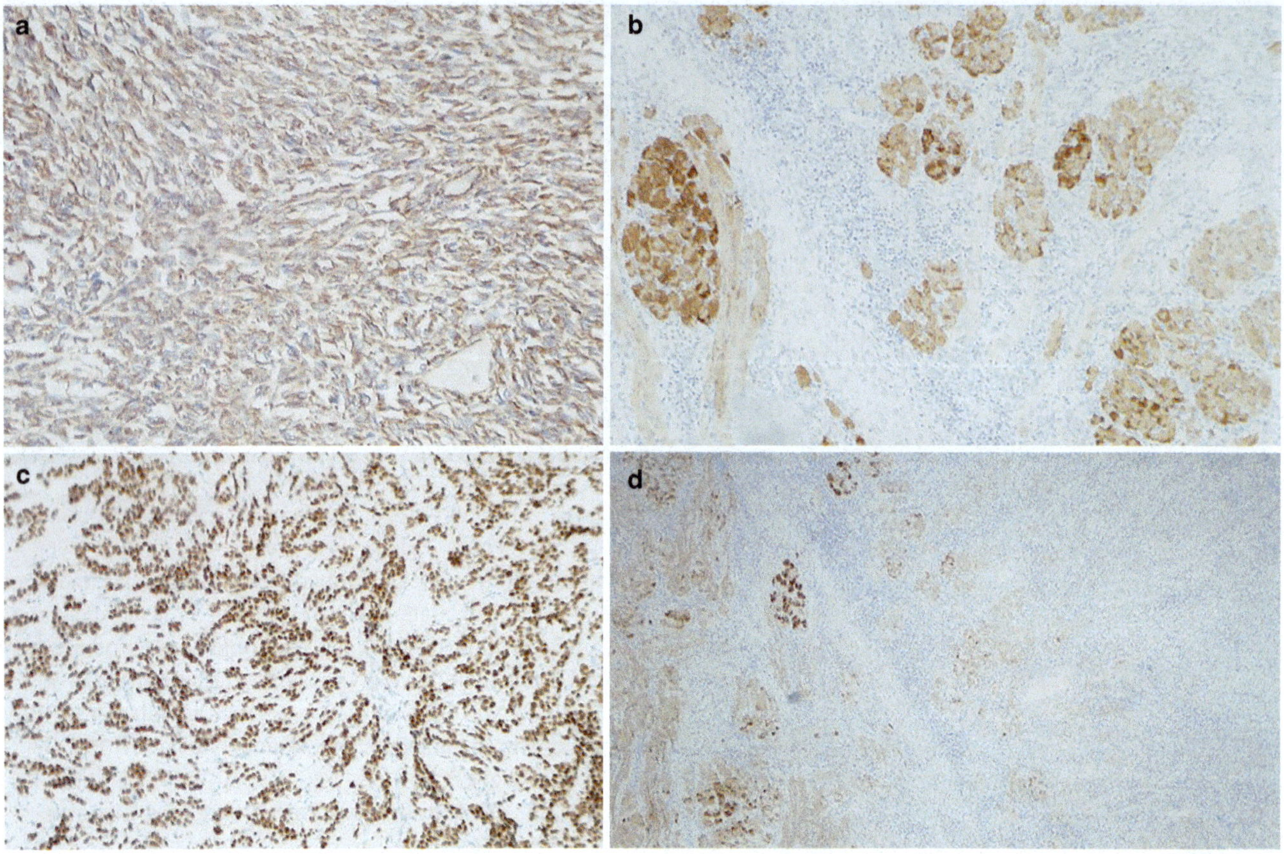

Fig. 33.8 Postoperative immunohistochemistry. **a** Positive Vimentin staining. **b** Positive Myoglobin staining. **c** Positive staining for MyoD1. **d** Positive staining for Myosin

33.2.3 Prognosis

The patient was discharged from the hospital 45 days after surgery. As of October, with a 3-month follow-up, the patient was in fair general condition, taking sunitinib, and no clear signs of tumor recurrence had been detected.

33.3 Case 45 Aggressive Fibromatosis Misdiagnosed as Recurrent GIST

Wenchang Yang and Weizhen Liu

33.3.1 Case Background

The patient, a 52-year-old man, presented to the Union Hospital, Tongji Medical College of Huazhong University of Science and Technology for investigation of right lower quadrant abdominal pain for 1 week, 11 months after surgery for a small intestinal GIST. The patient underwent surgical treatment for small bowel tumor resection at a local hospital in December 2018. Postoperative pathology showed small bowel GIST, size 5.2 cm × 4.5 cm × 3.0 cm, and mitotic count <5/50 HPF, the modified NIH risk classification was intermediate risk. Immunohistochemical staining showed that tumor cells were CD117 (+), DOG-1 (+), CD34 (−), SMA (+), S-100 (−). The genetic test results indicated a deletion mutation in *KIT* exon 11, and the mutation was p.M552_W557del. After the operation, the patient was treated with imatinib 400 mg/d adjuvant treatment, which was well tolerated. One week ago, the patient suffered pain in the right lower abdomen with no obvious cause. A plain CT scan of the abdomen at the local hospital revealed a space-occupying lesion in the small intestine of the right lower abdomen, and the surrounding lymph nodes were swollen. The patient then attended the Department of Gastrointestinal Surgery, Union Hospital, Tongji Medical

College, Huazhong University of Science and Technology for further diagnosis and treatment.

33.3.1.1 Past History and Family History

The patient was previously healthy, and reported no history of drug allergies. There was no similar medical history in the family.

33.3.1.2 Physical Examination

The patient's vital signs were stable, and the skin and mucous membranes were not yellowish or pale. The patient's abdomen was flat, no gastrointestinal or peristaltic waves were observed. Surgical scars were seen on the abdomen. The abdomen was soft, with no tenderness or rebound tenderness. Bowel sounds were normal.

33.3.1.3 Auxiliary Examination

Blood Routine WBC 3.67×10^9/L ↓, RBC 3.5×10^9/L ↓, Hb 102 g/L ↓, PLT 208×10^9/L ↑, NEUT% 64.6%, LY% 21.9%.

Blood Biochemistry TBil 11.9 μmol/L, DBil 4.0 μmol/L, TP 70.0 g/L, ALB 48.0 g/L, Cre 76.3 μmol/L, BUN 5.93 mmol/L, Na^+ 140.0 mmol/L, K^+ 3.93 mmol/L, Cl^- 101.3 mmol/L.

In November 2019, the upper and lower abdomen and pelvic plain scan and enhanced CT revealed postoperative changes of the small intestine on the right side of the middle and lower abdomen. An area of soft tissue density could be seen between the intestinal tubes and the mesentery area, approximately 7.1 cm × 6.0 cm in size, and there was uneven enhancement. There was an increase in small lymph nodes in the mesenteric area, which needed to be differentiated from reactive hyperplasia and neoplastic lesions. There were multiple cysts in the liver. Combined with the medical history, the possibility of tumor recurrence and incomplete intestinal obstruction after small bowel surgery should be considered (Fig. 33.9).

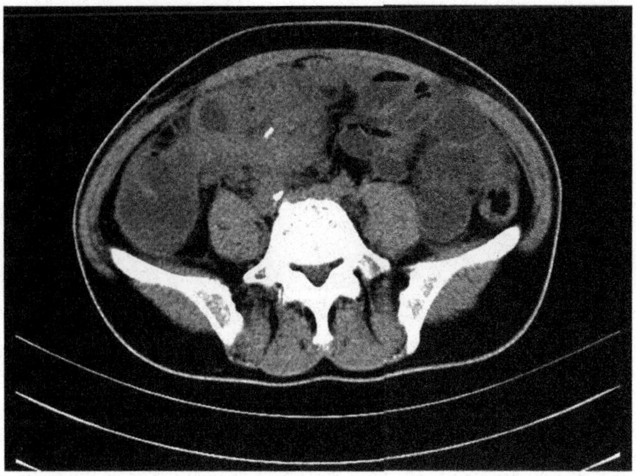

Fig. 33.9 CT showed multiple occupying lesions in the small intestine

33.3.1.4 Primary Diagnosis

1. Tumor recurrence after small bowel GIST resection
2. Incomplete intestinal obstruction

33.3.2 Therapy

33.3.2.1 Case Analysis

The patient was a middle-aged man. The tumor recurred during the standard-dose adjuvant treatment with imatinib after small bowel GIST. The recurrent tumor was assessed to be independent, resectable, and feasible for surgical treatment. Subsequent targeted therapy was to be administered based on pathology and genetic testing.

33.3.2.2 Treatment

Partial small bowel resection, partial colectomy and separation of intestinal adhesions were performed under general anesthesia on November 28, 2019. During the procedure, small intestinal wall segmental swelling and thickening. The portion of small intestine which was worst affected was that near the original anastomosis, and this was closely related to the colon and iliac blood vessels. There were no obvious metastases in the remaining organs, peritoneum, or pelvic cavity, and no ascites was observed. The patient recovered well after the operation and was discharged 6 days.

33.3.2.3 Postoperative Pathology

Pathological Diagnosis Terminal ileum and ascending colon mesenteric fibrosis adhesion, accompanied by a large number of acute and chronic inflammatory cell infiltrations and abscess formation. No residual tumor cells were seen on the slices. No tumor tissue metastasis was found on the sections of mesenteric lymph nodes. Combined with the immunohistochemistry, the mass was considered to be an aggressive fibroma.

Immunohistochemistry CD34, CD117 and DOG-1 did not indicate the presence of GIST. SMA and desmin staining showed that the fibrotic area contained a large number of proliferating fibers/myofibroblasts (Fig. 33.10).

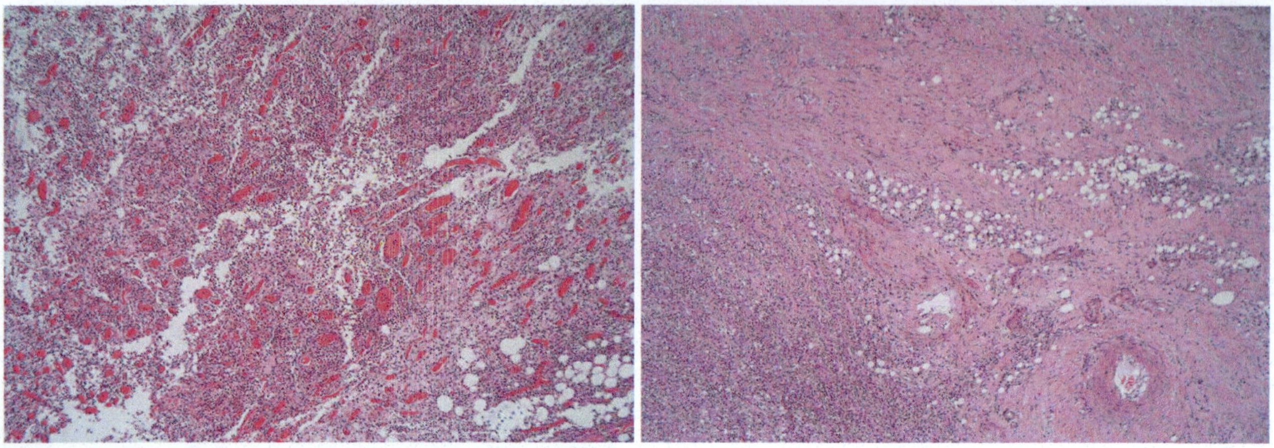

Fig. 33.10 Fiber/myofibroblast

33.3.3 Prognosis

The patient was discharged 6 days after the operation and resumed treatment with imatinib 400 mg/d 2 weeks after the operation. As of January 2022, there was no obvious discomfort or side effects, and the patient has survived without recurrence.

33.3.4 Experience of Diagnosis and Therapy

33.3.4.1 The Morbidity of GIST Combined with Desmoid Fibromatosis

Desmoid fibromatosis is commonly seen in location of surgery or traumatic lesions. GIST and desmoid fibromatosis rarely occur simultaneously. In 75% cases of GIST patients with desmoid fibromatosis, the latter developed after surgery for GIST [10].

33.3.4.2 The Diagnosis of Desmoid Fibromatosis

Desmoid fibromatosis is a rare soft tissue tumor with moderate malignancy which is prone to local recurrence, rather than distant metastasis [11]. The classification generally includes three types: outside-abdominal type, abdominal-wall type and intra-abdominal type [12]. Imaging often shows invasive growth, mostly with an unclear boundary, no capsule, and rarely with necrosis or calcification. There are no specific imaging characteristics, so this tumor is usually misdiagnosed. Intra-abdominal desmoid fibromatosis is easily misdiagnosed as GIST. Immunohistochemical markers are very helpful in identifying mesenchymal tumors in the gastrointestinal tract. The common markers are Vimentin, SMA, MSA, desmin, CD117, CD34, and S-100. Vimentin is commonly expressed in normal mesenchymal cells and mesenchymal tumors and is a marker to distinguish from epithelial tumors [13]. The overexpression of CD117 and CD34 is used for diagnosis of GIST, while SMA is used for diagnosis of smooth muscle tumors, except for some non-myogenic tumors with myoid phenotype, such as fibromatosis [14]. Desmin is widely distributed in skeletal muscle, smooth muscle, and myocardium, which is strongly expressed in benign muscle tumors. In addition, desmin is also expressed in myofibroblastoma and fibromatosis. S-100 protein is an acidic protein distributed in the nervous system and mainly used for diagnosis of neurological tumors, such as schwannomas, malignant nerve sheath tumors, and neurofibromas [15]. Therefore, the above markers lack specificity for fibromatosis. β-catenin is a multifunctional cytoplasmic protein, which is not only a key member of the Wnt signaling pathway for transcriptional regulatory function but is also an important component of the epithelial cadherin complex. The nuclear accumulation of β-catenin could be detected by immunohistochemistry, which expresses sensitively and specifically in desmoid fibromatosis [16]. So, β-catenin is one reliable marker for diagnosis of desmoid fibromatosis.

If an abdominal mass occurs after primary surgery for GIST, recurrence or metastasis ranks as the first diagnostic consideration. The patient in the case 43 was post-gastric GIST resection, and follow-up CT revealed a new mass in the small intestinal mesentery. In this case the possibility of GIST recurrence was first considered in the context of the medical history. However, reflecting on the diagnostic process of this case, the patient had an intermediate-risk GIST with a low recurrence rate during treatment with imatinib. Hence, the hidden face of clinical syndromes should be comprehensively revealed if the evidence is inconsistent with the train of thought on diagnosis and treatment. Careful analysis of imaging data and consideration of antidiastole could improve the accuracy of preoperative diagnosis for similar cases. The CT features of desmoid fibromatosis showed a single mass with clear boundaries, regular shapes, round or lobulated, and no invasive manifestations [17]. Owing to the enrichment of spindle-shaped fibrous cells in desmoid fibroma, the contrast medium cannot enter the lesion in a short time, resulting to mild enhancement during the arterial phase. In contrast, GIST is a blood-rich tumor, and its typical manifestation is obvious enhancement in the arterial phase.

33.3.4.3 The Therapy for Desmoid Fibromatosis

Surgery is the primary treatment for fibromatosis, but with a considerable postoperative relapse rate, about 20–30% [18]. Local radiotherapy is feasible for defined tumors, those undergoing repeat recurrence or losing the opportunity for radical resection. For advanced patients, methotrexate combined with vinblastine and pazopanib are used to achieve certain effects, proposed by some studies.

33.3.4.4 Rhabdomyosarcoma

Genetic secondary mutation is an important mechanism of drug resistance in GIST, but GIST usually retains its original morphological features and immunophenotype. It has been reported that some imatinib-treated GIST can transform from spindle cells to epithelial-like cells, showing various degrees of decreased KIT protein expression, deletion, or even chemotaxis, transdifferentiation, or dedifferentiation changes [19]. The histomorphology and immunophenotype of the patient's tumor in Case 44 underwent rhabdomyosarcoma differentiation after imatinib resistance, with absent KIT expression but positive expression of markers of rhabdomyosarcoma differentiation, such as myogenin. This may be related to the presence of GIST heterogeneity and its possible association with multidirectional differentiation after treatment, and the mechanism remains to be investigated. Therefore, this case suggests that in our clinical work, when some cases with good drug control suddenly present with rapid progression, we should think about this possibility. And if surgical intervention is possible, early surgical removal of the lesion will be beneficial to the patient's prognosis. It has also given me a deeper understanding of "treating different diseases together and treating the same disease differently" proposed by traditional Chinese medicine.

33.4 Expert Comments

Hui Cao

Ligamentoid fibromatosis (also called as desmoid tumor, DT) is a rare soft tissue tumor with moderate malignancy, characterized by invasive growth and local recurrence, but little distant metastasis. There are three categories of fibromatosis, grouped into abdominal-wall type, extra-abdominal type, and intra-abdominal type. Intra-abdominal and mesenteric fibromatosis can easily be mistaken for GIST. It requires more attention at the time of diagnosis owing to the specific targeted therapy for GIST, distinguished via pathological tests. Unlike GIST, DT cells, with smaller density and atypia, express β-catenin, but don't express CD117, CD34, or DOG-1. New single lesions in patients with a history of GIST should initially take the possibility of recurrent tumors into account. Since abdominal DT is closely related to GIST, it should be regarded as an important differential diagnosis. It has been reported that the following imaging findings should prompt consideration for intra-abdominal fibromatosis, without any evidence of biopsy: (1) A new single lesion appeared in the peritoneum around the surgical site; (2) Only one tumor grew out of control, while the other lesions are controlled well by imatinib; (3) CT clearly showed oval lesions, accompanied by delayed or mild enhancement, no necrosis, hemorrhage, or cystic changes; (4) PET indicated mildly raised or normal metabolic levels, contrary to the hyperactive metabolism of primary GIST.

In addition, rhabdomyosarcoma is a malignant tumor originating from rhabdomyoblasts or mesenchymal cells differentiated from rhabdomyoblasts and is the third most common soft tissue sarcoma after malignant fibrous histiocytoma and liposarcoma. In recent years, the development of rhabdomyosarcoma multiforme after targeted drug therapy for GIST has been occasionally reported, but the exact mechanism of its development needs to be further investigated.

When a new mass appears in the abdominal cavity after GIST resection, clinicians habitually consider it as recurrence or metastasis. Such mentality will lead to misdiagnosis of these cases. Therefore, these cases deserve more attention and introspection. The correct diagnosis and proper therapy for rare diseases or cases require rich knowledge and solid skills of doctors.

References

1. Koo DH, Ryu MH, Kim KM, Yang HK, Sawaki A, Hirota S, Zheng J, Zhang B, Tzen CY, Yeh CN, Nishida T, Shen L, Chen LT, Kang YK. Asian consensus guidelines for the diagnosis and management of gastrointestinal stromal tumor. Cancer Res Treat. 2016;48(4):1155–66. https://doi.org/10.4143/crt.2016.187.
2. Li J, Ye Y, Wang J, Zhang B, Qin S, Shi Y, He Y, Liang X, Liu X, Zhou Y, Wu X, Zhang X, Wang M, Gao Z, Lin T, Cao H, Shen L, Chinese Society of Clinical Oncology Csco Expert Committee on Gastrointestinal Stromal Tumor. Chinese consensus guidelines for diagnosis and management of gastrointestinal stromal tumor. Chin J Cancer Res. 2017;29(4):281–93. https://doi.org/10.21147/j.issn.1000-9604.2017.04.01.
3. Takehara Y, Yoshikawa K, Tokunaga T, Nishi M, Takasu C, Kashihara H, Yoshimoto T, Shimada M. Desmoid-type fibromatosis difficult to distinguish from GIST: a case report. J Med Investig. 2020;67(3.4):375–7. https://doi.org/10.2152/jmi.67.375.
4. Kim SW, Kim HC, Yang DM, Won KY. Gastrointestinal stromal tumours (GISTs) with a thousand faces: atypical manifestations and causes of misdiagnosis on imaging. Clin Radiol. 2016;71(2):e130–42. https://doi.org/10.1016/j.crad.2015.10.025.

5. Blay JY, Kang YK, Nishida T, von Mehren M. Gastrointestinal stromal tumours. Nat Rev Dis Primers. 2021;7(1):22. https://doi.org/10.1038/s41572-021-00254-5.
6. Mullen JT, Delaney TF, Kobayashi WK, Szymonifka J, Yeap BY, Chen YL, Rosenberg AE, Harmon DC, Choy E, Yoon SS, Raskin KA, Petur Nielsen G, Hornicek FJ. Desmoid tumor: analysis of prognostic factors and outcomes in a surgical series. Ann Surg Oncol. 2012;19(13):4028–35. https://doi.org/10.1245/s10434-012-2638-2.
7. Ceausu M, Socea B, Ciobotaru VP, Constantin VD, Enache S, Enache V, Bancu A, Socea LI, Serban D, Predescu D, Smarandache CG, Ceausu Z. A multidisciplinary approach in the diagnostic challenge of GIST. Exp Ther Med. 2021;22(4):1063. https://doi.org/10.3892/etm.2021.10497.
8. Starmans MPA, Timbergen MJM, Vos M, Renckens M, Grunhagen DJ, van Leenders G, Dwarkasing RS, Willemssen F, Niessen WJ, Verhoef C, Sleijfer S, Visser JJ, Klein S. Differential diagnosis and molecular stratification of gastrointestinal stromal tumors on CT images using a radiomics approach. J Digit Imaging. 2022;35(2):127–36. https://doi.org/10.1007/s10278-022-00590-2.
9. von Mehren M, Kane JM, Bui MM, Choy E, Connelly M, Dry S, Ganjoo KN, George S, Gonzalez RJ, Heslin MJ, Homsi J, Keedy V, Kelly CM, Kim E, Liebner D, McCarter M, McGarry SV, Meyer C, Pappo AS, Parkes AM, Paz IB, Petersen IA, Poppe M, Riedel RF, Rubin B, Schuetze S, Shabason J, Sicklick JK, Spraker MB, Zimel M, Bergman MA, George GV. NCCN guidelines insights: soft tissue sarcoma, version 1.2021. J Natl Compr Cancer Netw. 2020;18(12):1604–12. https://doi.org/10.6004/jnccn.2020.0058.
10. Dumont AG, Rink L, Godwin AK, Miettinen M, Joensuu H, Strosberg JR, Gronchi A, Corless CL, Goldstein D, Rubin BP, Maki RG, Lazar AJ, Lev D, Trent JC, von Mehren M. A nonrandom association of gastrointestinal stromal tumor (GIST) and desmoid tumor (deep fibromatosis): case series of 28 patients. Ann Oncol. 2012;23(5):1335–40. https://doi.org/10.1093/annonc/mdr442.
11. Wang J, Huang Y, Sun Y, Ge Y, Zhang M. Value of imaging findings in predicting post-operative recurrence of desmoid-type fibromatosis. Oncol Lett. 2020;19(1):869–75. https://doi.org/10.3892/ol.2019.11129.
12. Kim JH, Ryu MH, Park YS, Kim HJ, Park H, Kang YK. Intra-abdominal desmoid tumors mimicking gastrointestinal stromal tumors – 8 cases: a case report. World J Gastroenterol. 2019;25(16):2010–8. https://doi.org/10.3748/wjg.v25.i16.2010.
13. Scanlon CS, Van Tubergen EA, Inglehart RC, D'Silva NJ. Biomarkers of epithelial-mesenchymal transition in squamous cell carcinoma. J Dent Res. 2013;92(2):114–21. https://doi.org/10.1177/0022034512467352.
14. Miettinen M, Sobin LH, Sarlomo-Rikala M. Immunohistochemical spectrum of GISTs at different sites and their differential diagnosis with a reference to CD117 (KIT). Mod Pathol. 2000;13(10):1134–42. https://doi.org/10.1038/modpathol.3880210.
15. Langeh U, Singh S. Targeting S100B protein as a surrogate biomarker and its role in various neurological disorders. Curr Neuropharmacol. 2021;19(2):265–77. https://doi.org/10.2174/1570159X18666200729100427.
16. Tejpar S, Li C, Yu C, Poon R, Denys H, Sciot R, Van Cutsem E, Cassiman JJ, Alman BA. Tcf-3 expression and beta-catenin mediated transcriptional activation in aggressive fibromatosis (desmoid tumour). Br J Cancer. 2001;85(1):98–101. https://doi.org/10.1054/bjoc.2001.1857.
17. Suh J, Kang HJ, Kim SH. Differentiation of intra-abdominal desmoid tumor from peritoneal seeding based on CT and/or (18) F-FDG PET-CT in patients with history of cancer surgery. Abdom Radiol (NY). 2020;45(9):2647–55. https://doi.org/10.1007/s00261-020-02620-5.
18. Crago AM, Denton B, Salas S, Dufresne A, Mezhir JJ, Hameed M, Gonen M, Singer S, Brennan MF. A prognostic nomogram for prediction of recurrence in desmoid fibromatosis. Ann Surg. 2013;258(2):347–53. https://doi.org/10.1097/SLA.0b013e31828c8a30.
19. Liegl B, Hornick JL, Antonescu CR, Corless CL, Fletcher CD. Rhabdomyosarcomatous differentiation in gastrointestinal stromal tumors after tyrosine kinase inhibitor therapy: a novel form of tumor progression. Am J Surg Pathol. 2009;33(2):218–26. https://doi.org/10.1097/PAS.0b013e31817ec2e6.

SPRINGER NATURE

GPSR Compliance

The European Union's (EU) General Product Safety Regulation (GPSR) is a set of rules that requires consumer products to be safe and our obligations to ensure this.

If you have any concerns about our products, you can contact us on ProductSafety@springernature.com

In case Publisher is established outside the EU, the EU authorized representative is:

Springer Nature Customer Service Center GmbH
Europaplatz 3
69115 Heidelberg, Germany

The manufacturer's authorised representative in the EU is Springer
Nature Customer Service Centre GmbH, Europaplatz 3, 69115 Heidelberg,
Germany. If you have any concerns regarding our products, please
contact ProductSafety@springernature.com

Printed and bound by CPI Group (UK) Ltd, Croydon, CR0 4YY
30/09/2026
02225268-0001